Prenatal and Preimplantation Diagnosis

Joann Paley Galst • Marion S. Verp
Editors

Prenatal and Preimplantation Diagnosis

The Burden of Choice

Springer

Editors
Joann Paley Galst, PhD
New York, NY, USA

Marion S. Verp, MD
Department of Obstetrics and Gynecology
The University of Chicago
Chicago, IL, USA

Department of Human Genetics
The University of Chicago
Chicago, IL, USA

ISBN 978-3-319-18910-9 ISBN 978-3-319-18911-6 (eBook)
DOI 10.1007/978-3-319-18911-6

Library of Congress Control Number: 2015945168

Springer Cham Heidelberg New York Dordrecht London

Printed on acid-free paper

Springer International Publishing AG Switzerland is part of Springer Science+Business Media (www.springer.com)

This book is dedicated to my 3-Ds who have influenced my life in immeasurable ways.

JPG

To my children and grandchildren whose love and support have meant everything. May they always have choices.

MSV

Preface

In the past, a woman became pregnant and gave birth to a baby, navigating the pregnancy with little or no information about the fetus and unaware of problems that might be present until after delivery. More recently, thanks to advances in genetics, it has become possible to sequence individual human genomes and detect in a preimplanted embryo or a fetus the presence or absence of not only entire chromosomes but also single nucleotide variations. We have entered an era of rapidly expanding options for noninvasive prenatal screening and testing. Safe, reliable, and inexpensive screening is now available to women early in pregnancy as an alternative to invasive procedures such as amniocentesis and chorionic villus sampling. As a result of the availability of multiple options for prenatal information gathering, women and their partners are increasingly faced with decisions regarding whether to undergo preimplantation or prenatal screening and if so, which methods to choose.

Screening brings with it the possibility of receiving information indicating actual or potential fetal abnormality prior to transfer of an embryo to the uterus, or during an ongoing pregnancy. As prenatal screening becomes more routine not only for women above a particular age but also for all women, parents often perceive it as just another opportunity to confirm that all is well with the pregnancy; they do not necessarily understand that this testing is optional and fraught with downstream implications. This typical parental mindset underscores the need for pre-screening counseling in order to obtain truly informed consent. Post-screening counseling to address the need of some for additional diagnostic testing and to deal with their psychosocial needs must also be available as couples decide how to deal with the possibility or fact of a fetal anomaly.

After receiving information of an anomaly during an ongoing pregnancy, parents are forced to make decisions of enormous difficulty, including that of whether to continue the pregnancy. Complexity is added to these decisions as the severity of the problem is sometimes undeterminable while the fetus is in utero. For most parents this is experienced as a Sophie's Choice decision with no good option. Despite the availability in 2015 of more genetic information than ever before, some of the information still is of uncertain clinical significance, which only exacerbates parental uncertainty and anxiety.

Our purpose in editing this book has been to expand the awareness of professionals from multiple disciplines, including obstetricians, reproductive endocrinologists, clinical geneticists, genetic counselors, and mental health professionals, of the prenatal screening and diagnostic tests available, the information tests can provide as well as their limitations, and the emotional ramifications of prenatal/preimplantation diagnosis, prenatal decision-making, pregnancy interruption for fetal anomaly, multifetal reduction for high-order multifetal pregnancies, and preimplantation choices involving selection of only the "best" embryos. We believe this cross-fertilization among fields to be particularly important in light of the growing use of prenatal diagnostic techniques as well as the expansion of screening to include pregnant women of all ages and genetic backgrounds. It is our hope that professionals with enhanced sensitivity to these emotionally charged and potentially traumatic situations will be in a better position to assist and support patients in their decision-making and in coping after decisions have been made.

We have assembled a group of experts in their fields to inform our readers so they can better address fundamental questions, i.e., what tests are currently available and with what reliability and risks; how clinicians can best assist their patients in weighing the risks and benefits of screening and diagnostic testing; how the patient's values and preferences can be incorporated so the clinician and patient can collaborate in determining her optimal testing strategy; and how we can best support our patients during their decision-making process and after having made their decisions. Collaboration between patient and care giver is vitally important since there is no universal correct answer in prenatal genetic testing, only the answer that is right for each woman. She and her partner, if one is involved, are the ones who must live with the consequences of their decision. This reality presents professionals and their patients with both the justification for patient autonomy and its cost in decisions about pregnancies and pre-pregnancies with an anomaly.

Organization of the Chapters

Part I presents a medical perspective. We begin in Chapter 1 with a discussion by Dr. Verp of the details and recent innovations in the field of prenatal genetic screening and diagnosis, including the multiple new options for preconception carrier screening. Dr. Simpson continues this theme in Chapter 2, reviewing the evolution of preimplantation genetic diagnosis from traditional to novel indications, the unique diagnostic approaches required given the small amount of genetic material available at this stage, and the inherent ethical dilemmas.

Dr. Dungan (Chapter 3) explores the many factors influencing couples' choices about whether to terminate an abnormal pregnancy, and the frequency of termination with different chromosomal and single gene disorders. Differences in termination rates in different countries are also enumerated. In Chapter 4 Dr. Otaño and coauthors delineate the classification of anomalies used by dysmorphologists and geneticists, review ultrasound screening guidelines offered by professional organizations, and detail management and differential rates of termination for different structural abnormalities.

Dr. Evans and colleagues review in Chapter 5 the historical development of the procedure of fetal reduction, their own groundbreaking contributions as well as data and important contributions made by other centers, and the difficult choices and novel approaches possible. In Chapter 6, Dr. Derbyshire addresses the question of fetal pain, a controversial area much benefiting from his detailed knowledge of the science and his unbiased acknowledgement of the unknowns of this subject.

Dr. Lalor in Chapter 7 presents her research, conducted in a country (Ireland) where termination of pregnancy for fetal anomaly is not allowed, into typical patient assumptions during prenatal screening and diagnosis, and the effect of the unexpected finding of a fetal anomaly on the parents' assumptive world. She stresses the importance of both the language used by professionals in sharing information with their patients and the recognition of individual coping styles that patients use and with which they are most comfortable receiving diagnostic information. She offers guidance for most effectively approaching patients during initial sonograms and in the obstetrician's office when sharing troubling news.

In Part II (Chapter 8), Professor Koch presents an overview of the legal landscape of regulation and oversight of prenatal and preimplantation diagnosis across the United States.

Part III offers alternative social perspectives that may help the reader better understand patient values and preferences as they are factored into their decisions. Dr. Mahowald (Chapter 9) reviews bioethical principles of autonomy, nonmaleficence, beneficence, and justice that can guide individuals in making their decisions, along with an example of difficult decisions in preimplantation genetic diagnosis.

In Chapter 10 Professor Anderson explores the wide range of spiritual and religious beliefs, both across and within religions, on topics related to prenatal and preimplantation diagnosis. Summaries of original texts from the Hindu, Jewish, Islam, Catholic, and post-reformation Christian religions are offered.

The perspective of disability scholars and activists is presented in Chapter 11 by Professor Wasserman. While fully accepting a woman's right to choose, he raises concerns about the use of prenatal testing to select specifically against disabilities, as these decisions may be based on misconceptions that able-bodied people have about life as a disabled person. Dr. Blizzard (Chapter 12) presents a feminist perspective on prenatal and preimplantation diagnostic testing using bioethical concepts of patient autonomy and informed consent as a backdrop, suggesting that the availability of these tests, the information they offer and the subtle suggestions of the type of baby one "should" produce, adds pressure to women in making their reproductive choices.

Part IV offers a psychosocial perspective on making decisions after receiving a diagnosis of fetal abnormality and coping with those decisions. Dr. McCoyd (Chapter 13) suggests that decisions made after a diagnosis of fetal anomaly are highly contextual, driven by factors such as a woman's religious views, beliefs about quality of life, availability biases, access to support networks, and her sense of her ability to cope with the selected option. She stresses the inevitability of grief for any of the possible decisions that are made and offers strategies to provide care for the woman and her partner after a fetal anomaly is identified.

While women have the right to make choices regarding a pregnancy with a fetal anomaly, these choices, particularly to interrupt a wanted pregnancy, typically have emotional sequelae which can result in traumatic and/or complicated reactions. In Chapter 14 Dr. Galst discusses targeted psychotherapeutic interventions that mental health professionals can offer their patients, both after making their decisions and during a subsequent pregnancy. Dr. Bindeman (Chapter 15) stresses parents' need for support after making a termination decision and, because of the continuing stigma surrounding abortion, the additional difficult decisions regarding disclosure of their traumatic loss, depending on the support they expect to receive. Suggestions for communicating with existing children to help them process the experience of no longer having the expected new baby join their family are also presented.

The final Postscript of the book presents a patient's perspective of a pregnancy termination for fetal anomaly. The experience of being diagnosed with a fetal anomaly and the decision-making incorporating their religious beliefs and expectations as parents are just two of the multiple and complex factors that this author and her partner included in their thoughtful decision-making process. She discusses, as well, the shame she felt, imposed by the polarized political discussion of abortion in the United States, and the happiness she experienced with the birth of a healthy child, capable some day of making his own choices about living a fulfilling life.

Our hope is that this book will contribute to the discussion across multiple professional fields about prenatal testing and diagnosis. The many complex variables involved in patients' decisions about whether to undergo testing and how they deal with the burden of choices during a pregnancy make it clear that we must resist the temptation to assume that we understand what patients will want. Rather, we must listen for their unique values, preferences, coping styles, personal history, and other input regarding these ethical dilemmas, and respond with care and compassion. In this way, we can help these vulnerable patients with truly personalized health care, in hopes that, with time, they are able to find peace with the difficult decisions they have made.

New York, NY, USA — Joann Paley Galst, PhD
Chicago, IL, USA — Marion S. Verp, MD

Acknowledgements

Joann Paley Galst:

I would like to extend my deep gratitude to all of the chapter authors of this book for their dedication to this project and the depth of knowledge they have shared and integrated into their chapters.

Thanks also to Perry-Lynn Moffitt, my colleague at the *Pregnancy Loss Support Program* which is generously sponsored by the National Council of Jewish Women-NY Section, with whom I collaborated in initiating our first *Painful Choices in Pregnancy* Support Group to offer a healing community to this often overlooked group of parents.

I could not have completed the difficult task of shortening my rather lengthy, at times overly inclusive, individual chapter for this book without the help of my very dear friend and colleague, and expert "slicer and dicer," Dr. Judith Horowitz. With her infinitely generous heart, she was always willing to help.

I thank our Developmental Editor at Springer, Tracy Marton, who hung in with us from beginning to end and was always available to answer the many detailed questions which arose during the course of putting this book together. Her constancy is much appreciated.

I appreciate the ever-present support of my many colleagues, with particular gratitude to Dr. Madeline Licker Feingold, Dr. Judith Horowitz, Dr. E. Tobey Klass, and Dr. Julie Bindeman. Your insights have contributed to my growth as a clinician and I feel fortunate to have you all as a part of my life, both professionally and personally.

I am grateful to Sarah Dailey Galst who initially reminded me, during my own doubts and trepidation, that I really could take on this project and that I, in fact, do enjoy researching and writing, so "just do it," and to my touchstone and emotional rock, Jay Galst, who has always been there for me through it all.

Finally, I extend my heartfelt appreciation to my patients over the past many decades who both educated me and gave me the psychological benefit of witnessing their transformation and transcendence through their difficult and often heartbreaking choices.

Marion S. Verp:

I would first like to thank all of our contributors for both their fine chapters, and their professionalism including completing their work on schedule.

Central to my career development was my fellowship in Human Genetics at Northwestern University, supervised and mentored by Dr. Joe Leigh Simpson and Dr. Sherman Elias. Their continuing encouragement, support, and friendship could always be counted on. Dr. Albert Gerbie, a pioneer in the development of amniocentesis, was a wise guide to the worlds of academic obstetrics and gynecology and clinical genetics. I also want to thank all my long-time University of Chicago faculty colleagues for their collegiality and knowledge sharing, particularly the faculty in maternal—fetal—medicine, including Dr. Atef Moawad, Dr. Mahmoud Ismail, Dr. Laura DiGiovanni, and Dr. Deborah Boyle. And I must especially acknowledge the support and education I sought and was always kindly given by the genetic counselors I worked with most closely in perinatal medicine: Teri Hadro, Terri Knutel Lefler, Elyse Weber, and Bryanna Cox. My administrative assistant of many years, Gina Williams, always provided logistic support with much warmth.

Finally I must express my gratitude to the many patients whose trust in extremely difficult, emotional, situations enabled me to care for them as I wished to. Their grace in the most heartbreaking circumstances never ceased to amaze and to fill me with admiration.

Contents

Contributors

Horacio A. Aiello, MD Division of Obstetrics and Fetal Medicine Unit, Department of Obstetrics and Gynecology, University Hospital Italiano de Buenos Aires, Ciudad Autonoma de Buenos Aires, Argentina

Rebecca Rae Anderson, JD, MS, CGC College of Public Health, University of Nebraska Medical Center, Omaha, NE, USA

Stephanie Andriole, MS, CGC Comprehensive Genetics, PLLC, New York, NY, USA

Julie Bindeman, PsyD Independent Practice, Rockville, MD, USA

Deborah Blizzard, PhD Department of Science, Technology and Society, Rochester Institute of Technology, Rochester, NY, USA

David W. Britt, PhD FMFA, New York, NY, USA

Katherine Burns Brooklyn, NY, USA

Stuart W.G. Derbyshire, PhD Psychology and A*STAR-NUS Centre for Clinical Imaging, Faculty of Arts and Sciences, National University of Singapore, Singapore, Singapore

Jeffrey S. Dungan, MD Department of Obstetrics and Gynecology, Northwestern University Feinberg School of Medicine, Chicago, IL, USA

Shara M. Evans, MPH, MSc Comprehensive Genetics, PLLC, New York, NY, USA

Mark I. Evans, MD Department of Obstetrics & Gynecology, Mt. Sinai School of Medicine, New York, NY, USA

Joann Paley Galst, PhD New York, NY, USA

Valerie Gutmann Koch, JD IIT Chicago-Kent College of Law, Chicago, IL, USA

MacLean Center for Clinical Medical Ethics, University of Chicago, Chicago, IL, USA

New York State Task Force on Life and the Law, New York, NY, USA

Joan G. Lalor, PhD Trinity College Dublin, School of Nursing and Midwifery, Dublin, Ireland

Mary B. Mahowald, PhD Department of Obstetrics and Gynecology and MacLean Center for Clinical Medical Ethics, University of Chicago, Chicago, IL, USA

Judith L.M. McCoyd, PhD, LCSW School of Social Work, Rutgers University, Camden, NJ, USA

César H. Meller, MD Division of Obstetrics and Fetal Medicine Unit, Department of Obstetrics and Gynecology, University Hospital Italiano de Buenos Aires, Ciudad Autonoma de Buenos Aires, Argentina

Lucas Otaño, MD, PhD Division of Obstetrics and Fetal Medicine Unit, Department of Obstetrics and Genecology, University Hospital Italiano de Buenos Aires, Ciudad Autonoma de Buenos Aires, Argentina

Joe Leigh Simpson, MD Department of Research and Grants, March of Dimes Foundation, White Plains, NY, USA

Marion S. Verp, MD Department of Obstetrics and Gynecology, The University of Chicago, Chicago, IL, USA

Department of Human Genetics, The University of Chicago, Chicago, IL, USA

David Wasserman, JD, MA Clinical Center, Department of Bioethics, National Institutes of Health, Bethesda, MD, USA

Part I
Medical Perspective

Chapter 1
Prenatal Genetic Screening and Diagnostic Testing

Marion S. Verp

Prenatal evaluation for risk of a child with a chromosomal or genetic disorder or other birth defect is appropriate in all pregnancies. Evaluation begins with the health care professional obtaining a personal and family medical history from all women who present for prenatal care or who consult for preconception guidance.

Patients should be questioned regarding their age and that of their partner, their ethnic backgrounds, outcome of prior pregnancies, details regarding prior prenatal and postnatal losses and the health of their siblings, aunts and uncles, nieces and nephews, parents and grandparents. Consanguinity (descent from a common ancestor) of the patient and her partner should be ascertained. Screening questionnaires are useful but these should be reviewed with the patient to ensure she has correctly understood the questions and the medical terms.

Although prenatal and preconception screening and prenatal testing should be offered to all women, there are some risk factors that markedly increase a couple's chance of an affected child and therefore warrant especially careful consideration. In complicated cases consultation with a medical geneticist or genetic counselor is worthwhile.

M.S. Verp, M.D (✉)
Department of Obstetrics and Gynecology, The University of Chicago, Chicago, IL, USA

Department of Human Genetics, The University of Chicago, Chicago, IL, USA
e-mail: msverp@gmail.com

J.P. Galst, M.S. Verp (eds.), *Prenatal and Preimplantation Diagnosis*,
DOI 10.1007/978-3-319-18911-6_1

Preconception and Prenatal Indications for Screening and Diagnosis

Genetic Disorders

Prior History of Mendelian Disorder

Families that have had a child with an X-linked recessive, autosomal dominant, or autosomal recessive genetic syndrome are frequently at high risk for recurrence. For example, if one of the parents has an autosomal dominant genetic disorder (e.g., Marfan syndrome, neurofibromatosis), each fetus is at 50 % risk for inheriting the mutant parental allele. If the father has an X-linked disorder such as hemophilia, none of his sons but all of his daughters will inherit the gene and will be at high risk for affected offspring themselves. If a woman carries an X-linked mutation, each male offspring has a 50 % chance of inheriting the mutation and being affected. Each female offspring likewise has a 50 % chance of inheriting the mutation and being a carrier, like her mother. If both parents are carriers of a mutation for the same genetic disorder inherited in autosomal recessive fashion (e.g., cystic fibrosis, sickle cell anemia), each child has a 25 % chance of being affected with that disorder. On the other hand, if a child affected with an autosomal dominant or X-linked disorder has been determined to have a new mutation, not inherited from one of the parents, the recurrence risk is low. Therefore, it is important to identify patients with a family history of a genetic disorder, to obtain records to confirm the specific diagnosis, and to verify the pattern of inheritance of the disorder in their family.

Ethnic and Racial Background

In addition to families with known genetic disorders, many families at high risk are only identified by virtue of carrier screening. It is now standard to consider the expectant couple's racial and ethnic backgrounds in all pregnancies in order to decide on appropriate carrier screening.

Members of different ethnic and racial groups are at increased risk for specific disorders. Because almost all of these disorders are autosomal recessive in inheritance, prospective parents can be screened for the appropriate conditions once their ethnic/racial backgrounds are known. If both parents are found to be heterozygous (carriers) for the same condition, multiple options are available both prior to conception, i.e., avoidance of pregnancy, use of donor gametes, preimplantation diagnosis, and after conception, i.e., risk awareness and preparatory knowledge seeking, prenatal diagnosis, termination of affected pregnancies.

Screening the patient and then her partner consecutively takes time, and consideration of all options is best done before the patient is under the severe time constraint of the second trimester of pregnancy. In addition to the psychological burden of decision making at that point, the availability of pregnancy termination in the event of an abnormal fetus is more tenuous. Therefore, screening is optimally started prior to conception or at the first prenatal visit. If the patient presents for care later, it may be best to screen both members of the couple concurrently to avoid late discovery of a carrier couple.

African Background

Sickle cell disease (which includes SS disease, SC disease, and sickle cell/beta-thalassemia disease) occurs in 1 in 500 African Americans. Carrier frequency in the African-American population is 1 in 12. Mean corpuscular volume (MCV), a standard component of a complete blood count (CBC), and a hemoglobin electrophoresis are appropriate screening tests.

Ashkenazi Jewish Background

A number of conditions are more common in the Ashkenazi Jewish population. The most well known are Tay–Sachs disease, Canavan disease, and familial dysautonomia. Cystic fibrosis is found in Ashkenazi Jews at the same frequency as in other Caucasians.

In addition to the above disorders, screening is available for many other conditions which occur at increased frequency in this population, including Gaucher disease, Niemann–Pick disease type A, Bloom syndrome, mucolipidosis IV, and Fanconi anemia type C. Carrier frequencies range from 1/12 (Gaucher disease) to 1/110 (Bloom syndrome). Commercial laboratories offer a variety of screening panels that include some or all of the above conditions, with the option of screening for additional disorders. The method of screening for most of these disorders is by DNA mutation analysis; however, screening for Tay–Sachs disease may also require enzyme analysis depending on the type of DNA test selected.

Northern European Caucasian Background

Cystic fibrosis (CF) is most common among whites, particularly those of northern European origin. One in 2500 white newborns has cystic fibrosis, and 1 in 25 whites carries the CF trait. CF is also found in the Ashkenazi Jewish population. Standard screening is by DNA mutation analysis for a panel of ≥23 different mutations.

Mediterranean Background (also Southeast Asian, African)

Beta-thalassemia is common in a number of different ethnic groups. Carrier frequency varies depending on geographic origin. Screening is with MCV, followed by hemoglobin electrophoresis if the MCV is low. Normal iron studies and elevated hemoglobin A2 strongly suggest beta-thalassemia heterozygosity (carrier).

Southeast Asian Background

Alpha-thalassemia occurs most commonly in this group. Carrier frequency varies but may be as high as 1 in 20 in some populations. Screening is by measurement of MCV; if the MCV is normal or elevated, carrier status is excluded. If MCV is low, normal iron studies and a normal level of hemoglobin A2 on hemoglobin electrophoresis suggest alpha-thalassemia carrier status and that additional genetic studies are needed.

For all of the above, if one member of the couple is of the specific racial/ethnic background and the other is not, the former should be screened first. If he or she is positive for a trait (mutation), the partner should then be offered screening. For some of these conditions, the basic DNA screening tests (genotyping) have a lower detection rate in partners of a different racial/ethnic background, and consideration should be given to testing the partner with gene sequencing (see below) rather than with the screening test used in the population at higher risk.

Expanded Carrier Screening

Carrier screening for all of the conditions described above has traditionally been performed with individually designated tests. However, in the last few years commercial laboratories have developed microarrays that can screen for a large number of autosomal recessive conditions simultaneously, a much more cost efficient approach than that of screening for a few disorders individually (Lazarin et al. 2013). Microarrays can be customized such that the number of disorders and the particular disorders that one wants to screen for can be specified. Predetermined panels are generally offered by the laboratory and modified by the physician if desired. Focus is on mutations of known significance.

Patients should be made aware that the more disorders they are screened for, the more likely that they will be positive for at least one. If the latter occurs, specific counseling about the phenotype and range of expression of the disorder for which they are a carrier will be required. Screening of the reproductive partner must then be offered as well.

Disorders at increased frequency in many different racial/ethnic groups are included in these tests so knowledge of the specific background of the patient and her partner is less crucial during the initial screen, although that background will affect the detection rate and the patient's residual risk. However, most microarray panels and standard individual DNA screening tests are designed to detect the most common mutations in the population at greatest risk (genotyping). Therefore, the same screening panel may not provide good coverage of genetic variants for the carrier patient's partner, particularly if the partner is of an ethnic/racial background with a lower frequency (and different mutations) of the disorder in question. In these cases gene *sequencing*, a much more exhaustive search for mutations than genotyping, may be the better option. Unless the primary care provider is very familiar with the intricacies of such testing, referral to a geneticist or genetic counselor should be considered.

Finally, no matter how many screening tests are performed, patients must be reminded that carrier tests *reduce* but do not eliminate the possibility of a child with a genetic disorder (Grody et al. 2013).

Consanguinity

Consanguinity (descent from a common ancestor) is not uncommon in certain cultures and on occasion will be the reason couples present for genetic counseling. If one of the members of the couple is the result of a consanguineous union or has a close relative who is, it does not imply a greater risk to their offspring, as long as the individual in question is phenotypically normal and does not have a genetic disorder. However, if the couple itself is consanguineous, the exact degree of relatedness should be discussed. Offspring of first-cousin unions (in which the couple share 1/8 of their genes) have a twofold increase in risk for perinatal and childhood death, malformation, or intellectual disability, as compared to the general population risk (Bennett et al. 2002; Shieh et al. 2012). This assumes that both potential parents are phenotypically normal and there is no family history of a recessive disorder. If the family does have an autosomal recessive disorder, or if the ethnic background warrants, heterozygote (carrier) testing should be offered to the couple.

As the degree of relatedness decreases, the likelihood of the couple carrying identical mutant genes decreases sharply. The empiric risk to offspring of second or third cousins is not increased as compared to the general population (Bennett et al. 2002). Obviously if a known genetic disorder exists in the family, specific genetic counseling and testing should be offered.

Chromosomal Disorders

Parental Age

Well known to obstetricians and other providers of obstetrical care is that risk for chromosome abnormalities in offspring increases with maternal age (Table 1.1).

Risks are about 30 % higher at the time of amniocentesis as compared to those at livebirth (Hook et al. 1983). Risk in the first trimester is even higher, demonstrating the selective loss of chromosomally abnormal fetuses throughout gestation. Natural selection is greatest against fetuses with more severe chromosome abnormalities, e.g., trisomy 13 or 18, and much less so against those with the milder abnormalities of Klinefelter syndrome (47,XXY) or 47,XXX (Gardner et al. 2012).

Although the traditional approach of offering invasive testing (chorionic villus sampling, amniocentesis) based solely on the mother's age guided referrals for prenatal diagnosis for many years, the American College of Obstetricians and Gynecologists (ACOG 2007a) has endorsed the concept that neither is a specific age sufficient to require invasive diagnosis, nor should the option of invasive testing be

Table 1.1 Regression-derived rates of chromosome abnormalities[a] at birth, at amniocentesis, and at chorionic villus sampling

Maternal age	Risk of Down syndrome at birth	Risk of a chromosome abnormality at birth[b]	Risk of a chromosome abnormality at amniocentesis	Risk of a chromosome abnormality at CVS
20	1:1667	1:526		
21	1:1667	1:526		
22	1:1429	1:500		
23	1:1429	1:500		
24	1:1250	1:476		
25	1:1250	1:476		
26	1:1176	1:476		
27	1:1111	1:455		
28	1:1053	1:435		
29	1:1000	1:417		
30	1:952	1:385		
31	1:909	1:385		
32	1:769	1:323		
33	1:602	1:312		
34	1:482	1:253		
35	1:375	1:202	1:141	1:118
36	1:289	1:163	1:112	1:93
37	1:224	1:129	1:88	1:72
38	1:173	1:103	1:70	1:56
39	1:136	1:82	1:56	1:44
40	1:106	1:65	1:45	1:34
41	1:82	1:51	1:35	1:27
42	1:63	1:40	1:28	1:21
43	1:49	1:32	1:22	1:16
44	1:38	1:25	1:18	1:13
45	1:30	1:20	1:14	1:10
46	1:23	1:16	1:11	1:8
47	1:18	1:12	1:9	1:6
48	1:14	1:10	1:7	
49	1:11	1:8	1:6	

[a]Mosaics, balanced rearrangements, and invariably lethal abnormalities excluded. Data are taken from Hook (1981), Hook et al. (1983), Hook (1988), Hook et al. (1988)

[b]Estimated rates based on rate at amniocentesis and spontaneous loss rate of cytogenetically abnormal fetuses. For ages 20–32 years, 47, XXX is excluded (data not given)

Reprinted from Verp et al. (1993)

limited to those above a certain age. Rather, the care provider should be familiar with the risk for chromosome abnormalities at different ages and be able to provide initial counseling regarding screening and diagnostic options. There may be younger women who request a diagnostic procedure reasoning that their highest priority is avoidance of the birth of a child with a chromosome abnormality. In the latter case they may find the procedure-associated risks (see later) acceptable. On the other hand, some women in their late 30s and 40s may feel that under no circumstances do they want a test with any associated risk. Noninvasive screening would therefore be an appropriate choice for them.

Nonchromosomal congenital anomalies may also occur at slightly higher frequency in offspring of older women (Hay and Barbano 1972; Hollier et al. 2000). As cardiac defects comprise a substantial portion of these, a detailed ultrasound examination of the fetal heart in the second trimester is appropriate.

Less well known than maternal age effects is that advanced paternal age, while not significantly increasing the risk for autosomal aneuploidy, is associated with increased risk for a child with a new dominant mutation (e.g., Marfan syndrome, achondroplasia) (Vogel and Rathenberg 1975). The estimated level of risk is based on limited data but may be in the neighborhood of 0.3–0.5 % for offspring of men over 40 years (Friedman 1981). Thus, although elevated several fold compared to that of younger men, the risk for a new dominant mutation in the child of a father older than age 40 is still less than 1 %.

Structural chromosome rearrangements (Sloter et al. 2004) and cardiac defects (Olshan et al. 1994) may also be at slightly higher prevalence in the offspring of older men. Recent reports have shown elevated risks for autism and some psychiatric disorders (D'Onofrio et al. 2014). Although the manifestations of some dominant mutations and of cardiac defects can be visualized with ultrasound, prenatal screening/testing cannot at the present time exclude such an event or that of a neurodevelopmental disorder.

Previous Child, Stillborn or Spontaneous Abortions with Chromosomal Abnormality

After the birth of one child with either an autosomal trisomy or a sex chromosome abnormality, the likelihood that subsequent progeny will have a chromosomal abnormality has been considered increased, even if parental chromosome complements are normal. However, the risk for a second offspring with Down syndrome or another chromosomal abnormality appears to be substantially increased primarily for mothers 29 years of age or younger at the time of the affected pregnancy. Recurrence risks for women who were older than 30 years at the time of their affected pregnancy seem to be only 1- to 2-fold that of their current age risk (Gardner et al. 2012).

The same may be true for couples who have experienced a pregnancy loss with a chromosome abnormality. Although advancing maternal age is thought to account for the majority of recurrences, Warburton et al. (2004) demonstrated a small increased recurrence risk for a trisomic fetus following a trisomic pregnancy loss. The couple's second trisomic conceptus might not spontaneously abort, but rather continue to livebirth. Because chromosomal studies are not uniformly performed on abortuses and stillborn infants, in a particular case it is frequently unknown whether a couple with several abortuses or stillborns experienced recurrent aneuploid conceptions and are at increased risk for an aneuploid liveborn.

Table 1.2 Risk of an unbalanced rearrangement in a fetus whose parent has a balanced rearrangement (carrier)[a]

		Fetus		
Rearrangement	Sex of carrier	Normal	Carrier	Unbalanced
t(14q;21q)	Female	58	87	25 (14.7 %)
	Male	24	34	0
t(21q;22q)	Female	11	5	3 (15.8 %)
	Male	0	3	0
t(13q;14q)	Female	69	88	0
	Male	27	46	0
Reciprocal translocations (pooled)	Female	168	166	44 (11.6 %)
	Male	97	107	27 (11.7 %)
Inversions	Female	32	30	5 (7.5 %)
	Male	14	35	2 (3.9 %)

[a]Data Boué and Gallano (1984) and Mikkelsen (1986)
Reprinted from Verp et al. (1993)

Couples who have previously had a child or a loss with a chromosome abnormality are frequently anxious about the normality of another pregnancy and often request prenatal diagnosis or screening.

Parental Chromosome Rearrangement or Aneuploidy

Another, less common, cytogenetic indication for antenatal diagnosis is the presence of a balanced translocation or inversion in a parent. For example, about 4 % of Down syndrome is the result of a translocation between chromosome 21 and one of the other acrocentric (13, 14, 15, 21, 22) chromosomes. If a child has Down syndrome resulting from such a "Robertsonian" translocation, the rearrangement has been inherited from a parent with the balanced form of the rearrangement in 25–50 % of cases.

The theoretical risk that a parent carrying a balanced Robertsonian translocation will have a child with Down syndrome is 33 %. However, empirical risks are considerably less (0–14 %) and depend on which of the parents carries the rear rangement, and the particular chromosomes involved (Table 1.2) (Boué and Gallano 1984; Mikkelsen 1986).

In addition to the risk of an unbalanced translocation, carriers of Robertsonian translocations also have a small risk of uniparental disomy (UPD) in their offspring (<1 %). In UPD both copies of a chromosome are inherited from the same parent. This can result in an abnormal child if the UPD is of chromosomes 6, 7, 11, 14, 15, or 20.

Reciprocal translocations, which usually do not involve acrocentric chromosomes, are individually rare and specific empirical data for most reciprocal translocations are not available. Knowledge of the length of the translocated segment provides some guidance in predicting risk of a fetus with an unbalanced translocation as a longer translocation segment is associated with a lower risk. Ascertainment by an affected liveborn rather than a spontaneous abortion implies a higher risk for a nonlethal abnormality. Overall empirical risks for abnormal (unbalanced) offspring are approximately 10 % for either maternal or paternal carriers.

In a chromosomal inversion, the normal sequence of genes on the chromosome is altered. Individuals with such inversions are phenotypically normal; however, like those with balanced translocations, they may produce unbalanced gametes with certain genes duplicated and others deficient. Pericentric inversions and inversions involving long segments are more likely to be associated with anomalous offspring than are paracentric or short inversion segments. Empirical data are not available for specific inversions, but pooled data for all inversions indicate approximately a 3 % risk for abnormal progeny, with maternal carriers at greater risk than paternal carriers (Daniel et al. 1989). An exception is inv (9), which is a common variant and is without clinical significance. Couples experiencing repetitive abortions should undergo cytogenetic studies to exclude the presence of a parental translocation or inversion if the karyotype of one or more of their losses was not determined.

If a parent has a numerical chromosomal abnormality (aneuploidy), the risk to offspring is increased. For example, approximately 35 % (but not 50 %) of offspring of females with 47,XX, + 21 (Down syndrome) are aneuploid (Verp 1985); therefore, antenatal chromosomal studies are indicated in a pregnant female with Down syndrome. Males with Down syndrome are infertile. If a parent is mosaic for trisomy 21, antenatal diagnosis is again in order. Although risk figures are biased by the method of ascertainment, approximately 20 % of offspring of fertile 45,X; 45,X/46,XX; and 45,X/46,XX/47,XXX subjects are said to show abnormalities (Verp 1985). Women with 47,XXX or 46,XX/47,XXX also have produced children with chromosomal abnormalities, although almost always the offspring are normal. Theoretically, 47,XY Y men are also at increased risk for chromosomally abnormal offspring, and several abnormal offspring have been reported. Men with 47,XXY (Klinefelter syndrome) are sterile, but those with mosaicism (46,XY/47,XXY) may be fertile. Antenatal diagnosis should be offered to all aneuploid parents.

Previous Offspring with Isolated (Nonchromosomal) Structural Defect

Most congenital anomalies involving a single structure or organ system (e.g., neural tube defects [NTDs], cleft lip and palate) are ascribed to polygenic/multifactorial inheritance. This theoretical mode of inheritance postulates that "liability" for a disorder is contributed both by an individual's genetic inheritance and environmental exposures. If the fetus' total liability is beyond a (theoretical) threshold, the fetus will manifest the anomaly. Thus polygenic/multifactorial disorders will recur more frequently in families with an affected member than in the general population because the former must have a greater than average liability for the disorder.

Table 1.3 Polygenic/multifactorial disorders

Condition	Population incidence (%)	Sibling recurrence risks (%)
Cleft lip ± palate	0.1	3 (0.7 % for second degree relatives)
Ventriculoseptal defect	0.17	4.3
Patent ductus arteriosus	0.15	3.2
Atrial septal defect	0.1	3.2
Anencephaly or Spina bifida	0.1	4
Pyloric stenosis	0.3	4.5
Male proband		2.1
Female proband		9.9

Data from Fuhrmann and Vogel (1983), Bonaiti-Pellié and Smith (1974), Stevenson (1993)

Polygenic/multifactorial conditions recur in 2–5 % of siblings or offspring of affected individuals with, however, considerable variation in the risk depending on the particular disorder, the number of affected family members, the severity of the defect and the sex of the proband. Risks are significantly decreased for second degree relatives (Table 1.3).

Some of these conditions (e.g., neural tube defects) can be detected during pregnancy via maternal serum assay of alpha-fetoprotein, and others by ultrasound visualization (e.g., cardiac defects).

Prenatal Screening

Maternal Serum Screening

Maternal serum alpha-fetoprotein (MSAFP) screening was initially developed and continues to be used for detection of fetal neural tube defects (NTDs) and other open defects, e.g., gastroschisis, which are associated with elevated levels of MSAFP. AFP is a fetal-specific glycoprotein that is produced very early in fetal life, first in the yolk sac and later in the fetal gastrointestinal tract and liver. Concentration of AFP peaks in the fetal plasma and amniotic fluid at 12–14 weeks gestation and then gradually declines. AFP is also normally present in maternal serum, peaking at 28–32 weeks of gestation. The ratio of AFP in fetal plasma: amniotic fluid: maternal serum is roughly 50,000:250:1.

Screening for NTDs is based on detection of an abnormally elevated level of AFP in maternal serum. Screening is most effective at 16–18 weeks gestation and at that time detection of anencephaly can be close to 100 %, and approximately 80 % for open spina bifida (Milunsky et al. 1989). An abnormal serum screen should be followed by a basic ultrasound, if not already done, as incorrect gestational age, unrecognized multiple gestation, and fetal demise are frequent causes of apparently elevated MSAFP. If the elevated MSAFP is not explained by one of these conditions, a more detailed ultrasound should be performed. Not only NTDs, but other fetal defects, (e.g., omphalocele, gastroschisis, extensive open skin lesions, congenital nephrosis), and placental abnormalities (e.g., accreta), are also associated with elevated MSAFP. Most of these will be visible on ultrasound, but if there is no explanation for the elevated MSAFP, measurement of amniotic fluid AFP is an option. Elevation of AFP in amniotic fluid almost always indicates a fetal defect if confirmed by the presence of acetylcholinesterase (AChE) and absence of fetal blood in the sample. If, after amniocentesis or a detailed ultrasound, the etiology for an elevated MSAFP is still unexplained the patient can be counseled that most such pregnancies result in a normal outcome for mother and fetus, but the frequency of spontaneous abortion, low birth weight, and perinatal mortality are all elevated in this population (Milunsky et al. 1989).

The addition of other fetal–placental products (unconjugated estriol, human chorionic gonadotropin [hCG], and dimeric inhibin-A) to the second trimester MSAFP assay created the "Quad screen" which provides an estimate of risk for trisomy 21 (Down syndrome) and for trisomy 18. Optimally performed at 15–18 weeks gestation, MSAFP and estriol are decreased and hCG and inhibin increased in pregnancies of women carrying Down syndrome fetuses. At a false positive rate of 5 %, second trimester screening detects ~80 % of fetuses with trisomy 21 (Malone et al. 2005). Because MSAFP, unconjugated estriol and hCG are all significantly decreased in pregnancies with trisomy 18, the same assay can detect ~70 % of pregnancies with trisomy 18 at a false positive rate of 0.5 % (Palomaki et al. 1995). However, the detection rate and the false positive rate vary substantially with the age of the pregnant woman. That is, younger women have lower detection and false positive rates, the inverse is true for older women. Trisomy 13 is not detectable by second trimester aneuploidy screening but Turner syndrome (45,X) and triploidy will frequently be detected based on similarity to analyte patterns associated with trisomy 21 or trisomy 18.

At 11–13 weeks gestation, median total β-hCG (beta-human Chorionic Gonadotropin) and free β-hCG are elevated and pregnancy-associated plasma protein-A (PAPP-A) is decreased in women with Down syndrome fetuses; all three analytes are decreased with trisomy 18. These markers, combined with measurement of fetal nuchal translucency, are commonly used for the "first trimester screen" (FTS). The detection rate of FTS for Down syndrome is a little better (~85 %) (Malone et al. 2005) than that of second trimester screening with, again, higher detection and false positive rates as maternal age increases. Detection of non-Down syndrome aneuploidies (e.g., trisomies 18 and 13, 45, X, and triploidy) is close to 80 % with a false positive rate of 6 % (Breathnach et al. 2007). Patients who have FTS should still be offered screening for NTDs in the second trimester.

Another approach to screening for trisomies 21 and 18 has been to combine first and second trimester screens for one "integrated" result. Adding more parameters in this way can raise the detection rate for trisomy 21 to 95 % while maintaining a false positive rate of 5 % (Malone et al. 2005); similarly a detection rate of 90 % for trisomy 18 can be achieved at a false positive rate of 0.1 % (Palomaki et al. 2003). Nuchal translucency and PAPP-A are measured in the first trimester, and MSAFP, uE3, hCG, and inhibin A are assayed in the second trimester. Patients are either

Table 1.4 Relative frequency of various significant chromosome abnormalities in two high-risk prenatal populations

	#	%
Trisomy and Monosomy 13,18, 21, X and Y	274	68
Triploidy	17	4.2
Structural rearrangements	74	18.4
Other	38	9.4
Total	403	100

Evans et al. (1994), Norton et al. (2012)

informed of their results only after the second trimester assay has been completed (integrated test) or, in the "step-wise sequential" version, are alerted to their high risk status (if >1/50 for an affected fetus) after the first trimester portion of the screen. The latter approach allows the patient with a high risk to elect diagnostic testing in the late first trimester (CVS) or early second trimester (amniocentesis) without having to await the results of the second trimester portion of the screening test. Those with risks <1/50 after the first trimester portion of the screen complete the second trimester blood draw and receive final results when all of the parameters have been measured. Of course both the sequential and integrated tests have the disadvantage that they require most women to have two separate blood draws and to wait until at least 16 weeks gestation before receiving results.

Both first and second trimester serum screening have proved very useful for providing individual, patient-specific risk estimates for women younger than 35 years of age who traditionally were not offered prenatal diagnosis when the only option was invasive testing. Whether maternal serum screening should always precede amniocentesis or CVS for women 35 years of age and older has been a controversial issue. For example, if invasive testing were to be offered only to women with abnormal second trimester serum screens rather than to all women older than 34 years of age, the detection rate of fetal Down syndrome would be lower (89 %), but only 25 % of the older population would require amniocentesis. Conversely, if all older women were offered and accepted amniocentesis or CVS, the detection rate would be 100 % as would the procedure rate. Additionally, multiple marker screening is not highly sensitive in detecting chromosome abnormalities other than trisomy 21 and trisomy 18 (e.g., sex chromosome aneuploidies), some of which also increase with advancing maternal age. Thus, a significant number of aneuploidies are missed when using serum screening alone rather than invasive testing. Table 1.4 Awaiting the results of second trimester multiple marker screening before offering invasive testing also frequently results in delay in the diagnosis of chromosome abnormalities until approximately 20 weeks' gestation, rather than detection in the late first or early second trimester after CVS or amniocentesis. Moreover, screening is less sensitive in multiple gestations compared to singleton gestations. For these reasons, the advantages and limitations of both serum screening and invasive testing for cytogenetic abnormalities should be discussed carefully with patients before a choice is made (ACOG 2007a).

Cell Free Fetal DNA

In 1997 Lo et al. reported that a small proportion of cell free DNA in the blood of pregnant women was of fetal/placental origin. This non-maternal DNA is the result of apoptosis of placental cells. This observation has been exploited for the prenatal diagnosis of male fetuses (presence of Y chromosome DNA) (Devaney et al. 2011), and for detection of the gene for Rh D antigen (Rh positive) in fetuses of women who were RhD negative (Moise et al. 2013). Additionally, in 2008, Fan et al. and Chiu et al. reported detection of fetal Down syndrome from maternal blood samples, using massively parallel shotgun sequencing (MPSS).

MPSS is a process of first partially sequencing millions of fragments of DNA in a sample, then analyzing the nucleotide sequence and assigning each fragment to a specific chromosome of origin. Thus the relative number of fragments from each targeted chromosome can be quantified. Approximately 10 % of the free DNA in maternal blood is of fetal origin ("fetal fraction"). Software programs can differentiate the expected amount of free DNA derived from chromosome 21 in the blood of a pregnant woman with a euploid fetus from the amount found in a woman carrying a fetus with an extra copy of chromosome 21. The same approach is also used for detection of trisomies 18 and 13, and for quantitation of the number of sex chromosomes. The latter analysis results in diagnosis of fetal sex and detection of sex chromosome aneuploidies.

There are currently four commercial companies (Sequenom, Illumina, Ariosa, and Natera) offering cell free fetal DNA (cff DNA) tests in the USA. One of them, Natera, does not use MPSS but rather genotypes the fetus from a maternal blood sample and compares the *expected* frequency of certain single nucleotide polymorphisms (SNPs) to that *observed*. Overabundance of SNPs found on a particular chromosome implies an additional copy of that chromosome in the fetus. In contrast to the tests which employ MPSS, this technique also allows the detection of triploidy.

Several large scale studies of cff DNA testing in high-risk populations (advanced maternal age, prior history of an aneuploid fetus, known parental rearrangement, ultrasound suspicious for trisomy 21, 18, 13, abnormal screening test) have now been published (Bianchi et al. 2012; Nicolaides et al. 2013; Norton et al. 2012; Palomaki et al. 2011). All have shown a very high sensitivity and specificity, but the positive predictive value of the test is dependent on the a priori risk of the patient. For example, there is a higher chance that a 42-year-old woman with an abnormal cell free DNA screen for trisomy 21 is actually carrying a fetus with trisomy 21, compared to the chance of a 26 year old woman with the same screen result. This difference in positive predictive value has led to considerable discussion regarding whether the test is appropriate for patients without one of the high-risk indications.

In 2014, Bianchi et al. reported a study comparing detection of trisomies 21 and 18 via cff DNA testing versus first or second trimester serum screening with or without measurement of nuchal translucency. The study population was 1914 women with mean age of 29.6 years. The results showed that the detection rate (sensitivity) was equally high (100 %) with both approaches. However, the false positive rates with cff DNA testing (0.3 % for trisomy 21, 0.2 % for trisomy 18) were significantly lower compared to the serum screening tests (3.6 % and 0.6 % respectively). The positive predictive values (45.5 % vs. 4.2 % for trisomy 21, and 40 % vs. 8.3 % for trisomy 18) were superior in the cff DNA test.

Although the DNA test has a lower false positive rate and a higher positive predictive value than do the serum screening tests, one must recall that both false negatives and false positives do occur with cell free DNA tests. Some of the false positives may arise from karyotypic abnormalities confined to placental cells (Choi et al. 2013) or to the presence of a demised twin's DNA. Others may reflect maternal sex chromosome aneuploidy or mosaicism, for example of 47, XXX (Yao et al. 2012), or, rarely, the presence of a maternal cancer that is releasing cell free DNA into the maternal circulation (Osborne et al. 2013).

Because cff DNA tests are targeted to detect an abnormal quantity of only specific chromosomes, inevitably they do not detect balanced rearrangements, nor do they detect uncommon aneuploidies for chromosomes to which they are not directed. Compared to the diagnostic tests of CVS and amniocentesis, the detection rate for all aneuploidies with cff DNA is inferior as are the positive and negative predictive values. Table 1.4. Therefore cff DNA tests are most appropriately seen as improved screening tests rather than diagnostic tests equivalent to CVS or amniocentesis.

In addition, there can be technical difficulties in detecting enough fetal DNA in the blood of a pregnant woman, particularly if she is very obese. Almost 30 % of samples from women weighing >140 kg did not have adequate fetal DNA in one study (Wang et al. 2013). In such situations the blood sample will be rejected with no information obtained. A repeat blood draw may or may not be successful. Finally, the diagnostic efficacy in twin gestations is still uncertain with only a small number of published cases to date (Huang et al. 2014).

These considerations led the American College of Obstetricians and Gynecologists (ACOG) to opine in December 2012 that while cff DNA screening is appropriate for high-risk women in the setting of pretest counseling, review of the family history, and the patient's agreement, it is not yet appropriate for the general population nor for those with multiple gestations. However as more studies are published showing high sensitivity in low risk populations and the cost of the test comes down with acceptance by insurance companies, this may soon change. Providers will be responsible for patients' understanding that the positive predictive value of the test is <100 % and that a positive result should be confirmed prior to a pregnancy termination.

The same technology described for aneuploidy detection above also can be applied to the detection of paternally derived mutations and to new mutations not present in the mother. Single reports of detection of fetal Huntington disease, achondroplasia, myotonic dystrophy, and thanatophoric dysplasia with maternal blood samples have been published (Chitty et al. 2013; Wright and Burton 2009). In addition, some of the laboratories offering aneuploidy detection with cell free DNA have expanded their offerings to include detection of a few specific chromosomal deletions that are associated with clinical syndromes (DiGeorge, Cri-du-chat, del 1p36,

Prader–Willi, and Angelman) as well as trisomies 16 and 22. The latter aneuploidies do not result in livebirth but the information obtained with the screen could inform the etiology of a pregnancy loss. Clinical validation studies on the detection of deletions have not been reported yet (Vora and O'Brien 2014). In any case detection of these syndromes will be incomplete even if all pregnancies are studied as the etiology of these syndromes is not always a microdeletion.

Intact Fetal Cells

Initial attempts at fetal diagnosis using intact fetal cells in the maternal circulation were promising but ultimately confounded by the difficulty of consistently isolating sufficient fetal cells (Bianchi et al. 2002). More recently, individual *trophoblastic* cells in the maternal circulation were successfully recovered and analyzed, resulting in the accurate diagnosis of fetal cystic fibrosis and spinal muscular atrophy in 63 cases (Mouawia et al. 2012). Although still in early stages of investigation, the advantage of using intact cells rather than cell free DNA is that Mendelian disorders and chromosome aneuploidies can be analyzed simultaneously, and that some of the conditions causing false positive cff DNA results would not be pertinent.

Ultrasound

Trisomic fetuses, especially fetuses with trisomy 13 or 18, often show intrauterine growth restriction (IUGR) and structural anomalies, which may be clinically evident during the second trimester (Table 1.5). In addition, a number of ultrasonically detected fetal "markers" such as echogenic bowel, short femur, thickened nuchal fold, suggest a somewhat increased risk of a fetal chromosome abnormality. (See Chap. 4 for additional details.)

Antenatal chromosomal studies with chorionic villi or amniotic fluid cells are appropriate if an abnormal fetus is detected on ultrasound examination. In addition to a routine karyotype, particular defects suggest the need for more specific studies. For example, conotruncal heart defects are frequently associated with deletion of a small portion of chromosome 22 (del 22q.11.2) (DiGeorge/velocardiofacial syndrome). Fluorescent in situ hybridization (FISH) with specific probes will be diagnostic of this microdeletion that also implies the presence of other defects that may not be visible on ultrasound (see below).

In some cases, ultrasound abnormalities may be sufficiently specific that maternal serum screening with cell free fetal DNA would be a reasonable alternative, but in most cases an invasive procedure (CVS, amniocentesis) is more appropriate because it allows a much wider range of diagnoses to be assessed, both with a karyotype and a chromosomal microarray (see below).

Table 1.5 Association of chromosome abnormalities with abnormal ultrasound findings

Ultrasound finding[a]	% with chromosome abnormality
Cardiac abnormality	17.2
Cystic hygroma	61.8
Diaphragmatic hernia	11.2
Duodenal atresia	29.6
Gastroschisis	6.0
Genitourinary abnormality	9.7
Growth restriction or oligohydramnios	14.4
Holoprosencephaly	47.7
Hydrocephalus	13.7
Nonimmune hydrops without cystic hygroma	33.9
Omphalocele	24.5
Polyhydramnios	7.0

[a]Primary defect indicated by investigator. Multiple anomalies found in some cases
Ref: Verp (2008)

Ultrasound *screening* of second trimester pregnancies for "soft markers" (e.g., increased nuchal thickness, renal pyelectasis, short humerus or femur) has been used for many years as an adjunct, or an alternative, to maternal serum screening for aneuploidy. Although soft markers are indicative of an increased risk for a fetal chromosome abnormality, the finding of one or more soft markers is not diagnostic of a disorder.

Diagnostic Testing

Chorionic Villus Sampling

Technique

Chorionic villus sampling (CVS) is an outpatient procedure performed between 10 and 13 weeks gestation for the diagnosis of fetal chromosomal and genetic disorders. One of the advantages of first trimester testing is that for many patients earlier knowledge of a normal result is greatly reassuring. When the test results in an abnormal diagnosis, decision making about termination is generally easier in the first than in the second trimester. The safety of pregnancy termination is also greater earlier in pregnancy.

Prior to the procedure, ultrasound examination is performed to determine gestational age, viability, number of fetuses, location of the placenta, and cervical–uterine angle.

Tissue sampling is almost always through either the cervix or the abdomen; rarely is a transvaginal approach through the cul de sac required. In transcervical CVS a catheter is passed through the cervix into the uterus and directed to the placenta with ultrasound guidance. A small amount of chorionic villi are aspirated. The transabdominal approach also requires ultrasound guidance of an 18- to 20-gauge needle through the maternal abdominal wall and the uterus into the placenta.

The sample obtained by either approach is visualized to insure that adequate villus material (~10–25 mg) and not just maternal decidua has been obtained. Villi are identified by a characteristic branching morphology.

Chromosomal, biochemical, and DNA analyses can often be done directly on the freshly isolated villus tissue without the need to culture the cells (direct diagnosis). However, laboratories typically also culture villi to create a larger pool of cells for diagnosis, or to confirm the initial direct diagnosis. Fluorescence in situ hybridization (FISH) can be performed on uncultured chorionic villus cells in interphase, enabling rapid but specific detection of some chromosome abnormalities and microdeletion syndromes. CVS also can be performed on multiple gestations as long as the individual placentas can be distinguished and each sampled separately.

Some laboratories routinely collect a maternal blood sample from all CVS patients. If the CVS chromosome results are "normal female" (46,XX), DNA can be extracted from the villus sample and from the maternal blood sample. Polymorphisms in the maternal blood can be compared to those in the villus tissue. The latter should show variants unique to the fetus, thus excluding maternal contamination and misdiagnosis of the villus sample.

Origin of Chorionic Villus Cells

Aspirated chorionic villi (CV) consist of trophoblast and mesodermal cells. The trophoblast lineages differentiate from the trophoectoderm of the blastocyst independent of the inner cell mass that is destined to become the embryo, and the extraembryonic mesodermal primordial cells that evolve into the amniotic and chorionic membranes of the placenta. Because of this independent proliferation of trophoblastic, embryonic, and membrane precursor cells, aneuploidy may arise from non-disjunction in one of the lines but not the others. This then can yield a cytogenetic abnormality in the trophoblast, mesenchymal membrane cells, or both that are not present in the embryo but are present, usually in mosaic form, in the CVS sample.

A discrepancy between an abnormal mesodermal and a normal embryonic/fetal karyotype is called confined placental mosaicism (CPM). In cases of CVS-detected placental mosaicism, an amniocentesis is frequently required to determine if the abnormal cells are also present in amniotic fluid and, by inference, in the fetus, or, conversely, if the abnormal cells are confined to the placenta (CPM). CPM is usually associated with a normal pregnancy outcome but IUGR is more common in such cases (Verp et al. 1989).

Safety

A series of over 4000 women who underwent transcervical CVS showed no serious maternal complications (Rhoads et al. 1989). The few serious maternal infections reported to date have been limited to case reports. There is no evidence of clinically significant placental damage in ongoing pregnancies after CVS.

The fetal loss rate associated with CVS has been investigated in several large studies. Total loss rates from spontaneous abortion, induced abortion, and stillbirth, although generally a little higher in the CVS groups compared to patients having amniocentesis, were frequently not significantly different (Mujezinovic and Alfirevic 2007; Rhoads et al. 1989). More recent studies show a decreasing loss rate from CVS, likely related to operator and sonographer experience (Caughey 2006). Randomized comparisons of transcervical and transabdominal CVS by practitioners experienced in both approaches also did not show a significant difference in loss rates (Jackson et al. 1992). Importantly, despite several reports of limb reduction defects following transcervical CVS in the 1990s, an international CVS registry and studies by the US Center for Disease Control and Prevention did not support a statistically significant excess number of infants with limb reduction defects following CVS (Froster and Jackson 1996). In summary, the risk of loss associated with CVS, either transcervical or transabdominal, is similar to that of amniocentesis and probably <0.5 % when performed by experienced individuals.

Amniocentesis

In early gestation, amniotic fluid contains electrolytes present in concentrations similar to those found in maternal serum because the unkeratinized fetal skin allows passage of fluid, urea, creatinine, sodium, and chloride. Amniotic fluid also contains alpha-fetoprotein and other fetal proteins, as well as cells desquamated from amnion, fetal skin, and the bronchopulmonary, gastrointestinal, and genitourinary tracts. These cells can be cultured for fetal karyotyping, biochemical and molecular (DNA) analysis.

Cell number in amniotic fluid increases with gestation, although only 35 % of such cells are viable at 15–17 weeks' gestation. A traditional karyotype requires cultivation of viable cells to obtain mitotic figures. Amniotic fluid supernatant or uncultured cells may be sufficient for certain biochemical, DNA or chromosomal studies such as fluorescence in situ hybridization (FISH analysis).

Technique

Amniocentesis is an outpatient procedure traditionally performed at 15–20 weeks' gestation because at this stage at least 200 ml of amniotic fluid is present and the uterus is accessible by a transabdominal approach.

An ultrasound examination is performed immediately before amniocentesis to confirm gestational age, assess position of the placenta, identify the size and location of amniotic fluid pockets, confirm the presence of fetal cardiac activity or fetal movement, and quantify the number of fetuses. A 22-gauge needle is passed transabdominally into the amniotic fluid in aseptic fashion, avoiding the placenta if possible. Ultrasound monitoring is used to direct the course of the needle. Fifteen to thirty milliliters of amniotic fluid is aspirated; the amount withdrawn varies with individual laboratory requirements, indication for the procedure, and gestational age.

Grossly bloody amniotic fluid is aspirated on occasion and microscopic evidence of maternal erythrocytes can be found in most specimens; fortunately, blood usually does not adversely affect amniocyte growth. Gross blood may, however, interfere with biochemical or DNA assays because this usually reflects maternal cell contamination. Brown or green fluid is aspirated in <5 % of second trimester amniocenteses. Usually, such patients have a history of first trimester bleeding and the discoloration results from hemoglobin breakdown products in the amniotic sac. This does not reflect a technical problem and does not prevent amniocyte culture for diagnosis.

In experienced hands, failure to aspirate fluid during an amniocentesis occurs in <1 % of attempts, usually related to uterine contraction, maternal obesity or early gestational age.

Amniocentesis can be reliably performed on twin gestations by the injection of diluted indigo carmine into the first sac after aspiration of fluid. A second amniocentesis is then performed in the ultrasonographically determined location of the second sac. Aspiration of clear amniotic fluid without a blue-tinge confirms that the second sac has been entered correctly. In the case of a higher order gestation, the same dye can be added to each sac in succession until clear fluid has been aspirated from all sacs.

Safety

Although any invasive procedure involves risk to both mother and fetus, maternal risks of amniocentesis are very low. In a study conducted by the US National Institute for Child Health and Human Development (NICHD 1976), minor maternal complications such as transient vaginal spotting and minimal amniotic fluid leakage occurred in 2–3 % of cases while serious complications such as amnionitis occurred in only 1:1040 patients.

Potential fetal risks include needle puncture, umbilical cord hematoma and occlusion, placental separation, chorioamnionitis, and premature labor. Reported major injuries have been extremely rare and occurred primarily in the era before concurrent ultrasound guidance was employed. The question of increased fetal loss after amniocentesis has been addressed by several large studies that have shown the relative safety of the procedure. More contemporaneous studies (Eddleman et al. 2006; Mazza et al. 2007) have shown no significant difference in loss rate between patients undergoing amniocentesis and controls, or compared to the calculated background risk for spontaneous abortion in a large reference population. Although one clinical study and several animal studies suggested that respiratory problems occur more often in children born after amniocentesis, respiratory problems in offspring of women undergoing amniocentesis after 14 weeks gestation have not been observed by most investigators. Moreover, long-term follow-up for 7–18 years in children whose mothers had undergone amniocentesis have shown no increase in physical or neurodevelopmental problems (Baird et al. 1994). To summarize, the risk of fetal loss associated with amniocentesis is low. In counseling patients, we cite a 0.25 % risk of spontaneous abortion secondary to amniocentesis.

Early Amniocentesis

Some centers offer amniocentesis at 13–14 weeks of gestation. Because the number of viable amniotic fluid cells increases with gestational age, the number of culture failures and the time required for culturing prior to harvest is increased at earlier gestational ages. Amniocentesis at earlier gestational ages also has a higher failure rate in obtaining fluid on the first attempt. In addition, the total fetal loss rate (7.6 % vs. 5.9 %) and the incidence of clubfoot (1.3 % vs. 0.1 %) are significantly increased following amniocentesis prior to 13 weeks' gestation (Canadian Early and Mid-Trimester Amniocentesis Trial 1998). Therefore, the American College of Obstetricians and Gynecologists and others recommend that amniocentesis not be performed prior to 14 weeks' gestation (ACOG 2007b).

Fluorescence In Situ Hybridization (FISH)

Because the interval from CVS or amniocentesis to completed diagnosis is disconcerting to many patients, an approach that uses interphase cells without the need to await the mitotic cells required for karyotyping, offers significant advantages as the time spent culturing cells can be avoided. DNA probes can hybridize to specific regions on chromosomes irrespective of cell cycle phase. Incubation of amniotic fluid or chorionic villus cells with a fluorochrome labeled chromosome-specific DNA probe results in visible hybridization signals equal in number to the number of copies of that chromosome in the cell. Not only can the number of copies of one particular chromosome be counted, but cells can be probed simultaneously for several chromosomes (e.g., chromosomes 21, 18, 13, X, and Y), thereby detecting all the common aneuploidies seen in liveborns. Amniotic fluid cells, chorionic villus cells, fetal lymphocytes, and nucleated erythrocytes all are feasible targets for hybridization.

Many prospective studies of FISH analysis of amniotic fluid cells have reported good predictive values and results generally available in 1 day. However, not all samples are informative, and not all chromosome abnormalities are detectable with this approach. Evans et al. (1994) estimated that the FISH assay most commonly used in prenatal diagnosis would detect only 65 % of all chromosome abnormalities in their high-risk population (Table 1.4). Therefore, standard cytogenetic analysis must be performed in addition to FISH if the goal is detection of all chromosome abnormalities.

Fluorescently labeled DNA probes can also be used to determine the number of copies of short sequences unique to a specific region of the genome. Therefore, FISH can detect small deletions and duplications that are below the level of visualization of a karyotype. For example, deletion of a small region (q11.2) on chromosome 22 results in DiGeorge syndrome (cardiac defects, immunodeficiency, neurodevelopmental delay, hypocalcemia). Hybridization with a DNA probe for this region will reveal whether a fetus has the normal two, or only one, copy of the region. This is particularly useful in determining whether a fetus with an ultrasound detected cardiac defect typical of DiGeorge syndrome (tetralogy of Fallot, truncus arteriosus, abnormal aortic arch, ventricular septal defect), has an isolated cardiac defect, or the syndrome. FISH can also be used to clarify whether an apparently balanced de novo translocation actually is unbalanced at one of the breakpoints, and to identify the chromosomal origin of a marker (additional structurally abnormal) chromosome.

Chromosomal Microarray (Comparative Genome Hybridization)

Although a traditional karyotype performed on amniotic fluid cells or chorionic villi can detect most chromosome abnormalities in the prenatal population, small deletions and duplications (copy number variants [CNVs]) are not visible with this method. FISH testing can detect some of these structural changes but requires choosing a specific probe for a specific site. A microarray, on the other hand, can detect much smaller chromosomal abnormalities than those detected by a karyotype and allows much broader screening of the genome than that provided by individual FISH tests.

The technique of microarray analysis compares the DNA in a sample to that of a normal individual. There are a variety of "platforms" using thousands of either oligonucleotide or single nucleotide polymorphism (SNP) probes to interrogate the genome. In addition, different laboratories offer different numbers of targets on their platform.

Microarrays are most productive in diagnosing extra or missing material in fetuses with ultrasound visualized abnormalities. In several studies CNVs of clinical significance were found in approximately 6 % of anomalous fetuses with normal karyotypes (Callaway et al. 2013; Hillman et al. 2013; Wapner et al. 2012). The yield is lower in cases studied because of advanced maternal age (1.7 %) or parental anxiety, abnormal serum screen or history of chromosome abnormality (1.1 %). Microarrays can also be useful in determining etiology of intrauterine demise or stillbirth occurring in the second or third trimester.

However, because many targets throughout the genome are interrogated, and genetic variants are common in the general population, many variants are found in every sample. These can be benign polymorphisms, known pathogenic mutations, or variants of unknown significance (VOUS). In the latter case it is not known whether the variant is actually pathogenic and associated with a fetal defect, or a benign, fortuitous finding. Even if a variant is known to be pathological in some individuals, there may be incomplete penetrance (not all individuals with the genetic change express the disorder) and varied expression of the mutation in unrelated individuals and amongst family members. Therefore, while extremely useful in diagnosing pathologic small chromosomal changes in pediatric patients where the phenotype is known, interpretation of results is more problematic in the prenatal setting. Microarrays do not detect balanced chromosome rearrangements and some (oligonucleotide arrays) do not detect triploidy.

For many of the above reasons, ACOG (2013) has recommended the use of chromosomal microarray (CMA) analysis in patients with a fetus with a structural abnormality who are undergoing invasive prenatal diagnosis, and in cases of intrauterine demise, but not for first or second-trimester pregnancy losses. In patients who are having invasive prenatal diagnosis with a structurally normal fetus, CMA is an option, as is routine karyotyping. Obtaining consent for a microarray test requires detailed pretest genetic counseling to ensure the parents' understanding of the limitations of the test and that uncertain results may ensue. For some, the possibility of obtaining additional information about the fetal status justifies the test; for others, the potential additional anxiety of uncertain clinical consequences makes a microarray test undesirable.

Molecular Diagnosis of Mendelian Disorders

Diagnosis of Mendelian disorders is more difficult than chromosome diagnosis. For example, in contrast to most cytogenetic diagnoses, the specific Mendelian disorder sought must be absolutely identified prior to any invasive procedure. If a couple was ascertained because of a previously affected child, the correct diagnosis must be assured by review of old records and test results. Also, for a prenatal diagnosis to be possible the condition must be associated with a known gene mutation, gene location or an abnormal gene product that is expressed in chorionic villi, amniotic fluid cells, or fetal blood. If gene expression is key to the diagnosis, sampling of fetal/placental tissues should not be performed prior to the gestational age at which expression of the protein normally occurs, and gestational age matched controls may be necessary.

Now that the genetic mutation responsible for many Mendelian disorders has been identified, DNA obtained from amniotic fluid cells or from chorionic villi is commonly used for diagnosis of these single gene disorders. The mainstays of DNA diagnosis are polymerase chain reactions (PCRs), restriction enzymes and allele-specific oligonucleotide probes, which allow both direct mutation analysis and linkage analysis, each useful in different circumstances.

When the mutational basis of a condition in an affected family member is known, that mutation (autosomal dominant disorder, X-linked recessive disorder) or pair of mutations (autosomal recessive disorder) can be directly searched for in a sample of cells taken from amniotic fluid or chorionic villi. Diagnosis of cystic fibrosis and some hemoglobinopathies in a fetus are commonly performed in this manner. The same is true for hundreds of other Mendelian disorders.

If, on the other hand, the mutant gene is known but the specific mutation in the family has not been or cannot be identified, or when the gene in question is too large to sequence, indirect analysis with linkage can be performed in some cases. This approach requires identifying genetic markers that are located on the same chromosome as, and very close to (tightly linked), the disease gene. Participation of at least one affected family member is usually required for such studies. Because their genetic location is so close to the disease gene, the markers will usually segregate with the gene, rather than undergo recombination at meiosis. The presence or absence of these markers in the fetal cells can then be used to infer the presence of the abnormal gene.

Diagnosis of many rare Mendelian disorders is only available in a limited number of laboratories. Genetic counseling is almost always helpful in these complicated cases.

Future: Whole-Genome Sequencing (WGS)

Rather than interrogating or sequencing individual parts of the human genome, some far-sighted investigators have suggested sequencing the entire fetal genome (or just the coding portion: whole-exome sequencing [WES]) in an attempt to anticipate and, optimally, successfully treat genetic disorders. In 2012, two groups each reported sequencing a fetal genome from cell free fetal DNA in blood obtained from a pregnant woman (Fan et al. 2012; Kitzman et al. 2012). While certainly a scientific tour de force, the question of whether the information provided is clinically helpful is controversial (Feero 2014; Yurkiewicz et al. 2014). In addition to finding mutations associated with genetic conditions manifesting in childhood, mutations resulting in adult onset disorders are also detected with this approach. The advantage of knowledge of adult onset disorders in fetal life is questionable. In addition, WGS detects a huge number of genetic changes, some true de novo mutations, some inherited changes, and others errors due to technical issues. Many of the de novo mutations will not be known to be associated with a specific condition. This includes variants most often considered traits or benign changes, and variants of unknown significance (VOUS). For VOUS the disease implications and the penetrance of the genetic change are unknown.

As only a small minority of the findings will have known implications, the difficulty of explaining all of the revealed information to future parents seems almost insurmountable at this time. However, as the frequency of benign variants and the pathogenicity of others are revealed through further research studies, it may eventually be possible to identify which variants are of significance and which are not. At that point there may be real benefit in sequencing fetal genomes, and the financial, logistic, and ethical implications of WGS in the prenatal setting will have to be considered (Snyder et al. 2013).

References

American College of Obstetricians and Gynecologists. Screening for fetal chromosomal abnormalities. ACOG Practice Bulletin No. 77. Obstet Gynecol. 2007a;109:217–27.

American College of Obstetricians and Gynecologists. Invasive prenatal testing for aneuploidy. ACOG practice Bulletin No. 88. Obstet Gynecol. 2007b;110:1459–67.

American College of Obstetricians and Gynecologists. Noninvasive prenatal testing for fetal aneuploidy. Committee Opinion No. 545. Obstet Gynecol. 2012;120:1532–4.

American College of Obstetricians and Gynecologists. The use of chromosomal microarray analysis in prenatal diagnosis. Committee Opinion No. 581. Obstet Gynecol 2013;122:1374–7.

Baird PA, Yee IML, Sadovnick AD. Population-based study of long-term outcomes after amniocentesis. Lancet. 1994;344:1134–6.

Bennett RL, Motulsky AG, Bittles A, Hudgins L, Uhrich S, Lochner Doyl D, et al. Genetic counseling and screening of consanguineous couples and their offspring: recommendations of the National Society of Genetic Counselors. J Genet Couns. 2002;11:97–119.

Bianchi DW, Parker RL, Wentworth J, Madankumar R, Saffer C, Das AF, et al. for the CARE Study Group. DNA sequencing versus standard prenatal aneuploidy screening. N Engl J Med. 2014;370:799–808.

Bianchi DW, Platt LD, Goldberg JD, Abuhamad AZ, Sehnert AJ, Rava RP, on behalf of the MatErnal Blood IS Source to Accurately diagnose fetal aneuploidy (MELISSA) Study Group. Genome-wide fetal aneuploidy detection by maternal plasma DNA sequencing. Obstet Gynecol. 2012;119:1–13.

Bianchi DW, Simpson JL, Jackson LG, Elias S, Holzgreve W, Evans MI, et al. Fetal gender and aneuploidy detection using fetal cells in maternal blood: analysis of NIFTY 1 data. National Institute of Child Health and Development Fetal Cell Isolation Study. Prenat Diagn. 2002;22:609–15.

Bonaiti-Pellié C, Smith C. Risk tables for genetic counseling in some common congenital malformations. J Med Genet. 1974;11:375–7.

Boué A, Gallano P. A collaborative study of the segregation of inherited chromosome structural rearrangements in 1356 prenatal diagnoses. Prenat Diagn. 1984;4(spec iss):45–7.

Breathnach FM, Malone FD, Lambert-Messerlian G, Cuckle HS, Porter TF, Nyberg DA, et al. for the First and Second Trimester Evaluation of Risk (FASTER) Research Consortium. First- and second-trimester screening; detection of aneuploidies other than Down syndrome. Obstet Gynecol. 2007;110:651–7.

Callaway JL, Shaffer LG, Chitty LS, Rosenfeld JA, Crolla JA. The clinical utility of microarray technologies applied to prenatal cytogenetics in the presence of a normal conventional karyotype: a review of the literature. Prenat Diagn. 2013;33:1119–23.

Canadian Early and Mid-Trimester Amniocentesis Trial (CEMAT) Group. Randomized trial to assess safety and fetal outcome of early and midtrimester amniocentesis. Lancet. 1998;351:242–7.

Caughey AB. Chorionic villus sampling compared with amniocentesis and the difference in the rate of pregnancy loss. Obstet Gynecol. 2006;108:612–6.

Chitty LS, Khalil A, Barrett AN, Pajkrt E, Griffin DR, Cole TJ. Safe, accurate, prenatal diagnosis of thanatophoric dysplasia using ultrasound and free fetal DNA. Prenat Diagn. 2013;33:416–23.

Chiu RW, Chan KC, Gao Y, Lau VY, Zheng W, Leung TY, et al. Noninvasive prenatal diagnosis of fetal chromosomal aneuploidy by massively parallel genomic sequencing of DNA in maternal plasma. Proc Natl Acad Sci U S A. 2008;105:20458–63. doi:10.1073/pnas.0810641105.

Choi H, Lau TK, Jiang FM, Chan MK, Zhang HY, Lo PSS, et al. Fetal aneuploidy screening by maternal plasma DNA sequencing: "False positive" due to confined placental mosaicism. Prenat Diagn. 2013;33:198–200. doi:10.1002/pd.4024.

Daniel A, Hook EB, Wulf G. Risks of unbalanced progeny at amniocentesis to carriers of chromosomal rearrangements: data from United States and Canadian laboratories. Am J Med Genet. 1989;31:14–53.

Devaney SA, Palomaki GE, Scott JA, Bianchi DW. Noninvasive fetal sex differentiation using cell free fetal DNA. JAMA. 2011;306:627–36.

D'Onofrio BM, Rickert ME, Frans E, Kuja-Halkola R, Almqvist C, Sjölander A, et al. Paternal age at childbearing and offspring psychiatric and academic morbidity. JAMA Psych. 2014;71:432. doi:10.1001/jamapsychiatry.2013.4525.

Eddleman KA, Malone FC, Sullivan L, Dukes K, Berkowitz RL, Kharbutli Y, et al. Pregnancy loss rates after midtrimester amniocentesis. Obstet Gynecol. 2006;108:1067–72.

Evans MI, Ebrahim SAD, Berry SM, Holzgreve W, Isada NB, Quintero RA, et al. Fluorescent in situ hybridization utilization for high-risk prenatal diagnosis: a trade-off among speed, expense, and inherent limitations of chromosome-specific probes. Am J Obstet Gynecol. 1994;171: 1055–7.

Fan HC, Blumenfeld YJ, Chitkara U, Hudgins L, Quake SR. Noninvasive diagnosis of fetal aneuploidy by shotgun sequencing DNA from maternal blood. Proc Natl Acad Sci U S A. 2008;105:16266–71.

Fan HC, Gu W, Wang J, Blumenfeld YJ, El-Sayed YY, Quake SR. Non-invasive prenatal measurement of the fetal genome. Nature. 2012;487:320–6. doi:10.1038/nature11251.

Feero WG. Clinical application of whole-genome sequencing. Proceed with care. JAMA. 2014;311:1017–20.

Friedman JM. Genetic disease in the offspring of older fathers. Obstet Gynecol. 1981;57:745–9.

Froster UG, Jackson L. Limb defects and chorionic villus sampling: results from an international registry, 1992–4. Lancet. 1996;347:489–94.

Fuhrmann W, Vogel F. Genetic counseling. 3rd ed. Berlin: Springer; 1983.

Gardner RJM, Sutherland GR, Shaffer LG. Chromosome abnormalities and genetic counseling. 4th ed. Oxford: Oxford University Press; 2012.

Grody WW, Thompson BH, Gregg AR, Bean LH, Monaghan KG, Schneider A, et al. ACMG position statement on prenatal/preconception expanded carrier screening. Genet Med. 2013;15:482–3. doi:10.1038/gimi2013.47.

Hay S, Barbano H. Independent effects of maternal age and birth order on the incidence of selected congenital malformations. Teratology. 1972;6:271–80.

Hillman SC, McMullan DJ, Hall G, Togneri FS, James N, Maher EJ, et al. Use of prenatal chromosomal microarray: prospective cohort study and systematic review and meta-analysis. Ultrasound Obstet Gynecol. 2013;41:610–20.

Hollier LM, Leveno KJ, Kelly MA, McIntire DD, Cunningham FG. Maternal age and malformations in singleton births. Obstet Gynecol. 2000;96:701–6.

Hook EB. Rates of chromosome abnormalities at different maternal ages. Obstet Gynecol. 1981;58:282–5.

Hook EB. Evaluation and projections of rates of chromosome abnormality in chorionic villus studies (c.v.s.). Am J Hum Genet. 1988;43:A108.

Hook EB, Cross PK, Jackson LG, Pergament E, Brambati B. Maternal age-specific rates of 47, +21 and other cytogenetic abnormalities diagnosed in the first trimester of pregnancy in chorionic villus biopsy samples: comparison with rates expected from observations at amniocentesis. Am J Hum Genet. 1988;42:797–807.

Hook EB, Cross PK, Schreinemachers DM. Chromosome abnormality rates at amniocentesis and in live-born infants. JAMA. 1983;249:2034–8.

Huang X, Zheng J, Chen M, Zhao Y, Zhang C, Liu L, et al. Noninvasive prenatal testing of trisomies 21 and 18 by massively parallel sequencing of maternal plasma DNA in twin pregnancies. Prenat Diagn. 2014;34:335–40. doi:10.1002/pd.4303.

Jackson LG, Zachary JM, Fowler SE, Desnick RJ, Golbus MS, Ledbetter DH, et al. A randomized comparison of transcervical and transabdominal chorionic-villus sampling. N Engl J Med. 1992;327:594–8.

Kitzman JO, Snyder MW, Ventura M, Lewis AP, Qiu R, Simmons LE, et al. Noninvasive whole-genome sequencing of a human fetus. Sci Transl Med. 2012;4:137ra76. doi:10.1126/scitranslmed.3004323.

Lazarin GA, Haque IS, Nazareth S, Iori K, Patterson S, Jacobson JL, et al. An empirical estimate of carrier frequencies for 400+ causal Mendelian variants: results from an ethnically diverse clinical sample of 23,453 individuals. Genet Med. 2013;15:178–86. doi:10.1038/gim.2012.114.

Lo YM, Crobetta N, Chamberlain PF, Rai V, Sargent IL, Redman CW, et al. Presence of fetal DNA in maternal plasma and serum. Lancet. 1997;350:485–7.

Malone FD, Canick JA, Ball RH, Nyberg DA, Comstock CH, Bukowski R, et al. First-trimester or second-trimester screening, or both, for Down's syndrome. N Engl J Med. 2005;353:2001–11.

Mazza V, Pati M, Bertucci E, Re C, Ranzi A, Percesepe A, et al. Age-specific risk of fetal loss post second trimester amniocentesis: analysis of 5043 cases. Prenat Diagn. 2007;27:180–3.

Mikkelsen M. CVS Latest news! 1986 Dec 1;19:7–10.

Milunsky A, Jick SS, Bruell CL, MacLaughlin DS, Tsung Y-K, Jick H, et al. Predictive values, relative risks, and overall benefits of high and low maternal serum α-fetoprotein screening in singleton pregnancies: new epidemiologic data. Am J Obstet Gynecol. 1989;161:291–7.

Moise Jr KJ, Boring NH, O'Shaughnessy R, Simpson LL, Wolfe HM, Baxter JK, et al. Circulating cell-free fetal DNA for the detection of RHD status and sex using reflex fetal identifiers. Prenat Diagn. 2013;33:95–101. doi:10.1002/pd.4018.

Mouawia H, Saker A, Jais JP, Benachi A, Bussières L, Lacour B, et al. Circulating trophoblastic cells provide genetic diagnosis in 63 fetuses at risk for cystic fibrosis or spinal muscular atrophy. Reprod Biomed Online. 2012;25:508–20.

Mujezinovic F, Alfirevic Z. Procedure-related complications of amniocentesis and chorionic villous sampling. Obstet Gynecol. 2007;110:687–94.

NICHD National Registry for Amniocentesis Study Group. Midtrimester amniocentesis for prenatal diagnosis. Safety and accuracy. JAMA. 1976;236:1471–6.

Nicolaides KH, Syngelaki A, Gil M, Atanasova V, Markova D. Validation of targeted sequencing of single-nucleotide polymorphisms for non-invasive prenatal detection of aneuploidy of chromosomes 13, 18, 21, X, and Y. Prenat Diagn. 2013;33:575–9.

Norton ME, Brar H, Weiss J, Karimi A, Laurent LC, Caughey AB, et al. Non-invasive chromosomal evaluation (NICE) study: results of a multicenter prospective cohort study for detection of fetal trisomy 21 and trisomy 18. Am J Obstet Gynecol. 2012;207:137.e1–8.

Olshan AF, Schnitzer PG, Baird PA. Paternal age and the risk of congenital heart defects. Teratology. 1994;50:80–4.

Osborne CM, Hardisty E, Devers P, Kaiser-Rogers K, Hayden MA, Goodnight W, et al. Discordant noninvasive prenatal testing results in a patient subsequently diagnosed with metastatic disease. Prenat Diagn. 2013;33:609–11. doi:10.1002/pd.4100.

Palomaki GE, Haddow JE, Knight GJ, Wald NJ, Kennard A, Canick JA, et al. Risk-based prenatal screening for trisomy 18 using alpha-fetoprotein, unconjugated oestriol and human chorionic gonadotropin. Prenat Diagn. 1995;15:713–23.

Palomaki GE, Kloza EM, Lambert-Messerlian GM, Haddow JE, Neveux LM, Ehrich M, et al. DNA sequencing of maternal plasma to detect Down syndrome: an international clinical validation study. Genet Med. 2011;13:913–20.

Palomaki GE, Neveux LM, Knight GJ, Haddow JE. Maternal serum-integrated screening for trisomy 18 using both first- and second-trimester markers. Prenat Diagn. 2003;23:243–7.

Rhoads GG, Jackson LG, Schlesselman SE, de la Cruz FF, Desnick RJ, Golbus MS, et al. The safety and efficacy of chorionic villus sampling for early prenatal diagnosis. N Engl J Med. 1989;320:609–17.

Shieh JTC, Bittles AH, Hudgins L. Consanguinity and the risk of congenital heart disease. Am J Med Genet. 2012;158A:1236–41. doi:10.1002/ajmg.o.35272.

Sloter E, Nath J, Eskenazi B, Wyrobek AJ. Effects of male age on the frequencies of germinal and heritable chromosomal abnormalities in humans and rodents. Fertil Steril. 2004;81:925–43.

Snyder MW, Simmons LE, Kitzman JO, Santillan DA, Santillan MK, Gammill HS, et al. Noninvasive fetal genome sequencing: a primer. Prenat Diagn. 2013;33:547–54.

Stevenson RE. The genetic basis of human anomalies. In: Stevenson RE, Hall JG, Goodman RM, editors. Human malformations and related anomalies, vol. 1. New York, NY: Oxford University Press; 1993. p. 115–35.

Verp M. Antenatal diagnosis of chromosomal abnormalities. Glob libr. women's med., ISSN: 1756-2228. 2008; DOI: 10.3843/GLOWM.10221.

Verp MS. Chromosomal disorders in pregnancy. In: Gleicher N, editor. Principles of medical therapy in pregnancy. New York, NY: Plenum Publishing; 1985. p. 1223–9.

Verp MS, Rosinsky B, Sheikh Z, Amarose AP. Non-mosaic trisomy 16 confined to villi. Lancet. 1989;2:915–6.

Verp MS, Simpson JL, Ober C. Prenatal diagnosis of genetic disorders. In: Lin CC, Verp MS, Sabbagha RE, editors. The high-risk fetus. New York, NY: Springer; 1993. p. 181.

Vogel F, Rathenberg R. Spontaneous mutation in man. Adv Hum Genet. 1975;5:223–318.

Vora NL, O'Brien BM. Noninvasive prenatal testing for microdeletion syndromes and expanded trisomies. Obstet Gynecol. 2014;123:1097–9.

Wang E, Batey A, Struble C, Musci T, Song K, Oliphant A. Gestational age and maternal weight effects on fetal cell-free DNA in maternal plasma. Prenat Diagn. 2013;33:662–6. doi:10.1002/pd.4119.

Wapner RJ, Martin CL, Levy B, Ballif BC, Eng CM, Zachary JM, et al. Chromosomal microarray versus karyotyping for prenatal diagnosis. N Engl J Med. 2012;367:2175–84.

Warburton D, Dallaire L, Thangavelu M, Ross L, Levin B, Kline J. Trisomy recurrence: a reconsideration based on North American data. Am J Hum Genet. 2004;75:376–85.

Wright CF, Burton H. The use of cell-free fetal nucleic acids in maternal blood for non-invasive prenatal diagnosis. Hum Reprod Update. 2009;14:139–51.

Yao H, Zhang L, Zhang H, Jiang F, Hu H, Chen F, et al. Noninvasive prenatal genetic testing for aneuploidy detects maternal trisomy X. Prenat Diagn. 2012;32:1114–6. doi:10.1002/pd.3946.

Yurkiewicz IR, Korf BR, Lehmann LS. Prenatal whole-genome sequencing – is the quest to know a fetus's future ethical? N Engl J Med. 2014;370:195–7.

Chapter 2
Preimplantation Genetic Screening and Diagnostic Testing

Joe Leigh Simpson

Introduction

Since preimplantation genetic diagnosis (PGD) was first accomplished 25 years ago, thousands of in vitro fertilization (IVF) cycles with PGD have been performed worldwide (www.pgdis.org). The first 1000 PGD births occurred by 2004 (Verlinsky et al. 2004), and since then the pace has accelerated. PGD has evolved from simply an extension of traditional prenatal genetic diagnosis to a method with additional, novel, indications. In this update, we shall consider traditional and novel indications, approaches to obtaining cell(s) for PGD, diagnostic accuracy and methods to maximize accuracy, given the small sample available for diagnosis. That PGD obviates certain ethical dilemmas, yet poses novel controversies, will be discussed.

History

Although usually considered a recent idea, PGD has actually long been envisioned (see Harper (2009) for detailed history). In 1968, Gardner and Edwards biopsied a rabbit blastocyst and performed X-chromatin analysis, suggesting application to human X-linked recessive traits. Over the next decades, mouse geneticists demonstrated the ability to obtain metaphase chromosomes from murine blastomeres (Dyban 1991). However, progress in human PGD was unavoidably delayed until IVF, was successful in 1978 (Steptoe and Edwards 1978). Thereafter, animal studies paved the way for human PGD. Monk and various colleagues biopsied mouse

J.L. Simpson, M.D. (✉)
Department of Research and Grants, March of Dimes Foundation,
1275 Mamaroneck Avenue, White Plains, NY 10605, USA
e-mail: jsimpson@marchofdimes.com

J.P. Galst, M.S. Verp (eds.), *Prenatal and Preimplantation Diagnosis*,
DOI 10.1007/978-3-319-18911-6_2

blastomeres, showing feasibility for detecting a single-gene disorder (Monk and Handyside 1988). Pioneering work by Wilton and Trounson in Melbourne (1989) and by Nijs and Van Steirteghem (1987) in Brussels was especially noteworthy.

With the molecular diagnostic era of the late 1980s, polymerase chain reaction (PCR) made PGD practical. In Chicago, Verlinsky and colleagues developed polar body biopsy and showed clinical application, reporting in 1987 at an international IVF Congress (Verlinsky et al. 1987); their peer publication of this PGD diagnosis (alpha-1 antitrypsin) was delayed until 1990 (Verlinsky et al. 1990). In 1990, PGD for cystic fibrosis was reported by the same group (Strom et al. 1990), again using polar body biopsy. In the UK, Handyside and colleagues pursued blastomere biopsy on cleavage stage (3 day) embryos, in 1990 determining sex in a pregnancy at risk for ornithine transcarbamylase deficiency (OTC), an X-linked disorder (Handyside et al. 1990). This was soon followed by detection of cystic fibrosis, using nested primer PCR (Handyside et al. 1992).

Progress in detecting chromosomal abnormalities awaited development of fluorescence in situ hybridization (FISH) and chromosome-specific probes. In the UK, Griffin successfully performed FISH on blastomeres (Griffin et al. 1991), and in the USA, Grifo did so (Grifo et al. 1990, 1992a). Working with Cohen at Cornell Medical College (New York), a blastomere was subjected to X and Y FISH (Grifo et al. 1992b) to determine sex. Munné applied multicolor FISH to a single blastomere, setting the stage for aneuploidy testing (Munné et al. 1993). Munné also applied FISH for PGD of chromosomal translocations (Munné et al. 1998a, 2000). In the UK, Delhanty and Harper were performing rapid FISH (Harper et al. 1994), and in the USA, Verlinsky et al. (1995) independently applied FISH to polar bodies. These initial approaches permitted concurrent analysis of only a limited number of chromosomes (5–7). At present, chromosomal abnormalities are detected by array CGH or other 24 chromosome approaches to be discussed below.

Obtaining Cells for Preimplantation Genetic Diagnosis

PGD requires a nucleus (DNA) from gametes or from embryos prior to implantation (6 days after conception). There are three potential approaches: (1) polar body biopsy, (2) blastomere biopsy (aspiration) from the 3 day six- to eight-cell cleaving embryo and (3) trophectoderm biopsy from the 5- to 6-day blastocyst.

Polar Biopsy

The oocyte genome—chromosomes or genes—can be deduced by analysis of the first and second polar biopsy (Kuliev et al. 2014). If the first polar body from a heterozygous individual with a mutant allele is abnormal, it must be complemented by a primary oocyte having the normal allele. In such a situation, oocytes deduced to be genetically normal can be allowed to fertilize in vitro; the resulting embryo can be transferred for potential implantation. Conversely, a normal first polar body indicates an abnormal oocyte; thus, fertilization would not proceed. The same principle applies to cytogenetic analysis. If the first polar body does not show a chromosome 21, the oocyte must be presumed to have two number 21 chromosomes. If allowed to be fertilized by a normal (23 chromosomes) sperm, the result would be a trisomic zygote. The principle of complementation also dictates that if the first polar body were to have one number 21 chromosome, the oocyte would also have only one and, hence, be suitable for fertilization and transfer.

The obvious disadvantage of polar body diagnosis is the inability to assess paternal genotype, thus precluding application if the father has an autosomal dominant disorder. Polar body analysis is also less efficient in managing couples at risk for offspring with autosomal recessive disorders because even if the maternal allele is transmitted, the paternal allele might not be (normal sperm). In that case, the embryo would have been normal (heterozygous) like its parents but, not knowing the status of the paternal allele, this embryo would not be eligible for transfer. On the other hand, because chromosomal trisomy usually originates in maternal meiosis, in 90–95 % of all cases PGD is applicable for chromosome diagnosis.

PGD by polar body analysis must take into account recombination. At least one recombinational event occurs on each pair of chromosomes, thus maintaining orderly disjunction. If recombination were not to occur in the region or chromosome in question, the second polar body would be identical to the oocyte. If, however, crossing over were to involve the region containing the gene in question, the two chromatids of the single chromosome in the first polar body would differ and in aggregate show both alleles (heterozygosity). Given recombination, genotype of the oocyte could not be predicted without either biopsy of the second polar body or biopsy of the embryo *itself.* Actually, biopsy of polar bodies followed by biopsy of the embryo at the cleavage stage does not seem to decrease pregnancy rates compared to either alone (Cieslak-Janzen et al. 2006). In practice, both first and second polar bodies are typically biopsied unless a specific reason exists to the contrary. See below for one such an indication.

Cleavage Stage Embryo (8-Cell Blastomere Biopsy)

In the 3-day (8-cell embryo), a glycoprotein layer surrounds the embryo. This zona must be traversed by mechanical, laser or chemical means in order to extract a cell(s). The usual approach is to remove only one cell (blastomere). However, even one cell less reduces embryo survival, as manifested by a reduction in pregnancy rate; removal of two cells reduces the pregnancy rate further (Cohen et al. 2007). Practicing in an experienced center (Brussels) that once routinely removed two cells, DeVos et al. (2009) reported live birthrates of 37.4 % and 22.4 % after removal of one versus two cells, respectively.

Although beyond the scope of this chapter, a key diagnostic impediment in cleavage stage analysis is now recognized—mosaicism. This phenomenon can occur in any tissue, but is especially prone at this stage of embryogenesis. Presumably, the developing embryo is undergoing self-correction of some nature. The single blastomere removed may unwittingly be atypically aneuploid, unrepresentative of the remaining normal cells. However, because the euploid status of the remaining cells is unknown, the opportunity to transfer a normal embryo is lost.

Blastocyst (Trophectoderm Biopsy)

The trophectoderm can be biopsied in the 5- to -6 day, 120-cell blastocyst. More cells can be removed at this stage, potentially facilitating diagnosis. Because the trophectoderm is destined to form the placenta, embryonic cells per se are not removed.

Trophectoderm biopsy and analysis of blastocysts have long been envisioned (Dorkas et al. 1990; Carson 1991). Prior to development of PGD, Buster et al. (1985) recovered human blastocysts by uterine lavage. Lavage for blastocyst recovery was at that time considered an approach to obtain embryos for trophectoderm biopsy for genetic diagnosis. However, lavage and PGD were not pursued because of fear of retained (unexamined) embryos.

Decades later, blastocyst transfer in non-PGD assisted reproductive technology (ART) has become routine and shows high pregnancy rates. If biopsy is envisioned, the blastocyst is now seen as the preferred stage, facilitated by the use of laser for trophectoderm biopsy. The additional 2 or 3 days in culture beyond that required for transfer of an 8-cell embryo allows some selection against non-thriving embryos, but two-thirds of aneuploid embryos still continue until day 5 or 6. PGD is thus required to exclude remaining aneuploidies.

PGD for Traditional Prenatal Genetic Diagnostic Indications

Chromosomal Aneuploidy

The most common indication for PGD is detection of chromosomal abnormalities, most often aneuploidies. Although possible, it has never been possible to obtain a karyotype on a single cell reliably (Verlinsky and Evsikov 1999; Shkumatov et al. 2007). Therefore, PGD for cytogenetic analysis began by relying on FISH with chromosome-specific probes (Handyside et al. 2010; Simpson 2010). This was initially applicable for only a limited number of chromosomes, usually 5–9. No more than five different chromosome-specific probes could be subjected to hybridization per cycle, meaning 2–3 cycles were necessary even for interrogating 10–12 chromosomes. This required genuine expertise, which few laboratories were able to provide. FISH for PGD aneuploidy testing has now been largely replaced by genome-wide molecular approaches, namely single nucleotide polymorphisms (SNPs) from all chromosomes (Handyside et al. 2010) or array CGH (chromosomal microarrays) (Munné et al. 2010).

Array CGH is based on comparative genomic hybridization (CGH), a molecular cytogenetic technique that allows comprehensive analysis of the entire genome. The basis is the ability of single-stranded DNA from one source to anneal (hybridize) with a complementary single-stranded DNA from another source. Typically, normal (control) DNA is labeled with a fluorochrome of one color (e.g., green); test (patient) DNA is labeled with a fluorochrome of a different color (e.g., red). Once both test and control DNA are denatured (single stranded), hybridization can occur between the two. Provided that equal amounts of control and test DNA are present, the color of the hybridized mixture should be yellow if fluorochromes of the above two colors are used. If test DNA originates from a trisomic individual, the DNA of that chromosome is present in excess. Thus, the array would show more of the color used to connote test (patient) DNA.

In practice, small amounts of single-stranded DNA of known sequence are placed by photolithography onto a platform (array) in ordered fashion. The amount of DNA in each "spot" is small (i.e., micro = microarray). The number of sequences is chosen in advance but is expected to encompass the entire genome, with one sequence overlaying the adjacent one ("tiling"). Again, "control" DNA embedded by photolithography is labeled with a fluorochrome of one color, and exposed to single-stranded test DNA (e.g., patient) labeled with a fluorochrome of a different color as reasoned above. If control and test DNA are equal in quantity for a given sequence, or given chromosomes, the result is yellow. If test (patient) DNA is in excess (trisomy), that color predominates: If test DNA is deficient, the other color predominates.

Various commercial platforms all interrogate/sequences of DNA along every chromosome; however, sensitivity (coverage) varies. Arrays used to interrogate blood from liveborn infants or chorionic villi or amniotic fluid cells are designed to be more sensitive than those used for analysis in PGD. The latter are designed to detect only aneuploidies or large duplications or deficiencies. It is reasoned that the small amount of DNA available for PGD (6 pg per cell) precludes robust, more sensitive, diagnostic attempts. In addition, analysis based on a single cell (blastomere) shows a very high number of variants of uncertain significance. Given the high proportion of the latter, it can be assumed that not all convey untoward clinical significance because, if so, very few conceptions would yield viable pregnancies.

The array CGH typically used for PGD deserves special comment because it is based on bacterial artificial chromosomes (BACs) (BlueGnome)™. Only large chromatin segments are therefore interrogated because BAC arrays are large; thus only large (5 or 10 Mb: 5,000,000–10,000,000 base pairs) abnormalities are detected, much like a karyotype. The dilemma of disclosing or not disclosing smaller copy number variants (200 kb), which have increased likelihood of variants uncertain clinical significance (VOUS), does not arise in PGD diagnostics. Thus, PGD differs from prenatal genetic diagnosis; VOUS arises more often when analyzing chorionic villi or amniotic fluid cells. Of course, the downside is that microdeletions and other abnormalities smaller in magnitude are not sought in PGD.

Chromosomal Rearrangements

Chromosomal rearrangements (translocation or inversion) may result in unbalanced gametes and, hence, an unbalanced zygote. Many couples with balanced rearrangements are diagnosed after repeated spontaneous abortions, reflecting lethality often conferred by unbalanced gametes. Unbalanced rearrangements can be recognized by array CGH gains and/or losses involving two or more chromosomes. PGD not only reduces the number of abnormal liveborns but also obviates increased spontaneous abortions due to chromosomal imbalance. Reproductive efficiency is improved by transferring only cytogenetically normal or balanced embryos (Munné et al. 1998b, 2000). Because not all embryos are normal or balanced, clinical success requires a sufficient number of embryos from which the relatively few normal embryos can be identified. If pregnancy is attempted by natural conception, multiple attempts might be required to achieve conception with a normal embryo and, hence, continuing pregnancy (Fritz and Schattman 2008). Without PGD the necessary time required to achieve a pregnancy with a normal or balanced embryo might, for certain women, extend beyond the age realistic to achieve pregnancy. The mean time for translocation couples to achieve pregnancy naturally is 4–6 years (Goddijn et al. 2004; Stephenson and Sierra 2006; Sugiaura-Ogasawara et al. 2004). Using PGD, Otani et al. (2006) observed only 5.3 % abortions after PGD for translocations, far fewer than expected for women of comparable age. The lifetime cumulative pregnancy rate using PGD was 57.6 % involving an average of only 1.24 cycles.

One shortcoming of array CGH in couples with a balanced translocation is that it is not possible to distinguish between clinically normal embryos with or without the balanced translocation. Both have the same amount of DNA, the end point of array CGH. Breakpoint-specific probes could accomplish this, and were indeed employed in the early years of PGD translocation analysis (Munné et al. 1998a); however, costs were prohibitive. At present, haplotyping using SNPs could theoretically be applied. Current practice is simply to perform array CGH to exclude unbalanced embryos, transferring genetically normal embryos that may or may not be translocation carriers.

Single-Gene Disorders

Approximately one fourth of PGD cases are currently performed to detect a single mutant gene (ESHRE 2014). It is estimated that about 12,000 PGD cycles have been performed worldwide for this indication. The most frequent indications are hemoglobinopathies, cystic fibrosis, fragile X syndrome, and Duchenne muscular dystrophy. See Kuliev et al. (2014) and supplements to the ESHRE PGD Consortium (2014) for updated lists of disorders tested in US and European labs, respectively.

PGD can be performed whenever the chromosomal location of a given disease-causing gene is known. This holds even if the molecular basis of a causative mutation at the nucleotide level is not known. In that case, linkage analysis can be performed using polymorphic loci. Initially the polymorphisms were short terminal repeats or STRs, but SNPs can now also be used. Linkage analysis should, in fact, *always* be employed in PGD for single-gene disorders because of the phenomenon of allele drop out (ADO), to be discussed below.

In detecting single-gene disorders, one must amplify the small amount of DNA, using a technique called whole genome amplification (WGA). Efficiency does not exceed 90–95 % (Guidelines for Good Practice in PGD: programme requirements and laboratory quality assurance 2008). When amplification does not occur, ADO exists and no information (no result) is obtained. This presumably reflects stochastic phenomena by which probes fail to locate patient DNA, precluding hybridization and, hence, diagnosis. This is probably exacerbated when embryo damage has occurred in biopsy, resulting in loss of embryonic DNA. Diagnostic problems arise if ADO is not recognized. If only one allele is detected, it would not be known whether both alleles (identical) are in fact present or if one of two discordant alleles failed to amplify. If the mutant allele failed to amplify in a dominant disorder, a false negative result would exist. However, one can recognize ADO if linked markers both 5′ and 3′ to the mutant allele are interrogated. Linkage analysis is thus required in all PGD single-gene cases. Using this approach, Reproductive Genetics Innovation (RGI) has observed in a 20-year period only three errors in 2300 single-gene PGD cycles that resulted in over 500 babies (Kuliev et al. 2014). Liebaers and colleagues (2010) reported 0.6 % misdiagnosis in 581 single-gene PGD pregnancies studied. In the most recent ESHRE PGD Consortium report (December 2009–October 2010), there were no single-gene misdiagnoses in 1597 oocyte retrievals for single-gene disorders.

Prenatal Diagnosis Practical Only by PGD

Multiple At-Risk Single-Gene Conditions

PGD may be the only practical reproductive genetic diagnosis option when two different single-gene disorders are segregating in a given family, especially if the couple is older and has a limited interval to conceive. If a couple is at 50 % risk for an autosomal dominant disorder and independently for a non-linked autosomal recessive disorder (25 %), the likelihood that any given offspring (embryo) will be genetically normal is only $1/2 \times 3/4$ or $3/8 = 37.5$ %. Choosing from among multiple embryos enables the minority of embryos that are not affected to be identified and transferred.

Avoidance of Knowledge of Parental Genotype

PGD is the only practical approach if a person at risk for an adult-onset autosomal dominant disorder wishes to remain unaware of his/her status but nonetheless does not wish to burden offspring with a similar dilemma. This occurs when an ostensibly normal individual is the offspring of a mother or father who is affected with a disorder manifested only after reproductive age; risk is 50 % for the parent to be affected; and 25 % for each offspring (1/2 × 1/2 = 1/4). The prototypic indications are Huntington disease and early onset autosomal dominant Alzheimer disease. With PGD, multiple embryos can be tested to identify unaffected embryos suitable for transfer. If provider and patient agree *not* to disclose, the couple will be told no information in a given cycle other than that an embryo will or will not be available. The couple will not know the number of embryos retrieved or reason for no transfer if that situation arises. Failure to transfer could thus be speculated to be failure of embryonic development, aneuploid embryos (even if they lack the mutation), or embryos having the mutation for which they are at risk. Given these plausible options, a sham transfer is not necessary. Traditional prenatal genetic diagnosis using chorionic villus sampling (CVS) or amniocentesis theoretically could accomplish the same goal, but would involve terminations or subterfuge (e.g., claiming a trisomic fetus when the real diagnosis was the presence of the mutant allele).

A caveat in nondisclosure is that the scenario must be repeated in subsequent cycles, even if studies during the initial cycle proved the at-risk patient was actually unaffected. Otherwise, any at-risk patient could readily deduce his/her genotype (e.g., if they were told PGD was no longer indicated). The number of PGD cases performed for non-disclosure constitutes about 5–10 % of single-gene disorders in the ESHRE data collection and in two large US centers. With the new option of biopsies of multiple embryos, vitrification, and then transfer of a single embryo in subsequent natural cycles, a less unwieldy protocol is possible.

Selection of HLA-Compatible Embryos

One in four sibs is human leukocyte antigen (HLA)-compatible (identical), barring recombination that occurs in 5–10 % of cases. Having an HLA-compatible sibling could be invaluable if an older, moribund sibling with a lethal disease—genetic or nongenetic—could potentially benefit from stem cell transplantation to repopulate his/her bone marrow. Stem cell transplantation of HLA-compatible sibs is very successful (90–95 %), but much less so (60 %) if the individuals are not HLA-compatible. The ideal source of stem cells from a healthy sibling is umbilical cord blood. Given 25 % risk for an autosomal recessive disorder (e.g., β-thalassemia or Fanconi anemia), the obvious strategy for a couple wishing to avoid another genetically abnormal child is not only using PGD to exclude an affected embryo but also selecting an HLA-compatible embryo. Doing so would allow harvesting at birth of otherwise discarded umbilical cord blood to use for generating stem cells. If the latter are transplanted successfully into the older, moribund sib, he/she should survive and thrive.

Given that the pregnancy is also at risk for an autosomal recessive disorder, the likelihood of a genetically normal HLA-compatible embryo is low: 1/4 HLA-compatible × 3/4 unaffected with the disease = 3/16. If recombination occurs within the HLA locus, it is not possible to have a 100 % compatible match. Recombination found in a tested embryo indicates lack of suitability for transfer.

PGD for the purpose of transferring HLA-compatible embryos was first performed by Verlinsky and colleagues in a couple at risk for Fanconi anemia (Verlinsky et al. 2001). By 2004, 45 cycles for HLA typing had been performed (Kuliev and Verlinsky 2004a, 2004b, 2006; Verlinsky et al. 2004); 17.5 % of embryos were genetically suitable for transfer, very near the expected 18.7 % (3/16). In their 2014 report, Kuliev et al. (2014) tabulated 374 PGD cycles for HLA testing on 163 different patients.

In the USA and Turkey, PGD to obtain HLA-compatible embryos is performed not only for genetic indications but for nongenetic cases. The most common indication is leukemia in an older sib; transplantation of umbilical cord stem cells from a younger sib could be lifesaving. This was first shown by Kuliev and Verlinsky (2004a). PGD for HLA typing alone accounts for approximately one third of HLA matching PGD cases in the USA. This indication is much less common in the ESHRE PGD Consortium, save Turkey.

Aneuploidy testing is also recommended in couples desiring HLA-compatible embryos, as it is for all single-gene PGD. This is in particular true when a couple is relatively older. Rechitsky et al. (2009) reported that aneuploidy testing concurrent with HLA typing in 57 cycles yielded a 48.5 % pregnancy rate, twice that of age-matched HLA cases (<35 years) not undergoing aneuploidy testing.

Preconceptional PGD

The first polar body is extruded *before* fertilization. The second polar body, by contrast, is not extruded until the oocyte is fertilized (syngamy). Biopsy of the first polar body can, uniquely, provide *preconceptional* information. This is the only option for prenatal diagnosis in couples who do not wish to discard an abnormal embryo. First polar body PGD is also the only option if one must, for statutory reasons, limit the number of oocytes fertilized or embryos transferred. Biopsy of the first polar body allows, in the absence of recombination, normal oocytes to be identified. Thus, fertilizing only euploid oocytes can yield reasonable pregnancy rates, despite restrictive legislation as in Italy (Law 40) (Gianaroli et al. 2009).

Other Indications for PGD Aneuploidy Testing

Repeated Spontaneous Abortions

At least 50 % of first-trimester spontaneous abortions have numerical chromosomal abnormalities (aneuploidy). This is positively correlated with maternal age. A corollary, given that so many aneuploidies persist until clinical recognition of pregnancy, is that 50 % of *morphologically normal* embryos in women >35 years old are chromosomally abnormal and perhaps 25 % in younger women. Selecting an embryo optimal for transfer cannot be based solely upon morphology. Nonrandom distribution occurs in successive miscarriages; abortuses tend to be either successively aneuploid or successively euploid (Warburton et al. 2004). This stratification also occurs in preimplantation embryos tracked in successive cycles (Rubio et al. 2003).

Given the above, the rationale for performing PGD aneuploidy testing and transferring only euploid embryos in couples having experienced repeated abortions is unassailable. The rationale is strongest if at least one loss has been confirmed to be aneuploid. However, this information is not always known. If information regarding the chromosomal status of prior losses is not available, one can perform array CGH on archived specimens embedded in paraffin. If this also is not possible, the assumption should be that only half of couples with recurrent first trimester pregnancy losses will have experienced recurrent aneuploidy.

Randomized clinical trials (RCTs) have not been performed, but PGD in this circumstance has been repeatedly shown beneficial in descriptive studies (Gianaroli et al. 1999; Munné et al. 1999, 2005; Verlinsky et al. 2005; Verlinsky and Kuliev 2005a). One good surrogate involves comparison to objective criteria using the Brigham formula (Brigham et al. 1999), which takes into account maternal age and the number of prior abortions to derive the likelihood of a pregnancy loss. Munné et al. (2005) observed losses in only 13 % of couples who used PGD, compared to the expected rate (Brigham) of 33 %. Benefit was greatest for women older than 35 (expected 39 % vs observed 13 %; $p<0.001$). That is, the increased loss rate due to aneuploidy in older women is obviated by PGD aneuploidy testing.

PGD Aneuploidy Testing to Improve ART Pregnancy Rates

Ability to detect and transfer euploid embryos in ART should increase pregnancy rates in women who otherwise have no genetic indications for PGD. In Europe this is typically termed preimplantation genetic screening or PGS. Pregnancy rates in ART decline markedly beginning late in the fourth decade of a woman's life, primarily as a result of high embryonic losses due to aneuploidy. That endometrial factors are not paramount is evident by women in their fifth decade having successful pregnancies following transfer of donor embryos or use of a donor oocyte. Not only does aneuploidy increase with increasing maternal age, but miscarriage rates do as well. The decreasing ART pregnancy rate per maternal age is thus a mirror image of the increasing miscarriage rate. Based on success rates prior to and after PGD, favorable results were reported from experienced centers worldwide beginning in the late 1990s (Gianaroli et al. 1999, 2005; Munné et al. 1999, 2003; Verlinsky et al. 2005; Verlinsky and Kuliev 2005b, c). The same held when compared to historical expectations for age-matched women not undergoing PGD. Two smaller RCTs conducted in the USA (Mersereau et al. 2008; Werlin et al. 2003) showed improved pregnancy rates.

By the early 2000s, most larger PGD and ART centers in the USA and Europe were offering PGD to improve pregnancy rates in older women. However, the largest centers in the USA and Italy could never complete a RCT. Not only could such "embryo research" not be funded federally (National Institutes of Health) in the USA, but patients universally declined to participate when RCTs were attempted (Munné 2008, Study NCT 006646893). In the USA, the reality of self-funding and lack of adequate insurance coverage will doubtless continue to impede such trials, few patients agreeing to being assigned to the control arm given plausible rationale and now data favoring benefit of the PGD arm.

Given inability to conduct RCTs in larger centers, other European centers did conduct RCTs. With one exception, these centers had relatively little experience before initiating their RCT. None showed significant improvement in pregnancy rates (Debrock et al. 2010; Hardarson et al. 2008; Mastenbroek et al. 2007; Mersereau et al. 2008; Schoolcraft et al. 2010; Staessen et al. 2004, 2008). This author elsewhere has critiqued the RCTs of this era.

Since the RCTs mentioned above were performed (~2007), diagnostic approaches have greatly improved. The preferred way now is to obtain embryo DNA from trophectoderm biopsy of the 5–6 day blastocyst. This minimizes the pitfall of mosaicism that may occur if a single (unrepresentative) cell is analyzed in a cleavage stage 8-cell, 3-day embryo. Trophectoderm biopsy of the 5–6 day blastocyst also seems less difficult technically than blastomere biopsy of the 3-day cleavage stage embryo. Further, more than a single cell is obtained.

Irrespective of biopsy, the pivotal advance has been ability to interrogate all 24 chromosomes and to do so accurately, using either array CGH or a SNP-based method.

Recent RCTs have been performed by experienced labs, all showing statistically significant increased pregnancy rates. Schoolcraft and Katz-Jaffe (2013) reported the pregnancy rate to be 61 % for a single euploid blastocyst undergoing PGD but 41 % with an untested embryo; Yang et al. (2012) reported pregnancy rates of 69 % and 42 %. Scott et al. (2013) reported sustained implantation rates (leading to delivery) to be 66 % with quantitative PCR-based PGD and 48 % without PGD ($p=0.001$).

Of great public health impact, blastocyst PGD aneuploidy testing allows such good pregnancy rates that single embryo transfer can be defended with its benefit of avoiding multiple gestation. Forman et al. (2013) performed a RCT in which a single morphologically normal blastocyst embryo was subjected to PGD aneuploidy testing to confirm euploidy; the comparison arm involved two morphologically normal embryos that were transferred without PGD. Pregnancy rates in the two groups were not significantly different (61 % vs 65 %), but twin rates were strikingly different: 0 vs 53 %. (It should be remembered that not all embryos reach blastocyst stage; thus, the rates cited above are not per initiated cycle but per blastocyst transfer.) Multiple gestations carry significant morbidity due to preterm births with high economic costs (Chambers et al. 2014). Thus, it can be confidently predicted that interest in single embryo transfer will grow in order to decrease the frequency of multiple gestations and their neonatal complications, and PGD to select euploid embryos will be increasingly utilized.

Adult-Onset Disorders in Which One Parent Is Already Affected

Prenatal genetic diagnosis for adult-onset single-gene conditions was once not considered appropriate ("not ethical"). The reasoning was that prenatal diagnosis should not be offered and, hence, a diagnosis provided, if it could lead to termination for a disorder not associated with mental retardation nor manifested at birth. Given preimplantation genetic diagnosis, the situation has changed (Simpson 2002). Certainly this applies in the USA, although reticence still exists in much of Europe. Presumably the reason is that PGD to exclude transmission of an embryo with an autosomal dominant trait is more acceptable to at-risk families than first—or second—trimester prenatal diagnosis with its potential for clinical termination. Greater acceptance seems to exist if embryos and not fetuses are being tested and their results acted upon before a clinical pregnancy.

The first PGD case performed for a familial cancer syndrome involved Li–Fraumeni syndrome, a multisystem cancer syndrome due to a p53 perturbation (Verlinsky et al. 2001). Detection of other disorders rapidly followed (Rechitsky et al. 2002). BRCA1, multiple endocrine neoplasia, familial adenomatous polyposis (FAP), retinoblastoma, and von Hippel–Lindau (VHL) syndrome are the most common indications.

Safety of PGD

Removal of embryonic cells as required for PGD might logically be expected to adversely affect implantation or decrease survival and, hence, decrease ART pregnancy rates. However, the totipotential nature of embryonic cells at this stage of embryogenesis offers safety against organ-specific anomalies arising in liveborns. Loss of one or more cells prior to commitment to a given developmental pathway is considered mitigated by another cell with the biological capacity to accomplish that same purpose. Thus, the malformation rate should not differ from that in the general population, as shown conclusively in many animal experiments.

In humans, a confounder in assessing safety of embryo biopsy is that the rate of birth defects in non-PGD ART pregnancies is 30 % greater than in the general (non-ART) population (Hansen et al. 2005). It is unclear whether this increase is due to the ART protocol itself or rather due to the underlying infertility that necessitated ART. The latter seems the likely explanation, as best shown by Zhu et al. (2006) who observed a 20 % increase in birth defects in infertile couples who after 12 months of infertility eventually became pregnant without ART. Similar results were reported by Jacques et al. (2010) and Davies et al. (2012). The latter showed the odds ratio to be 1.2 for birth defects in offspring of women who underwent ART in one cycle but conceived spontaneously in a later cycle.

Irrespective of the background rate against which anomalies in PGD offspring should be compared, there seems to be no increased rate in anomalous liveborns after PGD. Liebaers et al. (2010) performed physical exams 2 months after birth in 563 PGD liveborns, 18 stillborns and 9 neonatal deaths. Anomalies were compared to those in a previously reported cohort study of intracytoplasmic sperm injection (ICSI) offspring who did not undergo PGD (Bonduelle et al. 2003). In approximately half the cohort studied by Liebaers et al. (2010), the indication for PGD was a single-gene disorder; in the other half the indication was aneuploidy testing. Structural malformations were found in 2.13 % in the PGD group and 3.38 % in the ICSI group. No differences were observed between the single-gene PGD group and the aneuploidy PGD group. In a smaller matched pair study ($N = 102$ in each arm), more in depth clinical assessment was performed, but still no statistical difference between PGD and ICSI offspring (Desmyttere et al. 2009) was observed.

In conclusion, it can be confidently stated that at present PGD seems safe (Simpson 2010). Given its efficacy and the increasing number of indications for which it is appropriate, it is reasonable to expect that PGD will become a common and desired component of IVF.

References

Bonduelle M, Ponjaert I, Steirteghem AV, Derde MP, Devroey P, Liebaers I. Developmental outcome at 2 years of age for children born after ICSI compared with children born after IVF. Hum Reprod. 2003;18:342–50.

Brigham SA, Conlon C, Farquharson RG. A longitudinal study of pregnancy outcome following idiopathic recurrent miscarriage. Hum Reprod. 1999;14:2868–71.

Buster JE, Bustillo M, Rodi IA, Cohen SW, Hamilton M, Simon JA, et al. Biologic and morphologic development of donated human ova recovered by nonsurgical uterine lavage. Am J Obstet Gynecol. 1985;53:211–7.

Carson S. Biopsy of blastocysts. In: Verlinsky Y, Kuliev A, editors. Preimplantation genetics. New York, NY: Plenum Press; 1991. p. 85–8.

Chambers GM, Hoang VP, Lee E, Hansen M, Sullivan EA, Bower C, et al. Hospital costs of multiple-birth and singleton-birth children during the first 5 years of life and the role of assisted reproductive technology. JAMA Pediatr. 2014;168:1045. doi:10.1001/jamapediatrics.2014.1357.

Cieslak-Janzen J, Tur-Kaspa I, Ilkevitch Y, Bernal A, Morris R, Verlinsky Y. Multiple micromanipulations for preimplantation genetic diagnosis do not affect embryo development to the blastocyst stage. Fertil Steril. 2006;85:1826–9.

Cohen J, Wells D, Munné S. Removal of 2 cells from cleavage stage embryos is likely to reduce the efficacy of chromosomal tests that are used to enhance implantation rates. Fertil Steril. 2007;87:496–503.

Davies MJ, Moore VM, Willson KJ, Van Essen P, Priest K, Scott H, et al. Reproductive technologies and the risk of birth defects. N Engl J Med. 2012;366:1803–13.

Debrock S, Melotte C, Spiessens C, Peeraer K, Vanneste E, Meeuwis L, et al. Preimplantation genetic screening for aneuploidy of embryos after in vitro fertilization in women aged at least 35 years: a prospective randomized trial. Fertil Steril. 2010;93:364–73.

Desmyttere S, Bonduelle M, Nekkebroeck J, Roelants M, Liebaers I, De Schepper J. Growth and health outcome of 102 2-year-old children conceived after preimplantation genetic diagnosis or screening. Early Hum Develop. 2009;85:755–9.

DeVos A, Staessen C, De Rycke M, Verpoest W, Haentiens P, Devroey P, et al. Impact of cleavage-stage embryo biopsy in view of PGD on human blastocyst implantation: a prospective cohort of single embryo transfers. Hum Reprod. 2009;24:2988–96.

Dorkas A, Sargent IL, Ross C, Gardner RL, Barlow DH. Trophectoderm biopsy in human blastocysts. Hum Reprod. 1990;5:821–5.

Dyban AP. Experimental cytogenetics of preimplantation development. In: Verlinsky Y, Kuliev A, editors. Preimplantation genetics. New York, NY: Plenum Press; 1991. p. 15–23.

Forman EJ, Hong KH, Franasiak JM, Scott Jr RT. Obstetrical and neonatal outcomes from the BEST Trial: single embryo transfer with aneuploidy screening improves outcomes after in vitro fertilization without compromising delivery rates. Am J Obstet Gynecol. 2013;210:157.e1–e6.

Fritz MA, Schattman G. Reply of the Committee: parental translocations and need for preimplantation genetic diagnosis? Distorting effects of ascertainment bias and the need for information-rich families. Fertil Steril. 2008;90:892–3.

Gardner RL, Edwards RG. Control of sex ratio at full term in the rabbit by transferring sexed blastocysts. Nature. 1968;218:346–9.

Gianaroli L, Magli MC, Ferraretti AP, Munné S. Preimplantation diagnosis for aneuploidies in patients undergoing in vitro fertilization with poor prognosis: identification of the categories to which it should be proposed. Fertil Steril. 1999;72:837–44.

Gianaroli L, Magli C, Ferraretti AP, Tabanelli C, Trengia V, Farfalli V, et al. The beneficial effects of PGD for aneuploidy support extensive clinical application. Reprod Biomed Online. 2005;10:633–40.

Gianaroli L, Magli MC, Lappi M, et al. Preconception diagnosis. 9th International Conference on Preimplantation Genetics, Miami, Florida, April 23–25. Reprod Biomed Online. 2009;18:S5.

Goddijn M, Joosten JHK, Knegt AC, van der Veen F, Franssen MTM, Bonsel GJ, et al. Clinical relevance of diagnosing structural chromosome abnormalities in couples with repeated miscarriage. Hum Reprod. 2004;19:1013–7.

Griffin DK, Handyside AH, Penketh RJ, Winston RM, Delhanty JD. Fluorescent in-situ hybridization to interphase nuclei of human preimplantation embryos with X and Y chromosome specific probes. Hum Reprod. 1991;6:101–5.

Grifo JA, Boyle A, Fischer E, Lavy G, DeCherney AH, Ward DC, et al. Preembryo biopsy and analysis of blastomere by in situ hybridization. Am J Obstet Gynecol. 1990;163(6 Pt 1): 2013–9.

Grifo JA, Boyle A, Tang YX, Ward DC. Preimplantation genetic diagnosis. In situ hybridization as a tool for analysis. Arch Pathol Lab Med. 1992a;116:393–7.

Grifo JA, Tang YX, Cohen J, Gilbert F, Sanyal MK, Rosenwaks Z. Pregnancy after embryo biopsy and coamplification of DNA from X and Y chromosomes. JAMA. 1992b;268:727–9.

Handyside AH, Kontogianni EH, Hardy K, Winston RM. Pregnancies from biopsied human preimplantation embryos sexed by Y-specific DNA amplification. Nature. 1990;244:768–70.

Handyside AH, Lesko JG, Tarin JJ, Winston RM, Hughes MR. Birth of a normal girl after in-vitro fertilization and preimplantation diagnostic testing for cystic fibrosis. N Engl J Med. 1992; 327:905–9.

Handyside AH, Harton GL, Mariani B, Thornhill AR, Affara N, Shaw MA, et al. Karyomapping: a universal method for genome wide analysis of genetic disease based on mapping crossovers between parental haplotypes. J Med Genet. 2010;47:651.

Hansen M, Bower C, Milne E, de Klerk N, Kurinczuk JJ. Assisted reproductive technologies and the risk of birth defects—a systematic review. Hum Reprod. 2005;20:328–38.

Hardarson T, Hanson C, Lundin K, Hillensio T, Nilsson L, Stevic J, et al. Preimplantation genetic screening in women of advanced maternal age caused a decrease in clinical pregnancy rate: a randomized controlled trial. Hum Reprod. 2008;23:2617–21.

Harper J. Preimplantation genetic diagnosis. 2nd ed. Cambridge: Cambridge University Press; 2009.

Harper JC, Coonen E, Ramaekers FC, Delhanty JD, Handyside AH, Winston RM, et al. Identification of the sex of human preimplantation embryos in two hours using an improved spreading method and fluorescent in situ hybridization using directly labelled probes. Hum Reprod. 1994;9:721–4.

Jacques AM, Amor DJ, Baker HW, Healy DL, Ukoumunne OC, Breheny S, et al. Adverse obstetric and perinatal outcomes in subfertile women conceiving without assisted reproductive technologies. Fertil Steril. 2010;94:2674–9.

Kuliev A, Verlinsky Y. Thirteen years' experience of preimplantation diagnosis: report of the Fifth International Symposium on Preimplantation Genetics. Reprod Biomed Online. 2004a;8:28–235.

Kuliev A, Verlinsky Y. Preimplantation HLA typing and stem cell transplantation: report of international Meeting, Cyprus, March 27-28, 2004b. Reprod Biomed Online. 2004b;9:205–9.

Kuliev A, Verlinsky Y. The future of preimplantation diagnosis. Exp Rev Obstet Gynecol. 2006;1:95–102.

Kuliev A, Rechitsky S, Verlinsky O. Atlas of preimplantation genetic diagnosis. 3rd ed. Boca Raton, FL: Taylor & Francis Group, LLC.; 2014.

Liebaers I, Desmyttere S, Verpoest W, De Rycke M, Staessen C, Sermon K, et al. Report on a consecutive series of 581 children born after blastomere biopsy for preimplantation genetic diagnosis. Hum Reprod. 2010;25:275–82.

Mastenbroek S, Twisk M, van Echten-Arends J, Sikkema-Raddatz B, Korevaar JC, Verhoeve HR, et al. In vitro fertilization with preimplantation genetic screening. N Engl J Med. 2007;357:9–17.

Mersereau J, Pergament E, Zhang X, Mila MP. Preimplantation genetic screening to improve in vitro fertilization pregnancy rates: a prospective randomized controlled trial. Fertil Steril. 2008;90:1287–9.

Monk M, Handyside A. Sexing of preimplantation embryos by measurement of X-linked gene dosage in a single blastomere. J Reprod Fert. 1988;82:365–8.

Moutou C, Goossens V, Coonen E, De Rycke M, Kokkali G, Renwick P, et al. ESHRE PGD Consortium data collection XII: cycles from January to December 2009 with pregnancy follow-up to October 2010. Hum Reprod. 2014;29:880–903.

Munné S, 2008. Comparison of embryo transfer with and without PGS for the indication of advanced reproductive age (37–42) in patients undergoing ART. NCT00646893, clinicaltrials.gov/show/NCT00646893.

Munné S, Lee A, Rosenwaks Z, Grifo J, Cohen J. Diagnosis of major chromosome aneuploidies in human preimplantation embryos. Hum Reprod. 1993;8:2185–92.

Munné S, Fung J, Cassel MJ, Marquez D, Weier HUG. Preimplantation genetic analysis of translocations case-specific probes for interphase cell analysis. Hum Genet. 1998a;102:663–74.

Munné S, Morrison L, Fung J, Marquez C, Weier U, Bahce M, et al. Spontaneous abortions are reduced after pre-conception diagnosis of translocations. J Assist Reprod Genet. 1998b;15:290–6.

Munné S, Magli C, Cohen J, Morton P, Sadowy S, Gianaroli L, et al. Positive outcome after preimplantation diagnosis of aneuploidy in human embryos. Hum Reprod. 1999;14:2191–9.

Munné S, Sandalinas M, Escudero T, Fung J, Gianaroli L, Cohen J. Outcome of preimplantation genetic diagnosis of translocation. Fertil Steril. 2000;73:1209–18.

Munné S, Sandalinas M, Escudero T, Velilla E, Walmsley R, Sadowy S, et al. Improved implantation after preimplantation genetic diagnosis of aneuploidy. Reprod Biomed Online. 2003;7:91–7.

Munné S, Chen S, Fischer J, Colls P, Zheng X, Stevens J, et al. Preimplantation genetic diagnosis reduces pregnancy loss in women aged 35 years and older with a history of recurrent miscarriages. Fertil Steril. 2005;84:331–5.

Munné S, Fragouli E, Colls P, Katz-Jaffe M, Schoolcraft W, Wells D. Improved detection of aneuploidy blastocysts using a new 12-chromosome FISH test. Reprod Biomed Online. 2010;20:92–7.

Nijs M, Van Steirteghem AC. Assessment of different isolation procedures for blastomeres from two-cell mouse embryos. Hum Reprod. 1987;2:421–4.

Otani T, Roche M, Mizuike M, Colls P, Escudero T, Munné S. Preimplantation genetic diagnosis significantly improves the pregnancy outcome of translocation carriers with a history of recurrent miscarriage and unsuccessful pregnancies. Reprod Biomed Online. 2006;13:879–94.

Preimplantation Genetic Diagnosis International Society (PGDIS). Guidelines for good practice in PGD: programme requirements and laboratory quality assurance. Reprod Biomed Online. 2008;16:134–47.

Rechitsky S, Verlinsky O, Chistokhina A, Sharapova T, Ozen S, Masciangelo C, et al. Preimplantation genetic diagnosis for cancer predisposition. Reprod Biomed Online. 2002;5:148–55.

Rechitsky S, Kuliev A, Sharapova T, et al. PGD impact on stem cell transplantation. 9th Annual International Conference on Preimplantation Genetics, Miami, Florida, April 23–25. Reprod Biomed Online. 2009;18:S2.

Rubio C, Simon C, Vidal F, Rodrigo L, Pehlivam T, Remohi J, et al. Chromosomal abnormalities and embryo development in recurrent miscarriage couples. Hum Reprod. 2003;18:182–8.

Schoolcraft WB, Katz-Jaffe MG. Comprehensive chromosome screening of trophectoderm with vitrification facilitates elective single-embryo transfer for infertile women with advanced maternal age. Fertil Steril. 2013;100:615–9.

Schoolcraft WB, Fragouli E, Stevens J, Munné S, Katz-Jaffe MG, Wells D. Clinical application of comprehensive chromosomal screening at the blastocyst stage. Fertil Steril. 2010;94:1700–6.

Scott Jr RT, Upham KM, Forman EJ, Hong KH, Scott KL, Taylor D, et al. Blastocyst biopsy with comprehensive chromosome screening and fresh embryo transfer significantly increases in vitro fertilization implantation and delivery rates: a randomized controlled trial. Fertil Steril. 2013;100:697–703.

Shkumatov A, Kuznyetsov V, Cieslak J, Ilkevitch Y, Verlinsky Y. Obtaining metaphase spreads from single blastomeres for PGD of chromosomal rearrangements. Reprod Biomed Online. 2007;14:498–503.

Simpson JL. Celebrating preimplantation genetic diagnosis of p53 mutations in Li-Fraumeni syndrome. Reprod Biomed Online. 2002;3:2–3.

Simpson JL. Preimplantation genetic diagnosis at 20 years. Prenat Diagn. 2010;30:682–85.

Staessen C, Plateau P, Van Assche E, Michiels A, Tournaya H, Camus M, et al. Comparison of blastocyst transfer with or without preimplantation genetic diagnosis for aneuploidy screening in couples with advanced maternal age: a prospective randomized controlled trial. Hum Reprod. 2004;19:2849–58.

Staessen C, Verpoest W, Donoso P, Haentiens P, Van der Elst J, Liebaers I, et al. Preimplantation genetic diagnosis does not improve delivery rate in women under the age of 36 following single-embryo transfer. Hum Reprod. 2008;23:2818–25.

Stephenson MD, Sierra S. Reproductive outcomes in recurrent pregnancy loss associated with a parental carrier of a structural chromosome rearrangement. Hum Reprod. 2006;21:1076–82.

Steptoe PC, Edwards RG. Birth after the reimplantation of a human embryo. Lancet. 1978;2:366.

Strom CM, Verlinsky Y, Milayeva S, Evsikoy S, Cieslak J, Lifchez A, et al. Preconception genetic diagnosis of cystic fibrosis. Lancet. 1990;336:306–7.

Sugiaura-Ogasawara M, Ozaki Y, Sato T, Suzumori N, Suzumori K. Poor prognosis of recurrent aborters with either maternal or paternal reciprocal translocation. Fertil Steril. 2004;81:367–73.

Verlinsky Y, Evsikov S. A simplified and efficient method for obtaining metaphase chromosomes from individual human blastomeres. Fertil Steril. 1999;72:1127–33.

Verlinsky Y, Kuliev A. Atlas of preimplantation genetic diagnosis. 2nd ed. Boca Raton, FL: Taylor and Francis; 2005a.

Verlinsky Y, Kuliev A. PGD and it's role in ART. In: Brinsden P, editor. Textbook of IVF and assisted reproduction. 3rd ed. London: Parthenon Publishing Group; 2005b.

Verlinsky Y, Kuliev A. Practical preimplantation genetic diagnosis. London: Springer; 2005c.

Verlinsky Y, Pergament E, Binor Z, Rawlins R. Genetic analysis of human embryos prior to implantation: future applications of in-vitro fertilization in treatment and prevention of human genetic diseases. In: Ferchlinger W, Kemeter P, editors. Future aspects in human in-vitro fertilization. Berlin: Springer; 1987. p. 262–6.

Verlinsky Y, Ginsberg N, Lifchez A, Valle J, Moise J, Strom CM. Analysis of the first polar body: preconception genetic diagnosis. Hum Reprod. 1990;5:826–9.

Verlinsky Y, Dozortsev D, Evsikov S. Visualization and cytogenetic analysis of second polar body chromosomes following its fusion with one-cell mouse embryo. J Assist Reprod Genet. 1994;11:123–31.

Verlinsky Y, Cieslak J, Freidine M, Ivakhneno V, Wolf G, Kovalinskaya L, et al. Pregnancies following pre-conception diagnosis of common aneuploidies by FISH. Hum Reprod. 1995;10:1923–7.

Verlinsky Y, Rechitsky S, Verlinsky O, Xu K, Schattman G, Masciangelo C, et al. Preimplantation diagnosis for p53 tumour suppressor gene mutations. Reprod Biomed Online. 2001;2:102–5.

Verlinsky Y, Tur-Kaspa I, Cieslak J, Bernal A, Morris R, Taranissi M, et al. Preimplantation testing for chromosomal disorders improves reproductive outcome of poor-diagnosis patients. Reprod Biomed Online. 2005;11:219–25.

Warburton D, Dallaire L, Thangavelu M, Ross L, Levin B, Kline J. Trisomy recurrence: a reconsideration based on North American data. Am J Hum Genet. 2004;75:376–85.

Werlin L, Rodi I, DeCherney A, Marello E, Hill D, Munné S. Preimplantation genetic diagnosis as both a therapeutic and diagnostic tool in assisted reproductive technology. Fertil Steril. 2003; 80:467–8.

Wilton LJ, Trounson AO. Biopsy of preimplantation mouse embryos: development of micromanipulated embryos and proliferation of single blastomeres in vitro. Biol Reprod. 1989;40: 145–52.

Yang Y, Zeng Y, Lv Z, Wan R, Tong M, Zhu H, et al. Abnormal development at early postimplantation stage in mouse embryos after preimplantation genetic diagnosis. Anat Rec. 2012;295: 1128–33.

Zhu JL, Basso O, Obel C, Bille C, Olsen J. Infertility, infertility treatment and congenital malformations: Danish national birth cohort. BMJ. 2006;333:679–83.

Chapter 3
Medical Reasons for Pregnancy Interruption: Chromosomal and Genetic Abnormalities

Jeffrey S. Dungan

Historical Perspectives

In the late 1960s, the feasibility of culturing amniotic fluid cells and obtaining a fetal karyotype was reported (Steele and Breg 1966). Shortly thereafter, the first report was published relating the prenatal detection of fetal aneuploidy via amniocentesis, with subsequent elective termination of the affected pregnancy (Valenti et al. 1968). A notable aspect of this and other early reports is that they predate the 1973 federal legalization of abortion in the USA.

Subsequent reports on similar clinical interventions appeared, but were limited in scope and were not oriented toward widespread use. One of the earliest series of "genetic amniocentesis" was reported by Nadler in 1968. The included cases covered a wide range of genetic risk factors, but demonstrated the possibility of enzymatic and chromosomal analyses. Successful amniotic fluid cell culture was achieved in 27/37 cases performed between 10 and 36 weeks; the most common indication was the evaluation of Rh incompatibility. In another of the earliest case series, Ferguson-Smith et al. (1971) tabulated a nearly 100 % termination rate of affected fetuses (39/41) from about 300 pregnancies that had been analyzed because of a variety of risk factors.

These early papers emphasized the significance of these medical developments, highlighting the advantage to couples who might otherwise have avoided pregnancy altogether because of their risk factors. Now a mechanism was available that would provide the option of having only healthy (genetically unaffected) children, by prenatal exclusion of the genetic disease in question.

J.S. Dungan, M.D. (✉)
Department of Obstetrics and Gynecology, Northwestern University Feinberg School of Medicine, 250 E. Superior St, Rm 05-2173, Chicago, IL 60611, USA
e-mail: jdungan@nmh.org

J.P. Galst, M.S. Verp (eds.), *Prenatal and Preimplantation Diagnosis*,
DOI 10.1007/978-3-319-18911-6_3

In the early 1970s, reports and discussion appeared on the feasibility of widespread prenatal "screening programs" for Down syndrome. The association between advanced maternal age and probability of giving birth to a child with Down syndrome was recognized and was now quantifiable. This would ultimately lead to proposals for large-scale prenatal testing, promulgated by a variety of public health experts (Huether 1983).

Also in this time period Hook published his landmark papers on birth incidence of Down syndrome stratified by maternal age. While the relationship between "advanced" maternal age and Down syndrome had been long recognized, his group was the first to calculate specific risk figures (Hook and Chambers 1977). These birth incidence numbers are still used today in counseling of women considering prenatal genetic testing or screening.

Widespread use of invasive prenatal testing did not really launch until several large international reports on safety and accuracy of amniocentesis were published in the early 1970s. Following these, the NICHD Consensus statement addressed this topic in 1979 (NIH Consensus Development Conferences 1979), supporting the routine use of amniocentesis in prenatal care of women at increased risk for genetic disorders in the fetus.

Notably, the NICHD amniocentesis registry (The NICHD National Registry of Amniocentesis Study Group 1976) included information on pregnancy terminations performed. Of the 19 women who had cytogenetically abnormal results, 16 (84.2 %) elected pregnancy termination, as did 11/15 (73.3 %) who had fetuses affected with a "metabolic" disorder. These percentages presaged with remarkable accuracy the rates of pregnancy termination reported subsequently in the context of fetal genetic disorders.

Counseling Issues

Prior to undergoing prenatal diagnostic testing, all women should undergo extensive counseling about the benefits and limitations of such testing. Many women voice their objections or hesitancy about pursuing prenatal testing because they would not terminate a pregnancy "no matter what." Women and couples are generally advised, or should be, that this testing is not a prelude to a recommendation for abortion. Having such knowledge prior to delivery prepares the patient and her partner for the arrival of a child who will have special needs, or potentially face a high chance of stillbirth or neonatal death, such as in the case of trisomy 18 or 13. Anecdotally, many of these women subsequently change their minds about TOP when faced with a diagnosis of fetal chromosome disorder.

Multiple authors have investigated reasons behind why women and couples choose to abort affected pregnancies as opposed to continuing the pregnancy (Hawkins et al. 2012; Pergament and Pergament 2012; Schechtman et al. 2002; Verp et al. 1988). The most commonly cited reasons for pursuit of abortion of a chromosomally abnormal pregnancy include

1. Severity of phenotype
2. Prospects for neurocognitive impairment

3. Need for surgical management/correction of structural abnormalities
4. Life expectancy
5. Family issues (impact on siblings)

The indication for prenatal testing and the gestational age at which this testing is performed also appear to play a role in the decision-making process. However, the specific aneuploidy and predicted phenotype carry the greatest relevance in most studies (Evans et al. 1996). Interestingly, women who undergo invasive diagnostic testing secondary to sonographic anomalies do not appear to be more likely to abort that pregnancy than are those who undergo "routine" prenatal testing, e.g., because of maternal age (Hawkins et al. 2012).

Many patients enter prenatal diagnostic testing with the preconceived plan of terminating the pregnancy if discovered to have a genetic abnormality. One important aspect of the counseling session is to address the limitations of prenatal diagnosis with respect to predicting phenotype. For example, the wide spectrum of intellectual disability in children with Down syndrome should be communicated.

Some couples benefit from a second counseling visit after an abnormal result is delivered. This is generally the time to have a more in-depth review of the results, with focus on anticipated phenotype. This visit also typically includes information about the abortion techniques available at a particular facility. Prior to the development of the surgical procedure of dilation and evacuation (D and E), most pregnancy terminations were accomplished by induction. Early techniques included hypertonic saline or urea, both known to have comparatively high complication rates. Modern pharmacologic agents, such as mifepristone and misoprostol, are now the primary agents used for induction abortion. Complication rates for induction are quite low. Nonetheless, surgical pregnancy termination remains the intervention of choice for the large majority of first- and second-trimester terminations (Centers for Disease Control and Prevention 2013). One caveat is the availability of trained and experienced providers, which limits access to surgical abortion in some areas of the USA.

Induction abortion is sometimes selected by parents who want to see or touch the delivered fetus. Surgical interventions preclude this option. Another reason cited for induction abortion is for more reliable autopsy results, should that be indicated. This scenario is most likely in the context of structural anomalies, as opposed to chromosomal or single-gene disorders. However, autopsy can play a role in pregnancies terminated for recognized syndromes if the patient desires getting maximal phenotypic information, confirmation of anomalies that posed high likelihood of lethal or grave prognoses, and other considerations (Papp et al. 2007). Some couples see consenting to autopsy as a way to achieve some benefit out of an otherwise tragic situation.

Some couples benefit from prolonged counseling over multiple sessions to work through the considerable psychosocial impact of this choice. Therapists specializing in such counseling can provide considerable benefit in these circumstances, as genetic counselors and obstetricians may have limited time or resources for such in-depth counseling.

Finally, patients are counseled about the impact of pregnancy termination on subsequent reproductive performance. They should be told of the relative safety of abortion, as reported from multiple sources (Centers for Disease Control and Prevention 2013). The majority of patients who desire another pregnancy after a genetic pregnancy termination are successful (Jackson et al. 2007). Experience also demonstrates that patients typically seek out earlier invasive prenatal testing if the incident pregnancy had been evaluated in the second trimester.

Common Trisomies

Down Syndrome

Trisomy 21 is the most common autosomal aneuploidy encountered prenatally and in newborns. It is the only full autosomal aneuploidy associated with long-term survival. It is also the chromosomal disorder most familiar to patients seeking prenatal testing. Accounting for over half of all cytogenetic abnormalities reported prenatally (Grati et al. 2010), it is the disorder for which essentially all prenatal aneuploidy screening programs have been implemented. It is also the most common single-chromosome disorder tracked by public health databases to monitor incidence, but this is only done by a small number of states in the USA.

History

The first reported case of elective pregnancy termination of a fetus affected with Down syndrome was in 1968 by Valenti et al. (1968). The diagnosis was made by amniocentesis in a woman known to have a D/G translocation (presumably between chromosomes 14 and 21) and one prior affected offspring. Amniocentesis confirmed an unbalanced translocation, and subsequently the pregnancy was terminated by hypertonic saline infusion, precluding postabortion cytogenetic confirmation secondary to tissue degradation. The fetus had phenotypic features of Down syndrome, which the authors used as presumptive evidence of a correct prenatal diagnosis. Following this report, other small series related the experiences of cytogenetic services incorporating prenatal testing. Such interventions for chromosome abnormalities were typically in patients deemed to be “at risk” by virtue of advanced maternal age, prior history of a chromosome disorder, or “anxiety.”

In the early 1970s, abortion was legal in only two states, New York and Hawaii, although some other states made allowances in the case of maternal rubella. During the late 1960s, experience with amniocentesis techniques was described by a number of researchers well before the national legalization of abortion. The federal legalization of abortion in 1973 happened to coincide with increased utilization of amniocentesis by women for genetic diagnosis.

Although some amniocenteses were reported to have been performed in the first trimester of pregnancy, it was generally deemed technically challenging at that gestational age. Alternative first-trimester diagnostic techniques in the form of placental biopsy (chorionic villi sampling [CVS]) were being developed contemporaneously with amniocentesis, but by fewer investigators. Early work by Chinese and Russian researchers ultimately culminated in the development of transcervical trophoblast biopsies. Chorionic villi could be cultured for karyotyping and other genomic studies, and CVS was ultimately made available on a widespread basis. While the advantages of first-trimester diagnosis are obvious, no center has reported higher rates of TOP following first-trimester diagnosis compared to obtaining the diagnosis in the second trimester.

Initial series of prenatally diagnosed cases of fetal chromosome disorders were reported primarily from single-center experiences. In reviewing pregnancy outcomes from several such series, Verp reported generally high rates of TOP of aneuploid pregnancies (Verp et al. 1988). Given that these cases were primarily patients seeking prenatal diagnosis secondary to maternal age concerns, the high rates are not surprising.

Data on abortion rates in the presence of prenatal Down syndrome diagnosis come from two primary sources: (1) hospital-based records, frequently from a single clinical genetics service, and (2) statewide or national birth defect registries. In the USA, the agency which has most frequently reported on birth prevalence of Down syndrome is the CDC (Centers for Disease Control and Prevention. National Center for Health Statistics 2014).

Virtually all reports examining induced abortion rates reveal high pregnancy termination rates in the face of fetal Down syndrome. Many of these studies have been included in a systematic review (Natoli et al. 2012). This review found that the overall rate for pregnancy termination for this indication was 67–85 %, depending on whether the data were from population-based data sets or collected from hospital-based sources. In this review, which included 24 studies, there were a roughly equal distribution of single-center results and population-based registries. Within the population-based studies, there were a total of approximately 2600 prenatal diagnoses of Down syndrome analyzed. From this cohort (spanning study years of 1986–2007), there were 1923 (74.2 %) that underwent pregnancy termination. These data may be somewhat limited in generalizability as they come from screening programs in three states: California, Hawaii, and Maine. Whether states in other regions of the USA would have different rates is a matter of speculation, as most states do not track birth incidence of Down syndrome.

This same systematic review also compiled data from single-center reports. In this dataset, there were 779 pregnancies with a prenatal diagnosis of Down syndrome and 663 (85.1 %) terminations of pregnancies. The range across the eight centers included in this compilation was 67.6–89.6 %. There was no stratification based on the mode of ascertainment (i.e., by indication for prenatal testing, such as age or sonographic anomaly). The authors of this review point out the lower overall termination rates compared to other studies, such as those from European registries, supporting an overall lower rate of TOP in the USA for Down syndrome. They also noted a trend toward lower rates of TOP in the more recent years of the study. Reasons for this trend are not clear, but some have conjectured that fewer women in increased-risk age strata are seeking prenatal diagnosis.

Population-based datasets extrapolate from the national birth incidence of Down syndrome as a proxy for rates of termination. One can calculate the expected number of cases of Down syndrome based on the number of total deliveries to women of a particular age group. The difference between this expected number and the *actual* number delivered, based on birth certificate data, approximates the number of terminations (correcting for background spontaneous loss rate of fetuses with Down syndrome). Using this approach, investigators demonstrated that roughly half the number of expected cases of Down syndrome were actually born in the USA during the interval 1989–2006 (Egan et al. 2011). This information however includes women who deliberately or inadvertently did not undergo screening or testing for Down syndrome prenatally. Therefore, using such national statistics is less informative for determining decision making by prospective parents when faced with a prenatal diagnosis of Down syndrome.

However, some interesting demographic differences were noted in this report. There appear to be regional and ethnic differences in live birth rates of infants with Down syndrome, which by inference reflect to some extent the prenatal decision making and subsequent TOP rates in these regions. For example, the western region of the USA had the lowest proportion of expected cases that were liveborn, suggesting higher termination rates in this region. The Midwest demonstrated the smallest difference between observed and expected (see Table 3.1), which likely reflects overall lower termination rates, but may also reflect regional differences in access to prenatal diagnostic services. In addition, there were proportionately fewer Down syndrome live births among African-Americans (37 % of expected) compared to whites (57 % of expected).

There appears to be conflicting data across different studies when examining the role of maternal race in elective pregnancy termination in the presence of an abnormal prenatal diagnosis. Part of this discrepancy may lie in the maternal age distribution among the various ethnic groups, and overall uptake of prenatal diagnosis. The relationship between maternal race and live birth incidence was also examined in metropolitan

Table 3.1 Percentage of expected Down syndrome live births that were actually born during 1989–2006 by maternal age group and geographic region in the USA

	Maternal age groups	
Region of the USA	15–34 years old (%)	35–49 years old (%)
Northeast	58.4	42.0
Midwest	74.2	59.0
South	59.1	42.5
West	53.4	35.4

Data from Egan JFX, Smith K, Timms D, et al. Demographic differences in Down syndrome livebirths in the US from 1989 to 2006. Prenat Diagn, 2011. 31:389–394

Atlanta utilizing data from the Metropolitan Atlanta Congenital Defects Program (MACDP) (Jackson et al. 2014). Overall, about a quarter of Down syndrome pregnancies ended in elective termination, and the rate was highest among non-Hispanic white women, at about 74 %. In this analysis, Hispanics and non-Hispanic blacks were about half as likely to undergo elective pregnancy termination compared to non-Hispanic whites when an abnormal cytogenetic result was obtained. This is despite a similar likelihood of undergoing prenatal diagnostic testing among blacks. Hispanic women were less likely to undergo prenatal testing by about 1/3 compared to the other two ethnic groups. Again, reconciling these discrepant conclusions is hampered by lack of a national database in the USA for tracking these types of testing and interventions.

Other countries do maintain such databases. For example, England and Wales maintain the National Down Syndrome Cytogenetic Register, which tracks all prenatal and postnatal cytogenetic laboratory results. A report from this database tracked trends in Down syndrome births from its inception in 1989 through 2008 (Morris and Alberman 2009). The number of live births with Down syndrome during this interval was relatively steady. However, with the temporal shift in maternal age distributions, the authors estimated that a 48 % increase in live birth prevalence would have occurred (after correcting for spontaneous losses) if not for prenatal diagnosis and TOP of affected cases. In their series, the TOP rate was about 92 % throughout the study interval.

Another assessment of Down syndrome incidence in Europe was estimated using the European Surveillance of Congenital Anomalies (EUROCAT) registers (Boyd et al. 2008). The countries participating in this voluntary register contribute a variable proportion of pregnancy outcomes. In addition, the countries participating also have different screening policies and regulations regarding pregnancy termination. Despite these shortcomings, this register provides useful data on the overall impact of prenatal screening and testing. In this series of >2300 Down syndrome pregnancies, the overall rate of pregnancy termination was 88 % (range 73–100 %).

The effect that sonographically detected structural anomalies have in decision making regarding management of Down syndrome pregnancies has not been widely examined. Perry et al. (2007) report an overall TOP rate of 73 %. Paradoxically, in their series of 59 affected pregnancies, the presence of any major or minor abnormal ultrasound finding was associated with a lower rate of TOP compared to pregnancies with normal sonographic findings; however, the number of fetuses with a major anomaly (typically cardiac) was small. The role of ultrasound in ascertaining the likelihood of Down syndrome prior to diagnostic testing undoubtedly plays a role in the decision making of some patients, but this aspect warrants further study.

The factors involved in decision making are myriad, and likely patient specific. Korenromp et al. (2007) explored this topic with an in-depth survey administered to 71 Dutch women who terminated their Down syndrome pregnancy. None of the fetuses had life-threatening anomalies detected by sonography. The survey was administered 4 months following the TOP. The survey responses were categorized as "related to the infant" or "related to the respondent or family." The women weighted the motivations "related to the infant" much higher than their own. The belief that the child would never be able to function independently was the highest scored factor. Interestingly, financial burden was one of the least impactful factors. Many of these women expressed doubt about the decision to terminate the pregnancy, mainly because the "reason" was in conflict with "feelings." Only about a third of the respondents expressed "no doubt at all" about the decision to terminate the pregnancy.

There are few data regarding differences in TOP rates depending on gestational age. Clinicians had predicted that first-trimester testing would result in higher pregnancy termination rates. Evans et al. (1996) reported TOP data from Wayne State, and found no difference in termination rates for abnormalities whether made in the first or second trimester, if the abnormality was considered "severe" (a category including the major autosomal trisomies). While not restricted to Down syndrome, or stratified based on specific trisomy, the pattern held across the 8-year study interval.

In summary, the rate of elective pregnancy termination secondary to prenatal detection of Down syndrome is variable, but hovers around 85–90 %. The impact on birth incidence of DS is more tempered, demonstrating that not all women avail themselves of prenatal diagnosis or screening. Most series relate that observed Down syndrome births are about 50 % lower than expected based on maternal age distribution. Data are conflicting as to the effect of maternal age, associated structural anomalies, and ethnicity.

Trisomy 18 and Trisomy 13

Data are sparse regarding TOP rates in cases of prenatally detected trisomy 18 and trisomy 13. There are few large-scale registries monitoring the birth incidence of these conditions, let alone information from tracking prenatal diagnoses and TOPs. Given the high lethality associated with these conditions, most centers reporting these results also report concomitantly high rates of pregnancy termination. On the other hand, some reports contain lower rates of TOP, but admit that ascertainment is likely incomplete. The large MACDP reviewed population-based statistics on trisomies 18 and 13 during the interval 1994–2003 (Crider et al. 2008). Termination rates overall were at 45–48 %. TOP rates collected via perinatal offices however were 75–89 %, which is likely a more accurate reflection of the experience in other prenatal diagnostic centers.

Tonks et al. (2013) report data from the West Midlands region of England, where a Congenital Anomaly Register is maintained. Their ascertainment was considered high, and the majority (95 %) of trisomy 18 and trisomy 13 pregnancies were known or suspected prenatally. For those cases with invasive prenatal testing, 84–88 % of affected pregnancies underwent TOP. The authors noted that overall prevalences of trisomy 18 and trisomy 13 in the population are increasing following the trend toward giving birth at older maternal ages.

Sex Chromosome Aneuploidy

It is not meaningful to collate TOP decision making for all sex chromosome aneuploidies (SCAs) as a group, given the wide spectrum of phenotypic consequences of SCA. Most patients make thoughtful and well-reasoned choices, and base their decisions on the expected phenotypes of the various SCAs. Given that most SCAs are not associated with structural anomalies (with the exception of 45,X), the phenotype is likely to be mild, and possibly considered normal in many circumstances. Screening programs for fetal aneuploidy have not typically included an assessment for SCA risks. Nonetheless, most reports addressing this question do indeed report on SCA as an entity rather than as individual conditions.

Much of the early reporting on TOP for SCA revealed quite high rates. This undoubtedly reflected the limited understanding of phenotypes associated with SCAs, as reported in Shaffer et al. (2006). Based on early and statistically suspect data, there was widespread belief that males with 47,XXY would be homosexual and mentally retarded. The (erroneous) phenotype associated with 47,XXX was of a tall and retarded female with psychiatric disease, and males with 47,XYY were likely to end up in prison and were violent.

With contemporary and longitudinal data on outcomes of children born with SCA, more accurate phenotype information is available for parents now (Lalatta and Tint 2013). Only 45,X (Turner syndrome) is consistently associated with structural abnormalities, and is associated with a relatively consistent phenotype. Many children with SCA go through life with no noticeable untoward effects. This evolution in understanding of the phenotypes associated with SCA has led to a general trend over time of diminishing rates of TOP in the presence of a prenatal diagnosis of most SCAs.

45,X

Unlike the other SCAs, Turner syndrome (TS) is commonly associated with structural malformations, especially cardiovascular. The fetal phenotype is frequently that of hydrops, and many of these early gestations do not survive in utero life. For this reason, the TOP rate is higher than for other SCAs. Many patients decide to terminate the pregnancy based on the prognosis associated with hydrops, and not the chromosome status per se. Reports on decision making about TOP with a prenatal diagnosis of 45,X typically do not stratify based on the sonographic findings.

In the large series from UCSF, Shaffer et al. (2006) report a TOP rate for 45,X of 65 % (34/52). This rate was steady over the 20-year study interval, and no specific demographic factors altered this finding. Jeon et al. (2012), in a systematic review of prenatal decision making associated with a variety of SCAs, related an overall TOP rate using data from nine studies of 76 %, but the range was wide (33–100 %).

Mansfield et al. (1999) performed a systematic review of 20 studies. The number of TS pregnancies was relatively small compared to other aneuploidies, but the rate of TOP was 72 %, with a range of 44–100 %. This review demonstrated no trend over time, with TOP rates remaining steady from 1987 to 1996.

Using data from a congenital anomaly register in Wales, Iyer et al. (2012) reported the outcomes of fetuses with TS over a 10-year interval. The overall TOP rate was 66 %. Most prenatal testing was performed as a result of sonographic abnormalities. These authors noted a decline in rates of TOP during the study interval. The TOP rate was also lower in instances of mosaicism.

A retrospective series from a collection of French cytogenetic services examined outcomes of TS over a 30-year interval (Gruchy et al. 2014). The indication for testing was an abnormal sonogram in 84 %, reflecting a more severe phenotype. The elective TOP rate was 81 % in this series. However, this rate was heavily weighted by those pregnancies with sonographic anomalies. When the diagnosis of 45,X was made incidentally (due to maternal age or serum screening, and with no abnormal sonographic findings), the TOP rate was 36 %. Similar to other reports, there was a lower TOP rate in cases of mosaicism.

In summary, the TOP rate for prenatally detected TS is relatively high, which seems attributable in large part to the coexistence of structural abnormalities visualized by sonography.

47,XXY

Klinefelter syndrome is a well-described syndrome of infertility and gynecomastia in adult males. There is no consistent phenotypic effect of the 47,XXY in prenatal life or in childhood, although higher rates of learning disabilities are reported. This prenatal diagnosis is generally an unanticipated result during testing performed secondary to maternal age or abnormal serum screening, as opposed to being specifically targeted by screening programs.

Gruchy et al. (2011) report the largest single series of pregnancy outcomes of prenatally diagnosed Klinefelter syndrome. Over a nearly 25-year span, this network of French cytogenetic labs collected 188 cases. TOP was elected in 24.3 % of cases. Some pregnancies had coexisting and unrelated mild sonographic anomalies, but this did not affect the overall TOP rate. In France, TOP for fetal anomalies must first be reviewed by a multidisciplinary prenatal diagnosis center (MDPC). This initiative, started in 1997, has had a large impact on TOP rates for cytogenetically abnormal pregnancies. Prior to the advent of these MDPCs, the TOP rate for 47,XXY peaked at around 75 %; it has since fallen to 0 %.

In the Jeon review (Jeon et al. 2012), seven studies which addressed Klinefelter syndrome were included. The overall TOP rate was 61 %, with a range of 44–85 %. Most of the included studies predate 2000, and no temporal trends were reported. From the UCSF cohort, the TOP rate for 47,XXY was 70 % (28/40). Boyd et al. (2011) reported that about 40 % of 47,XXY fetuses were terminated, and this rate did not vary by maternal age at diagnosis.

Compared to earlier small series from a variety of prenatal cytogenetic services, the rate of TOP for 47,XXY seems to be diminishing: while still over 50 % in some recent series, most centers report rates substantially lower.

47,XXX and 47,XYY

These sex chromosome trisomies are encountered less frequently in prenatal diagnosis, yet still frequently enough to pose challenges to the genetic counselor and other clinicians. Understanding of the typical phenotype has evolved dramatically over the years compared to what was believed 40 years ago.

The reader is referred to review articles that describe these generally mild phenotypes (Lalatta and Tint 2013). Counseling based on this updated information has generally led to a diminished rate of TOP for these SCAs.

Boyd et al. (2008) report, using EUROCAT data, that 50 % of 47,XXX pregnancies and 32 % of 47,XYY pregnancies were terminated in that series collated during 2000–2005. However, the proportions of SCA pregnancies that underwent TOP were lower in women over age 35 (23 % and 28 %, respectively). Jeon et al. (2012) reported a TOP rate for 47,XXX and 47,XYY of 32 %. In contrast, Shaffer et al. (2006) report that 57 % of 47,XXX pregnancies were terminated as were 40 % of 47,XYY in their series from UCSF.

The problems inherent in counseling about these disorders were noted early in the establishment of prenatal diagnosis techniques and results (Farrant and Hulten 1979). Specifically, erroneous prediction of the neurologic and psychological consequences of a 47,XYY chromosomal constitution was dramatic.

In summary, there appears to be a consistent trend toward continuation of pregnancies found to have a sex chromosome trisomy. However, a higher rate of TOP in the face of a prenatal diagnosis of 45,X is consistently reported, especially if sonographic abnormalities are seen. Additionally, most studies also report a lower rate of TOP for SCA among older women compared to younger women.

Of note, new testing and screening paradigms could potentially impact TOP rates for chromosome abnormalities. A new form of highly accurate, albeit imperfect, prenatal screening for fetal chromosome disorders called noninvasive prenatal testing (NIPT), will soon be available for all pregnancies. In high-risk pregnancies, such as women over age 35, detection rates of Down syndrome are reported to be 99–100 % with very high specificity. Studies addressing the impact of NIPT on birth incidence of Down syndrome and other chromosome disorders have yet to be reported.

Genomic Arrays

Genomic array technologies allow for a superior assessment of chromosomal state. Not only can numeric chromosome abnormalities be diagnosed, but submicroscopic deletions and duplications of chromosomal content can be detected.

There is increasing use of genomic arrays in prenatal testing. The increased resolution attainable with these technologies comes with a chance of uncovering variants of undetermined significance (VUS). The rate of VUS is around 1 %. Counseling about potential phenotypic effects of VUS is challenging.

Currently, most clinicians are using microarray testing in prenatal care on a limited basis, primarily in the presence of sonographic fetal abnormalities. Determination of TOP rates as a result of array abnormalities will thus be confounded by concomitant existence of structural anomalies in the fetus. Some of the array testing can uncover regions of the genome which, if disrupted, can predispose to developmental delay or autism spectrum disorders. However, precise quantification of the chance of these phenotypic effects is impossible at present. While this can pose difficult counseling dilemmas, such uncertainty is not new to prenatal diagnosis. Traditional cytogenetic analysis has always been associated with a small, but important, chance of ambiguity or uncertainty, such as in cases of mosaicism, marker chromosomes, or balanced structural rearrangements.

Little prospective data exist about pregnancy outcomes, including TOP, in women who undergo array testing. The largest array study in the USA was completed in 2012 (Wapner et al. 2012) but did not contain pregnancy outcome data. As additional experience is gained in the use of this new technology in prenatal medicine, more literature addressing TOP rates will likely be forthcoming.

Mendelian Disorders

Studies addressing TOP rates for any individual single-gene disorder are virtually nonexistent. As a group of diagnoses, Mendelian disorders comprise a minor fraction of all requests for prenatal diagnosis. Couples are typically identified as being at risk secondary to prior affected offspring, or through carrier screening. Those with previous affected children are sometimes targeted for surveys about prenatal diagnosis and potential TOP in subsequent pregnancies. This population represents a source of inherent ascertainment bias, and thus generalization about pregnancy decision making from these cohorts is limited.

Most reports are generated through surveys of affected patients or their parents, and typically contain hypothetical scenarios for the subject to address. While potentially useful from a needs assessment standpoint, clinicians in this field will recognize that the chasm between responses on a survey and real-life decision making, when faced with an actual prenatal diagnosis of a fetal abnormality, is wide and unpredictable.

Specific mention of select single-gene disorders will be presented here, but caution must be exercised about interpreting the conclusions in survey-based reports. As with data regarding TOP for chromosome disorders, those patients most likely to terminate an affected pregnancy for a Mendelian disorder are the ones who pursue prenatal testing to identify that disorder. Those couples who would not terminate a pregnancy for any reason frequently forego prenatal diagnosis.

Cystic Fibrosis

While long debated, universal prenatal screening to identify couples at risk for having a child with cystic fibrosis is now a routine part of prenatal care. Cystic fibrosis (CF) is an autosomal recessive disorder for which universal carrier screening during preconceptional or prenatal care is now endorsed by the American Congress of Obstetricians and Gynecologists (ACOG) and the American College of Medical Genetics and Genomics (ACMG). While classically thought of as a "lethal" disease, with death typically in childhood, the average life-span with modern care of a child with CF is 41 years (Cystic Fibrosis Foundation 2014). However, the medical burden of classic CF remains high.

Previously, couples seeking prenatal diagnosis for CF were those with a previously affected child, a factor that certainly would color decisions about the possibility of subsequent affected children. Now the majority of couples seeking CF testing are identified through parental carrier screening or by having an affected child identified through newborn screening, before becoming symptomatic. Most reported investigations into reproductive decision making come from surveys.

However, some sense of the rate of prenatal diagnosis with TOP of affected fetuses can be inferred from examining the liveborn incidence of CF. Unlike aneuploid pregnancies, there is no apparent increased risk of spontaneous pregnancy loss in cases of fetal CF.

In a review of CF liveborn incidence in Italy, Castellani et al. (2009) note an overall reduced incidence of CF with the advent of newborn screening (NBS) and prenatal diagnosis. The authors stratified their data by region of the country where routine prenatal carrier screening is performed, and noted a larger decrease in live birth incidence where screening was available. Additionally, they reported a TOP rate of affected pregnancies of about 75 %.

Scotet et al. (2008) examined reproductive decision making in western France among couples at risk for CF-affected offspring. Among 268 at-risk couples, including 195 with a previously affected child, there were 74 subsequent affected pregnancies. From this group, 70 chose to undergo TOP. In another set of 22 affected pregnancies identified secondary to echogenic bowel during prenatal ultrasonography, all were aborted.

In an interesting, albeit small, study of hypothetical versus real decision making, Sawyer et al. (2006) examined pregnancy outcomes among a cohort of Australian women who had a previously affected child. This cohort, by means of a survey, communicated that the majority (85 %) would use prenatal diagnosis in any future pregnancies, but only a little over half stated that they would terminate such a pregnancy. However, in the prospectively collected outcomes in subsequent pregnancies, all fetuses found to be affected (5/33) were terminated.

In most studies examining TOP rates in pregnancies affected with fetal CF, there appears to be a consistently high rate of TOP. Given that early medical intervention with intensive surveillance and treatment of affected children has prolonged life expectancy in individuals with CF, further investigation of TOP rates in more contemporary cohorts would be of interest.

Hemoglobinopathies

Screening programs to identify carriers of the thalassemias or sickle cell trait were some of the earliest developed. The majority of these diseases arise in geographic areas with less well-developed screening and prenatal care while most of what has been reported in the literature has been ascertained from examining opinions of at-risk populations within regions with more developed medical care.

However, some programs have published their experiences with prenatal diagnosis of a variety of hemoglobinopathies. Wang et al. (1994) published outcomes of a series of 500 prenatal diagnoses of sickle cell disease across a wide range of gestational ages and specific sickling syndromes. About 50 % of pregnancies affected with hemoglobin SS were terminated, whereas only 12 % of pregnancies affected with hemoglobin SC disease terminated. In addition, the authors noted a higher rate of TOP if the diagnosis was made prior to 20 weeks, with a 64 % TOP rate compared to 28 % if the diagnosis was made after 20 weeks.

Internationally, the experience is varied. Many areas of the world where hemoglobinopathies are endemic have few resources to offer their population prenatal diagnosis or TOP. There are also religious and political barriers to such testing and interventions in many nations. Nonetheless, where performed, rates of TOP are frequently high. As examples, all pregnancies affected with beta-thalassemia in an Egyptian series were terminated (El-Beshlawy et al. 2012) as were all pregnancies found to be affected in a Thai series (Tongsong et al. 2013). Both of these centers, however, also report a substantial proportion of at-risk pregnancies that do not undergo prenatal testing.

Deafness

Newborn screening for hearing loss is now routine across the USA. Given that over 50 % of congenital hearing loss is attributable to single-gene disorders, there has been increased attention to the potential for carrier screening (Ryan et al. 2003). However, little is known about the frequency of TOP if a fetus is tested and found to be affected. Part of the counseling difficulty has to do with the variability of hearing loss associated with many genes responsible for hearing loss.

The deaf community is generally opposed to prenatal testing for hereditary hearing loss [HHL] while being supportive of women's rights in general. It seems unlikely that there will be organizational endorsement of universal carrier screening for HHL. One study of attitudes toward prenatal testing with the option for terminating a fetus with HHL reported significant differences among hearing parents versus non-hearing parents, with the latter group almost unanimously opposed to TOP for a fetus with HHL (Stern et al. 2002).

Huntington Disease

Huntington disease (HD) is an adult-onset disorder that is highly penetrant and associated with severe, and ultimately lethal, neurologic deterioration. Much has been written about genetic counseling and presymptomatic testing for this disorder given the severe phenotype and lack of effective treatment. Prenatal testing for this disorder poses an added dimension in that individuals of reproductive age are generally younger than the typical age of onset of HD and so are usually unaware of their own personal mutation status. Under these circumstances, there can be undesired disclosure of the parental mutation status if direct fetal testing is performed. A novel approach to prenatal testing in these cases allows for "nondisclosure" by only assessing whether the fetus' chromosome #4, where the HD gene resides, was inherited from the affected grandparent. If so, this predicts a 50 % likelihood of the fetus being affected. Couples are expected to abort the pregnancy if the fetus is at 50 % risk (as opposed to the 0 % risk if the relevant chromosome came from the unaffected grandparent). While generally available, this approach is not undertaken by a large number of couples (8–18 %) (Richards and Rea 2005). There are scattered reports of uptake of prenatal diagnosis for HD, mostly after predictive testing in the parent at risk, which would allow a 0 or 100 % prediction of an affected fetus. Many such couples forego childbearing altogether. Overall the uptake for HD prenatal testing is low (Decruyenaere et al. 2007), but in the fraction that do pursue such testing, all affected (or at 50 % risk in nondisclosure testing) pregnancies have been terminated.

BRCA1/BRCA2

The presence of a mutation in the BRCA1 or BRCA2 genes connotes substantially increased risk for breast and ovarian cancers. There are no childhood phenotypic implications (except in the rare instance of homozygosity). While prenatal diagnosis for BRCA mutations is technically feasible to avoid transmission of the gene to offspring, there are no large-scale studies examining this topic. Since breast and ovarian cancer are adult-onset disorders with available treatments, there is little demand for prenatal testing (Derks-Smeets et al. 2014). Alternatively, many such patients opt for preimplantation genetic diagnosis. Reports of such interventions are also small in number.

Conclusions

Couples seeking prenatal diagnosis of fetal genetic disorders frequently do so with the preconceived plan for TOP in the event of an affected pregnancy. Studies examining rates of TOP for fetal genetic disorders will invariably have this inherent selection bias.

Prospective parents appear to generally be able to differentiate those disorders predicted to have a severe or lethal phenotype from those with milder or more variable manifestations, and TOP rates for various disorders reflect this. The advent of new and more widely available technologies for assessing fetal genetic and genomic disorders may play a role in prenatal decision making. Increasing state and federal restrictions on abortion rights may also well have an impact on TOP rates for fetal genetic disorders.

References

Boyd P, DeVigan C, Khoshnood B, et al. Survey of prenatal screening policies in Europe for structural malformations and chromosome anomalies, and their impact on detection and termination rates for neural tube defects and Down's syndrome. BJOG. 2008;115:689–96.

Boyd PA, Loane M, Garne E, Khoshnood B, Dolk H. Sex chromosome trisomies in Europe: prevalence, prenatal detection and outcome of pregnancy. Eur J Hum Genet. 2011;19:231–4.

Castellani C, Picci L, Tamanini A, et al. Association between carrier screening and incidence of cystic fibrosis. JAMA. 2009;302:2573–9.

Centers for Disease Control and Prevention. Abortion surveillance – United States, 2010. MMWR Surveill Summ. 2013;62:1–12.

Centers for Disease Control and Prevention. National Center for Health Statistics. 2014. http://www.cdc.gov/nchs/data/nvsr/nvsr62/nvsr62_09_tables.pdf. Accessed on September 11, 2014.

Crider KS, Olney RS, Cragan JD. Trisomies 13 and 18: population prevalences, characteristics, and prenatal diagnosis, metropolitan Atlanta, 1994-2003. Am J Med Genet. 2008;146A: 820–6.

Cystic Fibrosis Foundation. Patient Registry. 2014. http://www.cff.org/UploadedFiles/research/ClinicalResearch/PatientRegistryReport/2012-CFF-Patient-Registry.pdf. Accessed on September 12, 2014.

Decruyenaere M, Evers-Kiebooms G, Boogaerts A, et al. The complexity of reproductive decision-making in asymptomatic carriers of the Huntington mutation. Eur J Hum Genet. 2007; 15:453–62.

Derks-Smeets IAP, Gietel-Habets JJG, Tibben A, et al. Decision-making on preimplantation diagnosis and prenatal diagnosis: a challenge for couples with hereditary breast and ovarian cancer. Hum Reprod. 2014;29:1103–12.

Egan JFX, Smith K, Timms D, et al. Demographic differences in Down syndrome live births in the US from 1989 to 2006. Prenat Diagn. 2011;31:389–94.

El-Beshlawy A, El-Shekha A, Momtaz M, et al. Prenatal diagnosis for thalassaemia in Egypt: what changed parents' attitude? Prenat Diagn. 2012;32:777–82.

Evans MI, Sobiecki MS, Krivchenia EL, et al. Parental decisions to terminate/continue following abnormal cytogenetic prenatal diagnosis: "what" is still more important than "when". Am J Med Genet. 1996;61:353–5.

Farrant W, Hulten M. What is to be done with the XYY fetus? Br Med J. 1979;2(6182):131.

Ferguson-Smith ME, Ferguson-Smith MA, Nevin NC, Stone M. Chromosome analysis before birth and its value in genetic counseling. Br Med J. 1971;4:69–74.

Grati FR, Barlocco A, Grimi B, et al. Chromosome abnormalities investigated by non-invasive prenatal testing account for approximately 50% of fetal unbalances associated with relevant clinical phenotypes. Am J Med Genet. 2010;152A:1434–42.

Gruchy N, Vialard F, Blondeel E, et al. Pregnancy outcomes of prenatally diagnosed Turner syndrome: a French multicenter retrospective study including a series of 975 cases. Prenat Diagn. 2014;34:1133. doi:10.1002/pd.4439.

Gruchy N, Vialard F, Decamp M, et al. Pregnancy outcomes in 188 French cases of prenatally diagnose Klinefelter syndrome. Hum Reprod. 2011;26:2570–5.
Hawkins A, Stenzel A, Taylor J, Chock VY, Hudgins L. Variables influencing pregnancy termination following prenatal diagnosis of fetal chromosome abnormalities. J Genet Counsel. 2012; 22:238–48.
Hook EB, Chambers GM. Estimated rates of Down syndrome in live births by one year maternal age intervals for mothers aged 20-49 in a New York study – implications of the risk figures for genetic counseling and cost-benefit analysis of prenatal diagnosis programs. Birth Defects Orig Artic Ser. 1977;13:123–41.
Huether CA. Projection of Down's syndrome births in the United States 1979-2000, and the potential effects of prenatal diagnosis. Am J Public Health. 1983;73:1186–9.
Iyer NP, Tucker DF, Roberts SH, et al. Outcome of fetuses with Turner syndrome: a 10-year congenital anomaly register based study. J Matern Fetal Neonatal Med. 2012;25:68–73.
Jackson JE, Grobman WA, Haney E, Casele H. Mid-trimester dilation and evacuation with laminaria does not increase the risk for severe subsequent pregnancy complications. Int J Gynecol Obstet. 2007;96:12–5.
Jackson JM, Crider KS, Cragan JD, Rasmussen SA, Olney RS. Frequency of prenatal cytogenetic diagnosis and pregnancy outcomes by maternal race-ethnicity and the effect on the prevalence of trisomy 21, metropolitan Atlanta, 1996-2005. Am J Med Genet. 2014;164A:70–6.
Jeon KC, Chen L-S, Goodson P. Decision to abort after a prenatal diagnosis of sex chromosome abnormality: a systematic review of the literature. Genet Med. 2012;14:27–38.
Korenromp MJ, Page-Christiaens GCML, van den Bout J, Mulder EJH, Visser GHA. Maternal decision to terminate pregnancy after a diagnosis of Down syndrome. Am J Obstet Gynecol. 2007;196:149.e1–149.e11.
Lalatta F, Tint GS. Counseling parents before prenatal diagnosis: do we need to say more about the sex chromosome aneuploidies? Am J Med Genet. 2013;161A:2873–9.
Mansfield C, Hopfer S, Marteau TM. Termination rates after prenatal diagnosis of Down syndrome, spina bifida, anencephaly, and Turner and Klinefelter syndromes: a systematic literature review. Prenat Diagn. 1999;19:808–12.
Morris JK, Alberman E. Trends in Down's syndrome live births and antenatal diagnoses in England and Wales from 1989 to 2008: analysis of data from the National Down Syndrome Cytogenetic Register. BMJ. 2009;339:b3794.
Nadler HL. Antenatal detection of hereditary disorders. Pediatrics. 1968;42:912–8.
Natoli JL, Ackerman DL, McDermott S, Edwards JG. Prenatal diagnosis of Down syndrome: a systematic review of termination rates (1995-2011). Prenat Diagn. 2012;32:142–53.
The NICHD National Registry of Amniocentesis Study Group. Midtrimester amniocentesis for prenatal diagnosis – safety and accuracy. JAMA. 1976;236:1471–6.
NIH Consensus Development Conferences. Antenatal diagnosis – amniocentesis. Clin Pediatr. 1979;18:454–62.
Papp C, Szigeti Z, Joo JG, et al. The role of perinatal autopsy in the management of pregnancies with major fetal trisomies. Pathol Res Pract. 2007;203:525–31.
Pergament E, Pergament D. Reproductive decisions after fetal genetic counseling. Best Pract Res Clin Obstet Gynecol. 2012;26:517–29.
Perry S, Woodall AL, Pressman EK. Association of ultrasound findings with decision to continue Down syndrome pregnancies. Community Genet. 2007;10:227–30.
Richards FH, Rea G. Reproductive decision making before and after predictive testing for Huntington's disease: an Australian perspective. Clin Genet. 2005;67:404–11.
Ryan M, Miedzybrodzka Z, Fraser L, Hall M. Genetic information but not termination: pregnant women's attitudes and willingness to pay for carrier screening for deafness genes. J Med Genet. 2003;40:e80.
Sawyer SM, Cerritelli B, Carter LS, et al. Changing their minds with time: a comparison of hypothetical and actual reproductive behaviors in parents of children with cystic fibrosis. Pediatrics. 2006;118:e649–56.

Schechtman KB, Gray DL, Baty JD, Rothman SM. Decision-making for termination of pregnancies with fetal anomalies: analysis of 53,000 pregnancies. Obstet Gynecol. 2002;99:216–22.
Scotet V, Dugueperoux I, Audrezet M-P, et al. Prenatal diagnosis of cystic fibrosis: the 18-year experience of Brittany (western France). Prenat Diagn. 2008;28:197–202.
Shaffer BL, Caughey AB, Norton ME. Variation in the decision to terminate pregnancy in the setting of fetal aneuploidy. Prenat Diagn. 2006;26:667–71.
Steele MW, Breg Jr WR. Chromosome analysis of human amniotic fluid cells. Lancet. 1966; 1(7434):383–5.
Stern SJ, Arnos KS, Murrelle L, et al. Attitudes of deaf and hard of hearing subjects towards genetic testing and prenatal diagnosis of hearing loss. J Med Genet. 2002;39:449–53.
Tongsong T, Charoenkwan P, Sirivatanapa P, et al. Effectiveness of the model for prenatal control of severe thalassemia. Prenat Diagn. 2013;33:477–83.
Tonks AM, Gornall AS, Larkins SA, Gardosi JO. Trisomies 18 and 13: trends in prevalence and prenatal diagnosis – population based study. Prenat Diagn. 2013;33:742–50.
Valenti C, Schutta EJ, Kehaty T. Prenatal diagnosis of Down's syndrome. Lancet. 1968;2(7561):220.
Verp MS, Bombard AT, Simpson JL, Elias S. Parental decision following prenatal diagnosis of fetal chromosome abnormality. Am J Med Genet. 1988;29:613–22.
Wang X, Seaman C, Paik T, et al. Experience with 500 prenatal diagnoses of sickle cell diseases: the effect of gestational age on affected pregnancy outcome. Prenat Diagn. 1994;14:851–7.
Wapner RJ, Martin CL, Levy B, et al. Chromosomal microarray versus karyotyping for prenatal diagnosis. N Engl J Med. 2012;367:2175–84.

Chapter 4
Medical Reasons for Pregnancy Interruption: Structural Abnormalities

Lucas Otaño, César H. Meller, and Horacio A. Aiello

Classification of Structural Abnormalities

As the understanding of pathogenesis and etiology has increased, the classification of structural abnormalities has changed over time, and varies according to different perspectives. Thus, structural abnormalities can be classified according to the altered process in morphogenesis (dysmorphology), the etiology, or the clinical severity.

(a) **Dysmorphology**: classically the nomenclature of anomalies has been based on the type of problem in morphogenesis in (Jones et al. 2013; Siebert and Kapur 2001):

- *Malformation*: morphologic defect resulting from an intrinsically abnormal developmental process (structure is abnormal from its inception).
- *Deformation*: abnormal form, shape, or position of a structure, caused by mechanical factors.
- *Disruption*: morphologic defect resulting from extrinsic interference with a normal process.
- *Dysplasia*: abnormal organization of tissue.

Cases of multiple structural anomalies are usually grouped according a developmental pathology viewpoint:

L. Otaño, M.D., Ph.D. (✉) • C.H. Meller, M.D. • H.A. Aiello, M.D.
Division of Obstetrics and Fetal Medicine Unit, Department of Obstetrics and Gynecology, University Hospital Italiano de Buenos Aires,
Potosi 4135, Ciudad Autonoma de Buenos Aires C1199ACl, Argentina
e-mail: lucas.otano@hospitalitaliano.org.ar; cesar.meller@hospitalitaliano.org.ar; horacio.aiello@hospitalitaliano.org.ar

J.P. Galst, M.S. Verp (eds.), *Prenatal and Preimplantation Diagnosis*,
DOI 10.1007/978-3-319-18911-6_4

- *Syndrome*: "a recognizable pattern of anomalies which are known or thought to be causally related" (Khoury et al. 1994; Spranger et al. 1982), for example, chromosomal, monogenic, or environmental teratogen.
- *Sequence*: "pattern of anomalies derived from a known (or presumed) malformation or mechanical factor"
- *Complex*: "those groups of heterogeneous disorders with overlapping characteristics that are difficult to separate into specific conditions," e.g., facio-auriculo-vertebral spectrum, hypoglossia–hypodactylia (Martínez-Frías 1995)
- *Association*: "derivatives of causally nonspecific disruptive events acting on developmental fields" or "abnormal markers of normal embryologic relationships" (Lubinsky 1986). Developmental field is defined as basic biological units of individual development and of evolution, and association to represent the idiopathic occurrence of multiple congenital anomalies during blastogenesis (Opitz 1985). In a sense, this is a "wastebasket" category that should change with increasing understanding.

(b) **According to etiology**: structural anomalies can also be classified as:

- *Genetic*:
  - Chromosomal
  - Monogenic
- *Multifactorial*
- *Environmental*:
  - Infectious
  - Physical
  - Chemical
- *Unknown*

The knowledge of the etiology of any structural anomaly is of paramount importance in order to define the prognosis and the recurrence risk of the abnormality. However, in clinical practice it is not always possible to determine the cause of a fetal structural anomaly. The ability to determine the cause will depend on medical knowledge and availability and proper use of diagnostic tools.

For the purpose of this chapter, structural anomalies that are either isolated or occur as part of a genetic syndrome are considered.

(c) **According to clinical severity**: Structural anomalies have been usually classified as *minor* and *major* malformations. However, categorization as minor or major differs in the literature. The epidemiological surveillance program of congenital anomalies in Europe, EUROCAT, defines major anomalies as those that *require surgical treatment* (*medical*), *have serious adverse effects on health or development* (*functional*), *or have significant cosmetic impact* (*cosmetic*). Fetuses with two or more major malformations are classified as a polymalformed (EUROCAT 2011).

For major fetal structural anomalies, in turn, different subgroups are also described according to severity: lethal, severe major, and major.

- Lethal anomalies are those that almost always will cause death, but time of death will vary (prenatal, neonatal, or in infancy), and treatment does not prevent death.
- Severe major anomalies are those that are lethal without surgery or organ transplantation, those that severely affect quality of life and surgery is always needed, or those that always cause severe developmental delay or mental retardation.
- Major anomalies are those that are usually nonlethal or are lethal only very exceptionally but clearly affect quality of life, and surgery or other corresponding treatment is always needed, or always cause developmental delay or mental retardation of some degree.

When a fetal structural anomaly is detected, severity plays a central role in the prenatal counseling and, in some countries, in establishing when a TOP is possible. The Royal College of Obstetricians and Gynaecologists (RCOG) guidance on termination of pregnancy for fetal anomalies states that TOP may only be considered if there is a substantial risk that the child, if born, would suffer physical or mental abnormalities that would result in serious handicap (RCOG 2010). However there is no legal definition of substantial risk, and whether a risk is regarded as substantial may vary with the seriousness and consequences of the likely disability. Likewise, there is no legal definition of serious handicap. An assessment of the seriousness of a fetal abnormality should be considered on a case-by-case basis, taking into account all available clinical information (RCOG 2010).

Screening of Fetal Structural Abnormalities

In contemporary fetal medicine two dimensional ultrasound is the primary method for detection of fetal structural defects, and imaging modalities such as 3D or 4D ultrasound, and magnetic resonance, are diagnostic complements.

In order to standardize practice and improve the detection rate of fetal structural abnormalities, several professional associations have developed guidelines and recommendations for the use of ultrasound during pregnancy (International Society of Ultrasound in Obstetrics & Gynecology Education Committee (2007); International Society of Ultrasound in Obstetrics and Gynecology (2013); Salomon et al. 2011). The American Institute of Ultrasound in Medicine (AIUM), in conjunction with the American College of Radiology (ACR), the American College of Obstetricians and Gynecologists (ACOG) and the Society of Radiologist in Ultrasound (SRU), has developed guidelines that state the key elements of standard sonographic examinations in the first, second and third trimesters of pregnancy (AIUM 2013a).

All of these guidelines recommend, in order to evaluate the fetal anatomy, a mid-trimester scan between 18 and 22 weeks of gestation, the search for fetal malformations being one of the main goals.

The sensitivity of ultrasound for detection of major anomalies is variable, being higher in specialized centers, but surprisingly low at a general population level (Grandjean et al. 1999; Levi 2002; Saltvedt et al. 2006). Twenty years ago, a randomized controlled trial, the RADIUS, was performed in North America to assess the usefulness of ultrasound detection of fetal malformations for the perinatal outcome. This study compared the detection rate of major fetal anomalies in a general population with scheduled ultrasound evaluations at 15–20 weeks and at 31–35 weeks versus the anomaly detection rate in a population in whom ultrasound was done only for clinical indications. The incidence of fetal anomaly in this combined population of 15,281 women was 2.3 %. The anomaly detection rate in the scheduled ultrasound population was 35 % as compared to 11 % in the control group. A better detection rate was observed in tertiary care centers than in community based facilities. The study showed no difference in perinatal outcomes (Crane et al. 1994). Other series, however, showed a reduction in perinatal mortality following routine obstetric ultrasound, primarily because of an increase in the rate of TOP for congenital anomalies (Bucher and Schmidt 1993), the possibility of optimal antenatal care and referral to the required specialist level for delivery, and the anticipatory planning of the postnatal treatment of the newborn (Garne et al. 2005; Jaeggi et al. 2001).

(a) Second trimester screening of fetal structural abnormalities

A second trimester fetal anatomical survey has become an integral part of routine antenatal care (RANZCOG 2013; RCOG 2013). The objectives of this ultrasound scan are: to identify abnormalities associated with severe morbidity or that are incompatible with life, so that women and their partners can be offered a choice, within the constraints of the law, as to whether or not to terminate the pregnancy; to detect abnormalities which require early intervention following delivery or which may benefit, in a small number of cases, from intrauterine treatment (NHS 2012; RCOG 2010).

The second trimester ultrasound has been described by different professional associations and scientific societies, and it has different names: The "20 week" Anomaly Scan (RCOG 2013), Fetal Anatomic Survey (ACR 2013), Mid-trimester ultrasound for fetal structural abnormalities (RANZCOG 2013), The 18+0–20+6 weeks ultrasound scan (NHS 2012), Routine mid-trimester fetal ultrasound scan (Salomon et al. ISUOG 2011), Complete Routine Second Trimester Obstetrical Ultrasound Examination (18–22 weeks) (Cargill et al. SOGC 2009).

Most clinical guidelines recommend which patients should have a mid-trimester ultrasound, when it should be done (gestational age), who should perform it, what ultrasound equipment should be used and which standardized sonographic parameters should be measured. For example, Table 4.1 lists the recommended minimum requirements for a basic mid-trimester fetal anatomical survey and Fig. 4.1 shows some examples of standard views.

(b) First trimester screening of fetal structural abnormalities

Although the mid-trimester scan is considered the standard of care in the prenatal detection of fetal structural anomalies, routine prenatal ultrasound during the first trimester (11–13 weeks+6 days) is increasingly being offered in addition

Table 4.1 Recommended minimum requirements for basic mid-trimester fetal anatomical survey (Salomon et al. ISUOG 2011)

Head	Intact cranium
	Cavum septi pellucidi
	Midline falx
	Thalami
	Cerebral ventricles
	Cerebellum
	Cisterna magna
Face	Both orbits present
	Median facial profile[a]
	Mouth present
	Upper lip intact
Neck	Absence of masses (e.g., cystic hygroma)
Chest/ heart	Normal appearing shape/size of chest and lungs
	Heart activity present
	Four-chamber view of heart in normal position
	Aortic and pulmonary outflow tracts[a]
	No evidence of diaphragmatic hernia
Abdomen	Stomach in normal position
	Bowel not dilated
	Both kidneys present
	Cord insertion site
Skeletal	No spinal defects or masses (transverse and sagittal views)
	Arms and hands present, normal relationships
	Legs and feet present, normal relationships
Placenta	Position
	No masses present
	Accessory lobe

[a]Umbilical cord: Three-vessel cord

Reproduced from Salomon LJ, Alfirevic Z, Berghella V, Bilardo C, Hernandez-Andrade E, Johnsen SL, et al. ISUOG Clinical Standards Committee. Practice guidelines for performance of the routine mid-trimester fetal ultrasound scan. Ultrasound Obstet Gynecol. 2011;37(1):116–26, with permission of John Wiley & Sons

to the second-trimester scan (Salomon et al. 2013). Even though its primary focus has been aneuploidy screening (Nicolaides et al. 1994), the detection of some severe fetal structural abnormalities has also become a goal of the late first-trimester screen (Saltvedt et al. 2006).

In a review of the published literature between 2002 and 2008 the overall detection rate of structural anomalies in the first trimester (11–14 weeks scan)

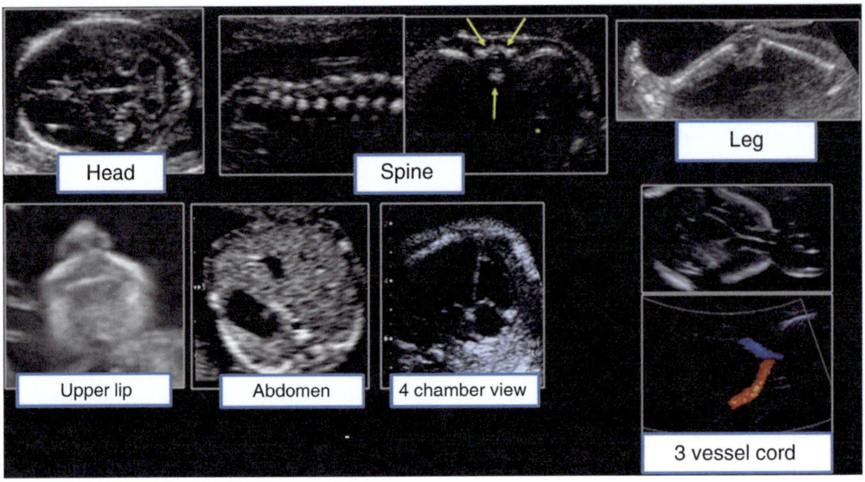

Fig. 4.1 Examples of standard views at the mid-trimester fetal anatomical survey

was 29 % (range 18–71 %) (Borrell et al. 2011). The most frequently detected anomalies (more than 65 %) were: holoprosencephaly, acrania, hydrops, omphalocele, gastroschisis, and megacystis (lower urinary tract obstruction).

In a specialized center, with highly trained operators and high quality equipment, the detection rate of major structural anomalies in fetuses with normal karyotypes was around 50 % with almost 100 % detection of the most severe anomalies (holoprosencephaly, acrania, megacystis, gastroschisis, ompholocele, and hydrops) (Grande et al. 2012; Syngelaki et al. 2011). Of note is the distribution of detection rates in different stages of pregnancy in a tertiary center: 49 % in the first trimester, 30 % in the second trimester, 15 % in the third trimester, and 6 % postnatally. Assessment of ultrasound "markers" associated with aneuploidy would improve the detection rate of structural abnormalities (Syngelaki et al. 2011). For example, increased nuchal translucency is associated with heart defects, skeletal dysplasias, and other major anomalies. Abnormal ductus venosus and tricuspid regurgitation are associated with heart defects (Borrell et al. 2011; Pereira et al. 2011).

It has been suggested that in the first trimester some anomalies are almost always detectable, some are potentially detectable, and some are undetectable:

- **Always detected**: body-stalk anomaly, anencephaly (Fig. 4.2a), alobar holoprosencephaly (Fig. 4.2b), exomphalos, gastroschisis, and megacystis (Fig. 4.2c).
- **Undetectable** in first trimester: microcephaly, agenesis of corpus callosum, ventriculomegaly (infection, hemorrhage), fetal tumors, ovarian cysts, duodenal atresia, hydronephrosis.
- **Potentially detectable**: spina bifida (Fig. 4.3a), facial clefting, cardiac defects, renal defects, limb defects and diaphragmatic hernia (Fig. 4.3b) (Syngelaki et al. 2011).

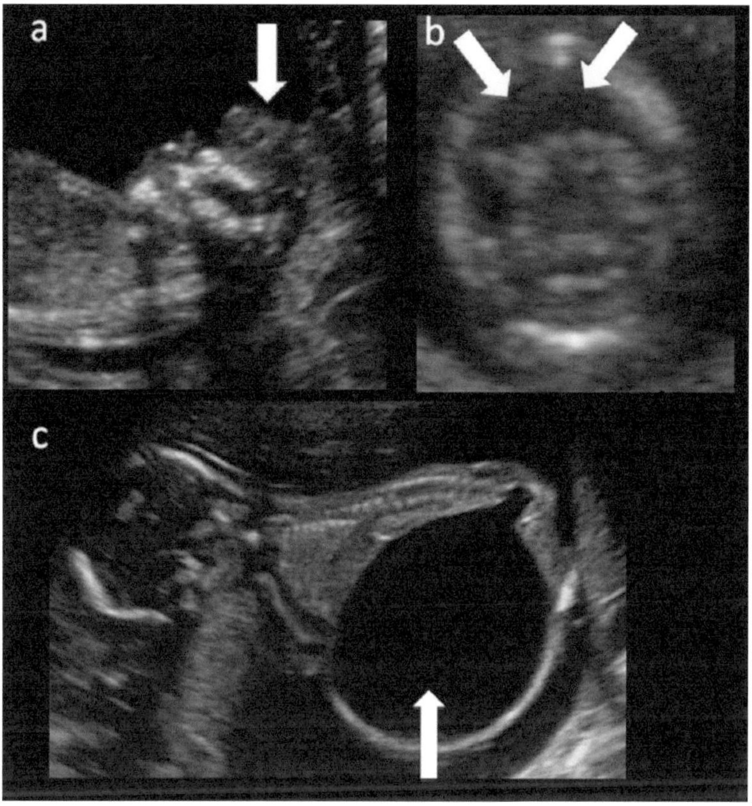

Fig. 4.2 Anomalies that should always be detected in the first trimester: (**a**) **Anencephaly**: 13 weeks fetus with absence of the skull and a disorganized brain floating in the amniotic fluid (*arrow*); (**b**) **Alobar holoprosencephaly**: the midline echo that should be present in a normal fetus is absent in alobar holorprosencephaly, and a single ventricle can be demonstrated (*arrows*); (**c**) **Megacystis** (*arrow*)

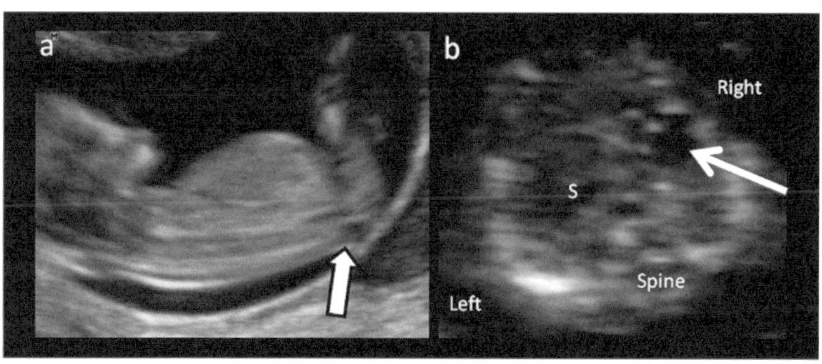

Fig. 4.3 Anomalies that are *potentially detectable* in the first trimester: (**a**) ***Spina bifida***: the *arrow* shows the defect in the spine in a 12 weeks fetus; (**b**) ***Congenital diaphragmatic hernia***: dextroposition of the heart (*arrow*) and the stomach (S) in the thorax

(c) Factors that affect ultrasound detection of fetal anomalies

- *Operator's skills and experience*: The performance of obstetric ultrasound is highly operator dependent (Bernaschek et al. 1996).
- *Fetal anomaly type*: The detection rate varies depending on the type of anomaly, being close to 100 % for anencephaly (Garne et al. 2005; Grandjean et al. 1999) and gastroschisis (NICE 2008), but less for major fetal cardiac defects and for facial oral clefts (25–60 %) (Gascard-Battisti et al. 2006; Hanikeri et al. 2006). The detection rate is significantly increased when multiple anomalies are present (Campaña et al. 2010; Calzolari et al. 2014). The detection rate further increases if the pregnancy is sequentially scanned for anatomic assessment in the first and second trimesters (Souka et al. 2006).
- *Gestational age*. The more severe the structural anomaly the earlier the gestational age at which it can be detected. As described before, 50 % of major structural abnormalities could be detected in the first trimester scan, 30 % in the second trimester and 15 % in the third.
- *Risk factors for fetal anomalies*. The detection rate for a specific anomaly improves substantially when risk factors are present, for example, a history of a previous affected fetus or family history of a multifactorial anomaly, exposure to environmental factors, maternal diseases such as pregestational diabetes (Yang et al. 2006), obesity (Watkins et al. 2003), or epilepsy. Risk is also increased in assisted reproductive technology pregnancies, and in monochorionic twins. Finally, positive serum or ultrasound markers may improve the detection rate because of a higher level of suspicion.
- *Imaging method and image quality*. The advances in ultrasound imaging methods, and color Doppler, have improved image quality and diagnostic accuracy.
- *Maternal factors*: Obesity is a well-known factor that impairs intrauterine visualization, and therefore detection rate of fetal anomalies is diminished (Hendler et al. 2005). Thus, it has been suggested for medicolegal reasons that the report describe whether image quality was compromised by maternal obesity.
- *Pregnancy factors*: Oligohydramnios, severe polyhydramnios, advanced gestational age, fetal position, and multiple pregnancy are factors that can affect visualization.
- *Baseline population risk*: Low risk or high risk population, referral center or primary care center.

Diagnosis and Management of Fetal Structural Abnormalities

(a) **Diagnosis**: The detection of a fetal structural abnormality is usually based on an abnormal ultrasound finding. One of the most important questions after the detection of a fetal structural abnormality is whether it is an isolated finding, it is associated with other anomalies, and if it is part of a genetic syndrome. Thus, the initial abnormal finding frequently is not the final diagnosis. The ultrasound detection of an omphalocele clearly illustrates the concept. This well-defined abdominal wall defect could be an isolated anomaly with an excellent prognosis, or it could be associated with lethal trisomy 18 or 13, or with any of several other syndromes of which omphalocele is one manifestation. Thus the diagnosis of a fetal structural anomaly is not just an abnormal ultrasound image, but a process, which is triggered by an ultrasound finding. After detection of a fetal structural anomaly, the patient should be referred to a specialist in fetal medicine (NHS 2012) or to a tertiary ultrasound unit as soon as possible to optimize therapeutic options (Gagnon et al. 2009). The process of diagnosis usually requires additional tests, e.g., a detailed ultrasound reassessment, echocardiography, invasive genetic testing with karyotyping, chromosomal microarrays (CMA) or other fetal tissue tests, magnetic resonance imaging, etc. (Gagnon et al. 2009; SOGC Committee Opinion 2009). Only after comprehensive evaluation may a final diagnosis be established or hypothesized.

A key step in the evaluation of a fetal structural abnormality is the genetic testing. The American College of Obstetricians and Gynecologists and the Society of Maternal–Fetal Medicine now recommend that chromosomal microarray analysis (CMA) be performed in lieu of karyotyping in pregnancies with an anomalous fetus undergoing invasive testing, or if the karyotype is normal (ACOG 2013; Donnelly et al. 2014; Hillman et al. 2013; Wapner et al. 2012). In other countries CMA is still considered a second-tier diagnostic test which can complement, but not replace, standard karyotyping in a selected group of pregnancies (Novelli et al. 2012). Concurrently, there are ongoing studies focusing on the "next step" in prenatal genetic diagnosis, e.g., the use of next generation sequencing and exome sequencing to determine if these will give more precise diagnostic and prognostic information on fetal structural anomalies (Hillman et al. 2015).

(b) **Prognosis and management of fetal structural anomalies**: The prognosis of a fetal anomaly is a major determinant for prospective parents considering TOP. An accurate diagnosis is needed for the severity of the condition to be assessed and the prognosis determined. This is reasonably clear-cut when the condition is deemed fatal and many such conditions will be identified before 22 weeks. It is when the anomaly is more likely to result in morbidity than mortality that problems in defining severity arise (RCOG 2010).

In cases of anomalies that are always *lethal* (e.g., renal agenesis, anencephaly), the clinical management should be directed to preventing maternal morbidity. Early diagnosis has potential benefits: termination is safer the earlier it is performed and earlier in pregnancy there may be greater access to surgical termination, which some women prefer (RCOG 2010) to induction termination. In later pregnancy, an important aspect of management is the induction of labor (unless contraindicated) when the cervix is favorable, and the avoidance of cesarean section for signs of fetal distress (Manning 2009).

There are severe anomalies that are compatible with limited survival but associated with severe neurologic disabilities (e.g., severe hydrocephaly). Management of these fetuses generally follows the same pathway as that of fetuses with lethal anomalies.

On the opposite end of severity, there are fetal anomalies, like oral clefts, that have limited functional sequelae and are amenable to repair in the postnatal period. Recent evidence shows that routine fetal anomaly scans decrease the gestational age at diagnosis of cleft lip and increase the detection rate, without a significant change in TOP rate (Ensing et al. 2014). The availability of methods to correct or ameliorate fetal structural defects has a significant impact on management. Most treatments are applied in the neonatal period. The usual goal of managing a fetus with a nonlethal anomaly for which there is a reasonable prospect of minimal postnatal disability is to delay delivery until the fetus is mature. Prenatal consultation with a neonatal team greatly facilitates care coordination and reduces mortality and morbidity (Manning 2009).

In highly selected cases, a fetal medical or invasive therapy to improve the perinatal prognosis may be available, thereby offering parents an alternative to termination or continuation of pregnancy with postnatal management. Examples of fetal medical therapy are the administration of steroids for microcystic congenital cystic adenomatoid malformation (Hui and Bianchi 2011; Witlox et al. 2011) or antiarrhythmic drugs delivered via the transplacental route for the treatment of fetal tachyarrythmias (Hui and Bianchi 2011; Jaeggi et al. 2011). Examples of invasive therapy are prenatal repair of myelomeningocele (Adzick et al. 2011), and endoscopic tracheal occlusion for congenital diaphragmatic hernia (discussed also in "Specific fetal structural anomalies") (Dekoninck et al. 2011; Ruano et al. 2012).

Unfortunately, many anomalies fall into a category in which the prognosis cannot be assigned with certainty. Accurate diagnosis and determination of prognosis for conditions such as isolated agenesis of the corpus callosum or mild ventriculomegaly poses problems due to difficulty in accurately detecting additional central nervous system abnormalities. The variable regression or progression of mild ventriculomegaly necessitates a repeat scan several weeks after the initial diagnosis (RCOG 2010) and the prognosis may be unclear until the natural course of the condition is followed.

(c) **Counseling**: The decision-making process for women and their partners after the diagnosis of fetal abnormality is a difficult one (Hern 2014). They must try to absorb the medical information they have been given, while in a state of emotional shock and distress, and work out a way forward that they can best live with (RCOG 2010). In such sensitive circumstances, women and their partners must receive appropriate counseling and support from the healthcare practitioners involved, including a trained genetic counselor and/or a maternal–fetal medicine specialist and/or a medical geneticist. Pregnant patients frequently receive conflicting information about the prognosis of a fetal anomaly, depending on the sometimes-narrow perspective of a subspecialist. Therefore, the diagnosis, counseling and management of a patient with a fetal anomaly requires multidisciplinary expertise from the different specialties involved: obstetrics, genetics, neonatology, pediatric surgery, pediatric subspecialties, etc. (Bianchi et al. 2010, preface). All staff involved in the care of a woman or couple facing a possible termination of pregnancy must adopt a nondirective, nonjudgmental, and supportive approach (RCOG 2010); counseling should be unbiased and respectful of the patient's choice, culture, religion, and beliefs (Gagnon et al. 2009). Counseling after prenatal diagnosis of a fetal anomaly depends mainly on the certainty and knowledge of the diagnosis. Women should receive information regarding the abnormal ultrasound findings in a clear, sympathetic, and timely fashion, and in a supportive environment that ensures privacy. Referral to the appropriate pediatric or surgical subspecialist(s) should be considered to provide accurate information concerning the anomaly or anomalies and the associated prognosis (Gagnon et al. 2009).

(d) **Factors that affect parental decision on TOP**: The prenatal diagnosis of major structural abnormalities is one of the main reasons for termination of pregnancy (TOP) worldwide. The decision to continue or terminate the pregnancy has been associated primarily with the severity of the malformation (Asplin et al. 2013; Nell et al. 2013) but also with other factors like gestational age at diagnosis (Tararbit et al. 2013), cultural issues, and the local legal status of TOP. Based on the EUROCAT registry, which provides useful data on overall impact of prenatal screening and testing, Garne et al. (2005) reported on prenatal diagnosis of severe structural congenital malformations in Europe. The study selected structural defects potentially detectable by prenatal ultrasound and sufficiently severe that termination of pregnancy would be considered as an option. Based on these criteria, 11 structural malformations were selected: anencephalus, encephalocele, spina bifida, hydrocephalus, transposition of great arteries, hypoplastic left heart, limb reduction defect, bilateral renal agenesis, diaphragmatic hernia, omphalocele and gastroschisis (Table 4.2).The study showed wide regional variation in the rate of prenatal diagnosis of these malformations, that may be explained by different screening policies, differences in pregnant women's attitudes to screening, differences in technology and skills, and differences in laws regarding the upper gestational age limit for pregnancy termination. The results also showed that with earlier diagnosis more pregnancies were terminated.

Gestational age at the time of diagnosis of an anomaly has a powerful impact on management decisions. As a general rule, the earlier the gestational age of diagnosis, the more severe the defect and the worse the prognosis. This association exists in part because the younger the fetus, the larger the defect must be to be recognized, and the larger the defect is, the greater the likelihood of damaging or disrupting both adjacent and remote tissues. In the mature fetus, delivery and postnatal evaluation may be the most appropriate management. In the immature (previable) fetus, termination of pregnancy is often selected, especially when the anomaly is associated with either a hopeless or very poor prognosis. Ultrasound at <14 weeks was associated with an earlier gestational age at abortion in pregnancies with structural fetal abnormalities (Chasen and Kalish 2013).

Table 4.2 Prenatal diagnosis, gestational age at discovery, and subsequent termination of pregnancy of 11 severe malformation in Europe (Garne et al. 2005)

Malformatiom	Cases (*n*)	Prenatal diagnosis (*n*)	Gestational age at diagnosis (%)			Termination of pregnancy (%)
			<24 weeks	≥24 weeks	Unknown	
Anencephalus	498	469 (94 %)	84	7	9	90
Encephalocele	162	128 (79 %)	62	26	12	84
Spina bifida	599	405 (68 %)	69	26	5	78
Hydrocephalus	816	626 (77 %)	52	40	8	63
Transpositionof great arteries	324	89 (27 %)	53	43	4	40
Hypoplastic left heart	289	164 (57 %)	62	31	7	69
Limb reduction defects	694	251 (36 %)	73	22	5	67
Bilateral renal agenesis	257	201 (78 %)	74	17	9	79
Diaphragmatic hernia	377	197 (52 %)	55	39	6	35
Omphalocele	355	275 (77 %)	81	11	8	64
Gastroschisis	196	175 (89 %)	79	15	6	30
Total malformations	4567	2980 (65 %)	69	24	7	67
Total cases	4366	2806 (64 %)				66
Genitalia:	Male or female[a]					

[a]Optional component of checklist: can be evaluated if technically feasible

Reproduced from Garne E, Loane M, Dolk H, De Vigan C, Scarano G, Tucker D et al. Prenatal diagnosis of severe structural congenital malformations in Europe. Ultrasound Obstet Gynecol. 2005; 25: 6–11, with permission of John Wiley & Sons

Another factor that may affect parental decision is local professional practice and attitudes regarding fetal abnormalities. Maternal–Fetal Medicine and Fetal Care Pediatrician specialists' counseling attitudes differ for fetal abnormalities (Brown et al. 2012).

(e) **Specific fetal structural anomalies**: Most congenital malformations visible at birth have also been diagnosed prenatally, but it is beyond the scope of this chapter to consider the entire spectrum of fetal structural anomalies. Thus, the most prevalent and significant fetal anomalies, severe enough for considering the option of TOP, are discussed. Table 4.2 shows the prenatal detection rate, gestational age at diagnosis and the TOP rate of these structural abnormalities.

Neural Tube Defects (NTD)

Neural tube defects are the second most prevalent defect in the USA, behind cardiac malformations, and include:

(a) **Anencephaly**

One of the most common NTD and the first congenital malformation detected by ultrasound (Campbell et al. 1972) (Fig. 4.4).

- **Definition**: Complete or partial absence of the forebrain, overlying meninges, skull and skin.
- **Incidence**: Highly variable and dependent upon geographic location, race, and sex. The prevalence in the USA prior to the introduction of folic acid supplementation for the prevention of neural tube defects was 1 in 1000 births.
- **Diagnosis**: Sonographic diagnosis is very accurate from 12 weeks gestation and there are almost no false positive diagnoses. In a normal fetus, echogenic areas can be seen that correspond to calcification of the cranial bones at 11 weeks gestation. If calcification is absent, exencephaly should be considered (Bianchi et al. 2010)
- **Long-term outcome**: Uniformly fatal.
- **Termination of pregnancy rate**: Very high, close to 90 % (Garne et al. 2005; Johnson et al. 2012)

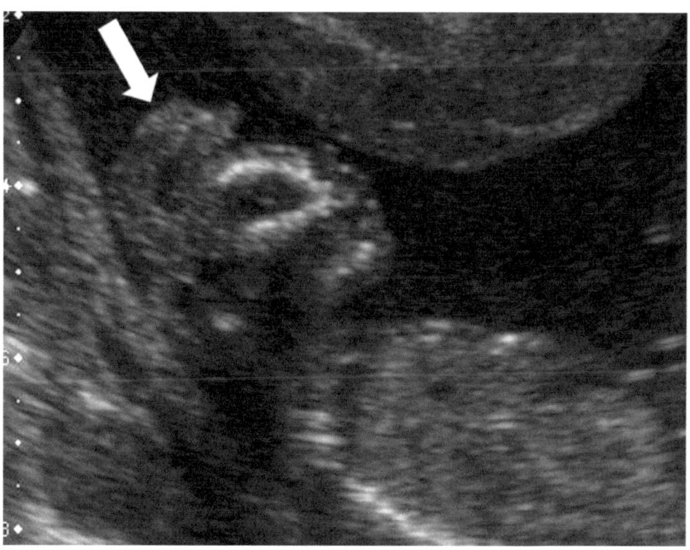

Fig. 4.4 Anencephaly: Fetal profile demonstrating the absence of the skull. The disorganized brain is floating in the amniotic fluid (*arrow*) and the orbits appear prominent

(b) **Open spina bifida**
The most common type of NTD.

- **Definition**: The defect results from the failure of the neural tube to fuse during early embryogenesis, with no closure of the vertebral arches and protrusion of the neural structures and meninges (myelomeningocele) through the defect.
- **Incidence**: Geographic and population dependent; ranges from 1:500–1: 2000 live births.
- **Diagnosis**: Ultrasonographic diagnosis is based upon direct visualization in the second trimester of the vertebral defect and protruding meninges and neural structures (Fig. 4.5a), but more than 50 % of affected cases are missed using these findings only. As a consequence of the spinal dysraphism, cranial changes occur during gestation that can be easily detected by ultrasound. These abnormal central nervous system sonographic findings are due to Arnold–Chiari malformation type 2 and include a smaller than expected biparietal diameter and head circumference, the "***lemon sign***," and the "***banana sign***," the effacement of the cisterna magna, and ventriculomegaly (Fig. 4.5b). These ***intracranial signs*** are present in more than 95 % of the fetuses with spina bifida at 18–22 weeks of gestation (Bianchi et al. 2010).
- **Long-term outcome**: Although not considered a lethal defect, 35 % of live-borns die within the first 5 years and 50 % of individuals have an IQ less than 80. Long-term sequelae include impairment in neuromuscular and urologic function, and sexual dysfunction. Hindbrain herniation is the main cause of death during the first year of life. The typical consequences of spina bifida that affect overall prognosis are full or partial paralysis, loss of sensation in the skin, urinary incontinence, bowel dysfunction, birthmarks, skin discoloration or dimpling, hydrocephalus, infections such as encephalitis or meningitis, and nerve damage.

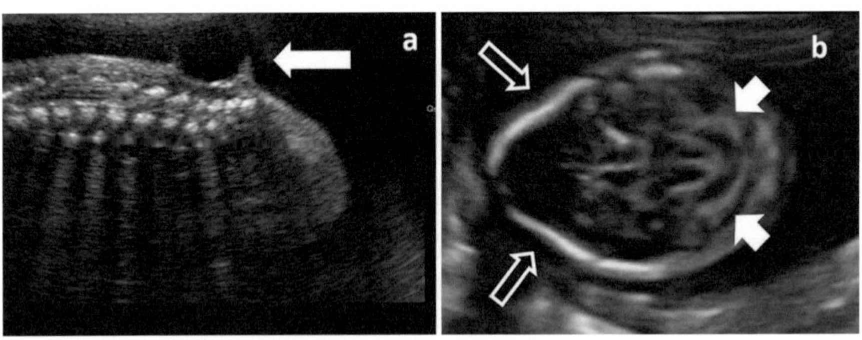

Fig. 4.5 (**a**) Sagittal section of the spine showing a large ***meningocele*** (*white arrow*) with intact sac below L5 level. (**b**) The head is bilateral flattened (*open arrows*), giving the typical appearance of the "lemon" sign. The cistern magna is obliterated and the cerebellum is rounded to form the "banana sign" (*white arrows*)

- At the milder end of these findings, e.g., birthmarks, the prognosis is far more positive than it is for those who develop extensive nerve damage or infections. The wide range of manifestations makes it difficult to formulate prenatally any one-size-fits-all prognosis. The degree of handicap depends mainly on the size and level of the affected spinal segments. The lower the spinal level, the better the prognosis.
- Recently it has been shown that in utero correction of spina bifida in selected cases reduced the need for postnatal shunting and improved motor outcomes at 30 months of life, but open fetal surgery is associated with maternal and fetal risks (Adzick et al. 2011).
- **Termination of pregnancy rate**: 65–80 % (EUROCAT 2005; Johnson et al. 2012).

(c) **Encephalocele**
A less common NTD than anencephaly and spina bifida.

- **Definition**: Herniation of cranial contents through defects in the skull (Bianchi et al. 2010). In western countries, more than 80 % of the defects are in the occipital region.
- **Incidence**: 1:2000–1:4000 live births. The cause is unknown, but encephaloceles are the result of a failure of neural tube closure in the cranial region during the first month of embryonic development. Unlike anencephaly and spina bifida, encephaloceles are frequently associated with other brain and non-neural abnormalities. This anomaly has been described as one finding in more than 30 disorders, including chromosomal abnormalities, Mendelian and sporadic conditions.
- **Diagnosis**: The sonographic appearance of encephalocele is diverse. The best diagnostic clue is the presence of a bony defect with a paracranial mass (Fig. 4.6). The mass could be cystic, solid or mixed. The defect has been noted to have a unique "cyst within a cyst" or "target sign" which is created when the fourth ventricle herniates into the encephalocele. Ventriculomegaly

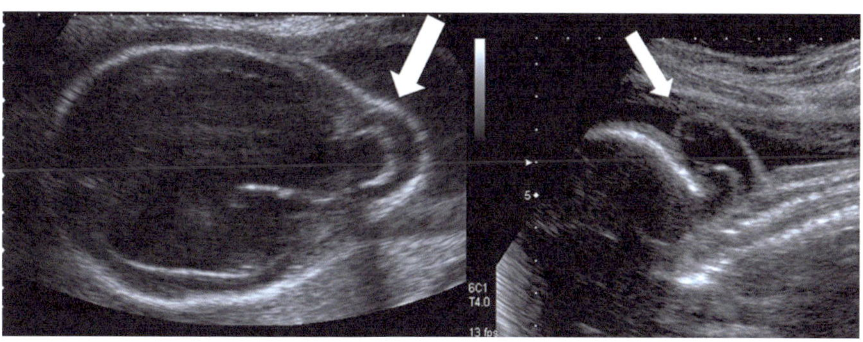

Fig. 4.6 Axial view (*left*) and posterior sagittal section of the head in a fetus with ***encephalocele***. Note the occipital bone defect and the "target sign" (*arrow*)

is present in 70–80 % of the fetuses, and microcephaly in 25 %. Intracranial signs observed in fetuses with open spina bifida (lemon sign, banana sign, obliteration of cisterna magna) are often present in cases with encephalocele and Arnold–Chiari Type 3 malformation (cerebellar herniation through the occipital defect). Both polyhydramnios and oligohydramnios are described. Genetic syndromes with renal compromise like Meckel–Gruber Syndrome (encephalocele, polycystic kidneys, and polydactyly) may have anhydramnios. In these cases, magnetic resonance imaging (MRI) can help in the diagnosis. Prenatal detection rate by ultrasound and MRI is high, near 80 %.

- **Long-term outcome**: it is almost uniformly poor, and varies with the amount of brain tissue in the defect and the presence of associated malformations. Mortality rates reach 80 % in fetal series and 40 % in neonatal series. Isolated cranial meningocele without brain herniation has a better prognosis. Nevertheless, 80 % of survivors show neurologic impairment, with developmental delay, often significant, and seizures.
- **Termination of pregnancy rate**: around 85 % (Garne et al. 2005).

Hydrocephalus

(a) **Definition**: A pathological increase of intracranial cerebrospinal fluid (CSF) volume, which results in **ventriculomegaly** (VM), a condition in which the atrium of the lateral ventricles is dilated. The etiology is heterogeneous, and includes obstruction of CSF flow (Arnold–Chiari malformation, Aqueductal stenosis, tumors, congenital infections, and intracranial hemorrhage), maldevelopment of ventricles (corpus callosum agenesis, porencephaly), and genetic syndromes (chromosome abnormalities and Mendelian disorders).

(b) **Incidence**: The incidence of isolated VM is 0.5–1 of 1000 pregnancies (Bianchi et al. 2010; Garne et al. 2010).

(c) **Diagnosis**: Prenatal diagnosis is based on the diameter of the ventricles. The diameter of the lateral ventricle is measured from inner edge to inner edge, perpendicular to the long axis of the ventricle at the glomus of the choroid plexus. The lateral ventricle measurement should be less than 10 mm throughout gestation, although male fetuses may have slightly larger ventricles than female fetuses. Many authors define mild VM as ventricular diameter ≥10 and ≤12 mm, and moderate VM with ventricles of 13–15 mm. Values ≥15 mm are always considered severe VM (Fig. 4.7).

(d) **Long-term outcome**: The most important prognostic factor is the presence of associated abnormalities. Ventriculomegaly is often associated with CNS and non-CNS malformations (Garne et al. 2010). This association is higher (≥60 %) in VM greater than 15 mm and lower (10–50 %) in cases of borderline VM (10–15 mm). Even when other malformations are not present on ultrasound, aneuploidies are found in 3–15 % of borderline VM.

VM is the most common false positive diagnosis at ultrasound screening for fetal malformations. One study reported that VM accounted for 12 % of 76 false

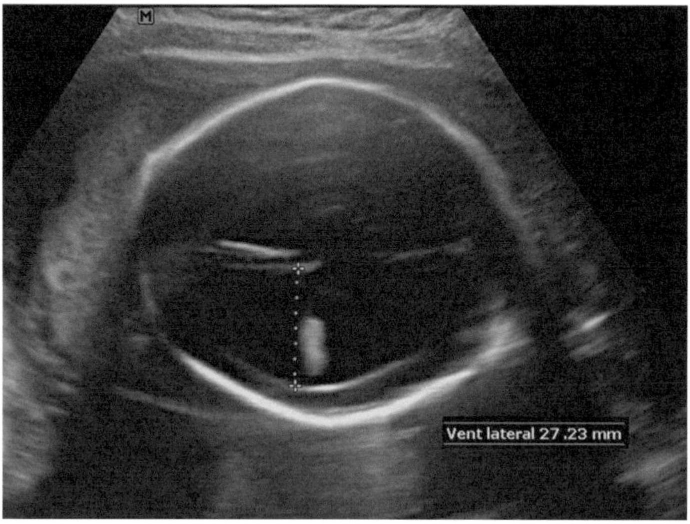

Fig. 4.7 Axial section of the head in sever ***hydrocephalus***, with lateral ventricle greater than 27 mm, and the hanging choroid sign

positive diagnoses (Martinez-Zamora et al. 2007). Prenatal sensitivity for VM is near 75 %, and 90 % in severe cases (Grandjean et al. 1999) with more than 50 % detected before 24 weeks of gestation (Gaglioti et al. 2005). The outcome of fetuses with VM and chromosomal or other structural (CNS or non-CNS) malformations is uniformly poor and defined by the type of associated anomaly. With isolated VM, the incidence of perinatal and neonatal death is higher in cases of severe (>15 mm) and moderate (12–15 mm) VM: about 25 % and 10 %, respectively; with mild VM (10–12 mm) mortality is comparable to the general population (Pagani et al. 2014). Developmental delay is observed in up to 90 % of severe cases, 25 % of moderate cases and 5 % of those with mild VM (Gaglioti et al. 2005).

(e) **Termination of pregnancy rate**: Around 65 %. In a series, TOP was more common in the presence of associated anomalies (76.9 % compared with 51.9 % in isolated cases) (Hannon et al. 2012).

Omphalocele

(a) **Definition**: An abdominal wall defect characterized by absent abdominal muscles, fascia and skin, with herniation of organs, e.g., small bowel or liver, and covered by membranes that consist of amnion and peritoneum.
(b) **Incidence**: 1 in 4000–1 in 7000 at birth, but higher during the fetal period, reflecting the increased risk of intrauterine fetal death (Bianchi et al. 2010).

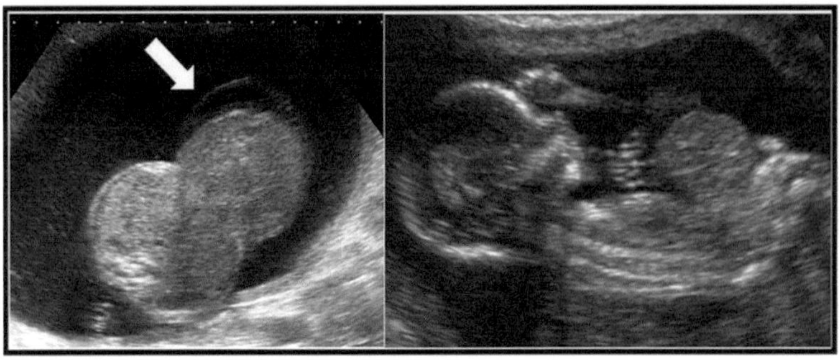

Fig. 4.8 Axial (*left*) and sagittal (*right*) views of the abdominal wall show the typical appearance of a large ***omphalocele*** containing bowel and liver. The surrounding membrane covering the defect is seen (*arrow*)

(c) **Diagnosis**: Ultrasonographic findings include a smooth mass protruding from the abdominal wall with a covering membrane, with the umbilical cord insertion into the membrane at a location distant from the abdominal wall (Fig. 4.8). Polyhydramnios is common and ascites may be present.

(d) **Long-term outcome**: Omphalocele can present as an isolated defect or as part of a syndrome. The most important prognostic variable is the presence of associated malformations, present in 25–60 % of the cases, or chromosomal abnormalities, most commonly trisomy 18 and trisomy 13, present in about 30 % of cases (Fratelli et al. 2007; Springett et al. 2014). In some cases, especially in giant omphaloceles, there may be pulmonary hypoplasia or tracheobronchial malacia with severe respiratory problems, and gastroesophageal reflux is common. The 1-year survival rate of live born babies with an isolated exomphalos is 90 %, compared with 80 % in cases with multiple anomalies and 25 % in cases with chromosomal anomalies (Springett et al. 2014).

(e) **Termination of pregnancy rate**: Around 65 %, but it varies according to the prognosis: higher if the omphalocele is associated with a chromosomal anomaly (around 85 %), and lower if it is an isolated defect.

Gastroschisis

(a) **Definition**: Bowel herniation through a right paramedian abdominal wall defect. The umbilical cord insertion is normal. The defect is small and compromises all layers of the abdominal wall, with bowel loops floating freely in the amniotic cavity.

(b) **Incidence**: Around 1 in 3000 live births. Young maternal age and maternal smoking are associated with an increased risk of gastroschisis (David et al. 2008).

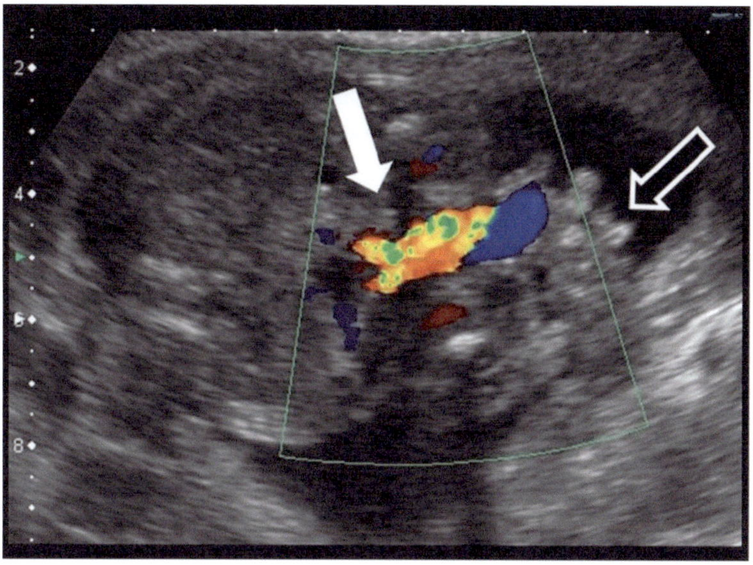

Fig. 4.9 ***Gastroschisis***: axial ultrasound of a second trimester fetus shows loops of small bowel floating freely in the amniotic cavity (*open arrow*). This is right sided to the normal umbilical cord insertion (*arrow*). Oligohydramnios is present

(c) **Diagnosis**: Prenatal diagnosis of gastroschisis is very high, around 90 %, and it is based on the visualization of extra-abdominal bowel loops floating in the amniotic cavity without a covering membrane. Color Doppler assists in demonstration of normal umbilical cord insertion with the herniation of bowel to the right of the umbilical cord (Fig. 4.9).The majority of the cases are isolated (Lepigeon et al. 2014).

(d) **Long-term outcome**: Gastroschisis is not associated with chromosomal abnormalities or structural defects. The duration of postnatal hospitalization is directly related to the degree of gastrointestinal compromise, and postoperative complications are responsible for the 4–10 % mortality rate in the postnatal period (Lepigeon et al. 2014). Although there are many studies that have tried to predict prenatally the extent of gastrointestinal damage, the prognostic value of intra- and extra-abdominal bowel dilatation, gastric dilatation, bowel wall thickness, and other markers (Lepigeon et al. 2014; Tower et al. 2009) is still controversial. The majority of patients eventually have a quality of life not different from the general population.

(e) **Termination of pregnancy rate**: As gastroschisis is usually an isolated defect, the rate of termination of pregnancy is lower than with other abdominal wall defects: 5–30 % (Fratelli et al. 2007, Garne et al. 2005).

Congenital Diaphragmatic Hernia (CDH)

(a) **Definition**: Defect in the formation of the diaphragm, with abdominal contents herniating into the thorax, and associated pulmonary hypoplasia. Bochdalek hernia (posterior and left defect in diaphragm) is the most common type in fetuses.
(b) **Incidence**: Between 1 in 2000 and 1 in 3000 live births, and left sided hernias represent more than 85 % of cases. Up to 40 % of CDH are nonisolated, including chromosomal abnormalities in 10–20 % of cases and other multiple malformation syndromes, e.g., Cornelia de Lange syndrome, Fryns syndrome, and Beckwith–Wiedemann syndrome.
(c) **Diagnosis**: Prenatal diagnosis by ultrasound and MRI is based on visualization of abdominal contents in the thorax. In left sided CDH, the four classic sonographic signs described are the presence of a fluid filled mass (stomach) in the thorax at the same level as the four chamber view, non-visualization of the stomach in the abdomen, mediastinal shift to the right, and bowel loops in the thorax (Figs. 4.10 and 4.11). Polyhydramnios may be present, too. Overall detection

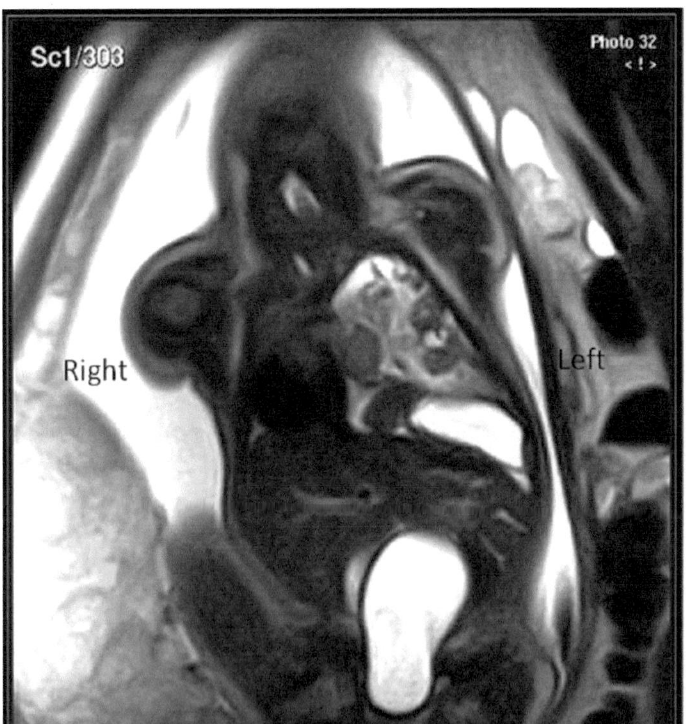

Fig. 4.10 Fetal MRI demonstrating the ***left congenital diaphragmatic hernia*** with cardiac shift to the right, and the presence of bowel loops and stomach in the left side of the chest. Liver is not herniated

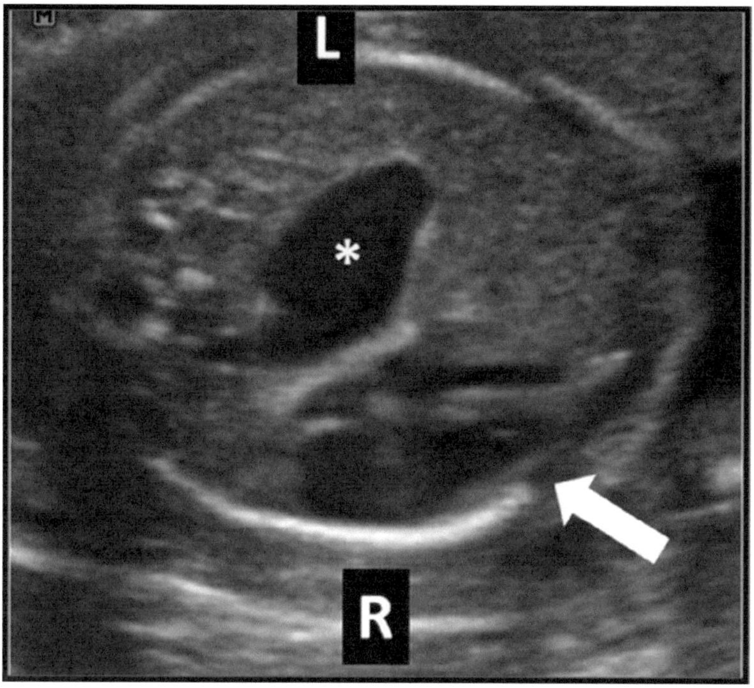

Fig. 4.11 Axial ultrasound of the chest in a fetus with ***left sided congenital diaphragmatic hernia***. The stomach (*) is present at the same level of the four-chamber view of the heart, and mediastinal shift with dextroposition is observed (*arrow*). *L* left, *R* right

rate of CDH is 60 %, but there is a significant difference in the detection rate of isolated CDH (around 50 %) compared with CDH associated with multiple malformations, karyotype anomalies or syndromes (72 %) (Garne et al. 2002).

(d) **Long-term outcome**: Perinatal prognosis is highly affected by the existence of associated malformations and karyotype anomalies. In isolated cases, mortality is highly dependent on the degree of lung hypoplasia and the position of the liver. The long-term outcome depends on the severity of pulmonary hypoplasia and the degree of bronchopulmonary dysplasia resulting from long-term ventilator support. There is also a high incidence of neurologic problems (Bianchi et al. 2010).

(e) **Termination of pregnancy rate**: The overall TOP rate is 20–35 %, but it is greater in CDH with chromosomal abnormalities and other genetic syndromes (more than 50 %). If an ongoing randomized trial in Europe of fetal intervention with fetoscopic balloon tracheal occlusion, the TOTAL trial (www.totaltrial.eu), demonstrates better outcomes for patients with CDH, the rate of TOP may fall.

Congenital Heart Disease (CHD)

(a) **Definition**: CHD is a group of defects in the structure of the heart and great vessels that is present at birth (Figs. 4.12 and 4.13).

(b) **Incidence**: CHD are among the most common birth defects and are the leading cause of birth defect-related deaths. The reported total prevalence of CHD is 8.0 per 1000 births, including live births, fetal deaths and TOP (Dolk et al. 2011), and the prevalence of severe cases is 1.5 per 1000 live births (Egbe et al. 2014). CHD are frequently associated with chromosomal defects, single gene mutations, and teratogens, although most cardiac malformation are isolated defects inherited in a multifactorial fashion without specific risk factors (Manning 2009).

(c) **Diagnosis**: Antenatal recognition of cardiac defects is today based on the systematic evaluation of cardiac structures, according to the ISUOG guidelines for cardiac screening in midgestation (Carvalho et al. 2013). The cardiac screening examination should include both the four-chamber and outflow tract views (left and right ventricular outflow tracts, three vessel view, and three vessels and trachea view). A fetal echocardiogram should be performed by specialists who are familiar with the prenatal diagnosis of CHD if CHD is suspected, if the normal four-chamber and outflow tract views described above cannot be obtained at the time of screening or if recognized risk factors indicate increased risk for CHD (American Institute of Ultrasound in Medicine 2013b). The ultrasound detection rate of CHD is variable but in general surprisingly low, around 20 % (Dolk et al. 2011), and varies significantly between countries even with the same screening recommendations. The presence of associated malformations significantly increases the prenatal detection rate. In order to evaluate the effect of introduction of a 20 week scan in the detection rate of CHD in the

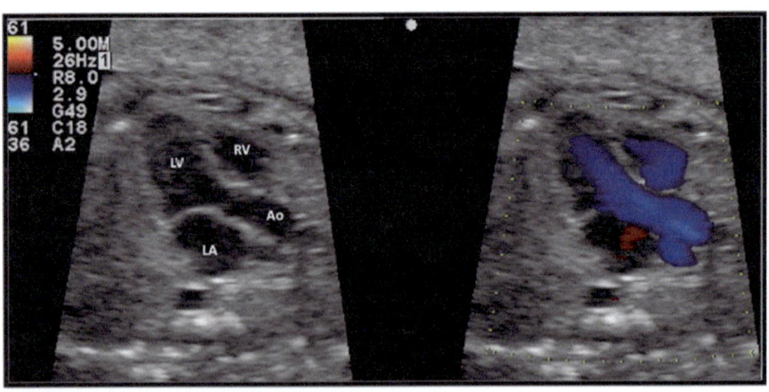

Fig. 4.12 Fetal echocardiographic view of normal left ventricular outflow tract with 2D-US (*left*) and color Doppler (*right*). Note the ascending aorta arising from the left ventricle. *Ao* aorta, *LA* left atrium, *LV* left ventricle, *RV* right ventricle

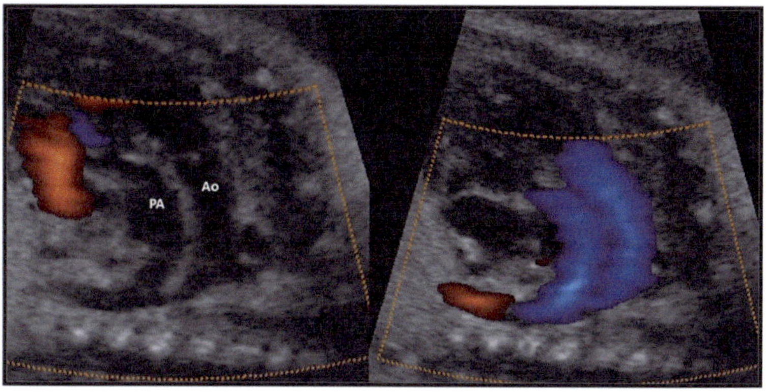

Fig. 4.13 Fetal echocardiographic view of ***transposition of the great arteries*** with 2D-US (*left*) and color Doppler (*right*). Note that aorta and pulmonary artery run parallel to each other instead of crossing. *Ao* aorta, *PA* pulmonary artery

Netherlands in 2007, Baardman et al. (2014) compared the prenatal detection rate and TOP rate between the periods 2001–2005 and 2007–2011. The prenatal detection rate increased from 34.6 to 84.8 % ($p<0.001$) in CHD with abnormal four-chamber view, and from 14.3 to 29.6 % ($p<0.04$) in CHD with normal four-chamber view. The TOP rate also increased between periods from 15.4 to 51.5 % ($p<0.001$) in the group with abnormal four-chamber view.

(d) **Long-term outcome**: Severe cardiac abnormalities have a reasonably predictable outcome. Once an abnormality has been identified, pediatric cardiologists can offer fairly accurate information on whether the anomaly can be corrected (to normal anatomy) or whether a palliative procedure is required, with the much greater risk of long-term morbidity (RCOG 2010). Prenatal diagnosis has been shown to improve preoperative morbidity in newborns with CHDs, but there are conflicting results regarding mortality (Oster et al. 2014). Many variables are related to perinatal outcome: the severity of the defect, the association with chromosomal abnormalities or single gene disorders, and the success of neonatal treatment. This suggests that it may not be possible to extrapolate data on mortality from one specific region or country to another (Dolk et al. 2011).

(e) **Termination of pregnancy rate**: TOP varies according to the severity of the CHD and the time of diagnosis (Table 4.2). Parents opted for TOP more often in cases with highly complex cardiac and extracardiac malformations (70–80 %) compared to less severe cases (Baardman et al. 2014; Nell et al. 2013). In addition to the severity of the congenital heart disease (CHD), ethnicity, gestational age at diagnosis, and chromosomal abnormalities influence parental decision regarding pregnancy continuation or interruption (Chenni et al. 2012).

Bilateral Renal Agenesis

(a) **Definition**: Congenital absence of both kidneys due to a complete failure of the kidney to form.
(b) **Incidence**: 1 in 3000 live births (Cardwell 1988, Droste et al. 1990).
(c) **Diagnosis**: Antenatal detection is greater than 90 % with the mid-trimester scan (Wiesel et al. 2005), and the sonographic findings are anhydramnios in the second trimester, failure of visualization of the bladder because it is empty, and failure of visualization of the kidneys. Color Doppler should be used to support the diagnosis, demonstrating the absence of the renal arteries (Fig. 4.14).
(d) **Long-term outcome**: Lethal in 100 % of the cases.
(e) **Termination of pregnancy rate**: Around 80 % (Table 4.2)

Limb Defects

(a) **Definition**: Group of heterogeneous conditions. The etiology of limb abnormalities is very complex, and it may involve single gene disorders, chromosomal abnormalities, intrauterine factors, vascular events, maternal diseases, and teratogens. In many cases, the etiology is unknown.
(b) **Incidence**: Approximately 6 in 10,000 live births. The incidence is higher in the upper limbs than in the lower limbs; unilateral abnormalities are more frequent than bilateral, and are more prevalent on the right than on the left side (Gramellini et al. 2005)

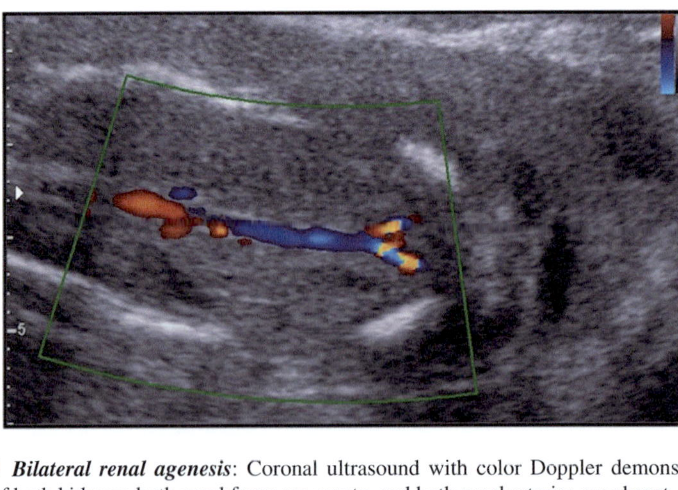

Fig. 4.14 ***Bilateral renal agenesis***: Coronal ultrasound with color Doppler demonstrating the absence of both kidneys: both renal fossa are empty, and both renal arteries are absent

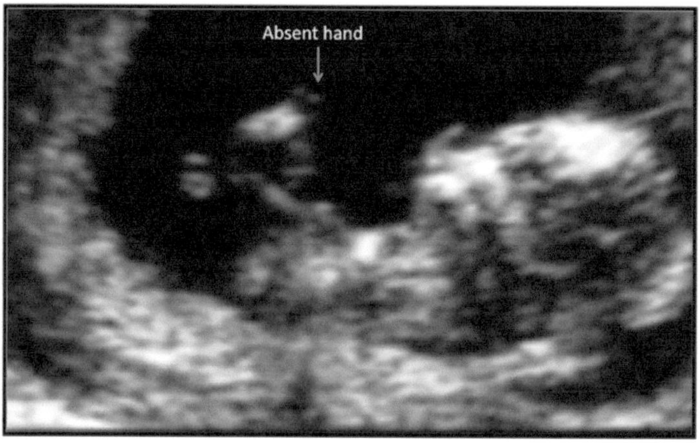

Fig. 4.15 Limb reduction defect: 14 week fetus with absent hands

(c) **Diagnosis**: During the second trimester scan, characteristics of the upper and lower limbs should be documented routinely (Fig. 4.15). A comprehensive scan evaluation should be performed if any abnormality is suspected. Prenatal detection rate of limb reduction defects varies in relation to the different ultrasound screening policies of different countries, ranging from 20.0 to 64.0 %. For instance, Holder-Espinasse et al. (2004) report a detection rate of 45 %. As expected, the detection rate is higher in the presence of associated malformations than with isolated limb reductions (49 % vs. 25 %) (Stoll et al. 2000)
(d) **Long-term outcome**: Perinatal and long-term outcomes depend not on the limb reduction itself, but on the associated malformation(s) or genetic syndrome, if any.
(e) **Termination of pregnancy rate**: In severe cases of limb reductions, 50–70 % of pregnancies were terminated (Garne et al. 2005; Gramellini et al. 2005). An increase in TOP rate has been observed over time in different countries associated with improvement in prenatal diagnosis (Ephraim et al. 2003).

Future Challenges in Prenatal Diagnosis of Structural Abnormalities

The future challenges in prenatal diagnosis of structural abnormalities are at all levels of prevention. In primary prevention, the current challenge is to reach the whole population with known proved interventions, i.e., folic acid supplementation, and the search for novel interventions. In secondary prevention, early, precise, and noninvasive prenatal diagnosis of fetal anomalies, a better knowledge of the natural history, and the development of optimal management strategies represent the main goals.

References

ACR–ACOG–AIUM–SRU Practice Guideline for the Performance of Obstetrical Ultrasound. American College of Radiology - American College of Obstetricians and Gynecologists -American Institute of Ultrasound in Medicine-Society of Radiologists in Ultrasound. 2013. http://www.acr.org/~/media/ACR/Documents/PGTS/guidelines/US_Obstetrical.pdf

Adzick NS, Thom EA, Spong CY, Brock III JW, Burrows PK, Johnson MP, et al. A randomized trial of prenatal versus postnatal repair of myelomeningocele. N Engl J Med. 2011;364(11): 993–1004.

American College of Obstetricians and Gynecologists Committee on Genetics. Committee Opinion No. 581: the use of chromosomal microarray analysis in prenatal diagnosis. Obstet Gynecol. 2013;122(6):1374–7.

American Institute of Ultrasound in Medicine. AIUM practice guideline for the performance of fetal echocardiography. J Ultrasound Med. 2013a;32(6):1067–82.

American Institute of Ultrasound in Medicine. AIUM practice guideline for the performance of obstetric ultrasound examinations. J Ultrasound Med. 2013b;32:1083–101.

Asplin N, Wessel H, Marions L, Ohman SG. Pregnant women's perspectives on decision-making when a fetal malformation is detected by ultrasound examination. Sex Reprod Healthc. 2013;4(2):79–84.

Baardman ME, du Marchie Sarvaas GJ, de Walle HE, Fleurke-Rozema H, Snijders R, Ebels T, et al. Impact of introduction of 20-week ultrasound scan on prevalence and fetal and neonatal outcomes in cases of selected severe congenital heart defects in The Netherlands. Ultrasound Obstet Gynecol. 2014;44(1):58–63.

Bernaschek G, Stuempflen I, Deutinger J. The influence of the experience of the investigator on the rate of sonographic diagnosis of fetal malformations in Vienna. Prenat Diagn. 1996;16(9): 807–11.

Bianchi DW, Crombleholme TM, D'Alton ME, Malone FD, editors. Fetology, diagnosis and management of the fetal patient. 2nd ed. New York, NY: McGraw Hill; 2010.

Borrell A, Robinson JN, Santolaya-Forgas J. Clinical value of the 11- to 13+6-week sonogram for detection of congenital malformations: a review. Am J Perinatol. 2011;28(2):117–24.

Brown SD, Ecker JL, Ward JR, Halpern EF, Sayeed SA, Buchmiller TL, et al. Prenatally diagnosed fetal conditions in the age of fetal care: does who counsels matter? Am J Obstet Gynecol. 2012;206(5):409.e1–11.

Bucher HC, Schmidt JG. Does routine ultrasound scanning improve outcome in pregnancy? Meta-analysis of various outcome measures. BMJ. 1993;307(6895):13–7.

Calzolari E, Barisic I, Loane M, Morris J, Wellesley D, Dolk H, et al. Epidemiology of multiple congenital anomalies in Europe: a EUROCAT population-based registry study. Birth Defects Res A Clin Mol Teratol. 2014;100(4):270–6.

Campaña H, Ermini M, Aiello HA, Krupitzki H, Castilla EE, López-Camelo JS. Latin American Collaborative Study of Congenital Malformations Study Group. Prenatal sonographic detection of birth defects in 18 hospitals from South America. J Ultrasound Med. 2010;29(2):203–12.

Campbell S, Johnstone FD, Holt EM, May P. Anencephaly: early ultrasonic diagnosis and active management. Lancet. 1972;2(7789):1226–7.

Cardwell MS. Bilateral renal agenesis: clinical implications. South Med J. 1988;81:327–8.

Cargill Y, Morin L, Bly S, Butt K, Denis N, Gagnon R, et al. Content of a complete routine second trimester obstetrical ultrasound examination and report (SOGC Clinical Practice Guideline). J Obstet Gynaecol Can. 2009;31(3):272–5. 3.

Carvalho JS, Allan LD, Chaoui R, Copel JA, DeVore GR, Hecher K, et al. ISUOG practice guidelines (updated): sonographic screening examination of the fetal heart. Ultrasound Obstet Gynecol. 2013;41:348–59.

Chasen ST, Kalish RB. Can early ultrasound reduce the gestational age at abortion for fetal anomalies? Contraception. 2013;87(1):63–6.

Chenni N, Lacroze V, Pouet C, Fraisse A, Kreitmann B, Gamerre M, et al. Fetal heart disease and interruption of pregnancy: factors influencing the parental decision-making process. Prenat Diagn. 2012;32(2):168–72.

Crane JP, LeFevre ML, Winborn RC, Evans JK, Ewigman BG, Bain RP, et al. A randomized trial of prenatal ultrasound screening: impact on detection, management and outcome of anomalous fetuses. The RADIUS Study Group. Am J Obstet Gynecol. 1994;171:392–9.

David AL, Tan A, Curry J. Gastroschisis: sonographic diagnosis, associations, management and outcome. Prenat Diagn. 2008;28(7):633–44.

Dekoninck P, Gratacos E, Van Mieghem T, Richter J, Lewi P, Ancel AM, et al. Results of fetal endoscopic tracheal occlusion for congenital diaphragmatic hernia and the set up of the randomized controlled TOTAL trial. Early Hum Dev. 2011;87(9):619–24.

Dolk H, Loane M, Garne E. European Surveillance of Congenital Anomalies (EUROCAT) Working Group. Congenital heart defects in Europe: prevalence and perinatal mortality, 2000 to 2005. Circulation. 2011;123(8):841–9.

Donnelly JC, Platt LD, Rebarber A, Zachary J, Grobman WA, Wapner RJ. Association of copy number variants with specific ultrasonographically detected fetal anomalies. Obstet Gynecol. 2014;124(1):83–90.

Droste S, Fitzsimmons J, Pascoe-Mason J, Shepard TH, Mack LA. Size of the fetal adrenal in bilateral renal agenesis. Obstet Gynecol. 1990;76(2):206–9.

Egbe A, Uppu S, Lee S, Ho D, Srivastava S. Changing prevalence of severe congenital heart disease: a population-based study. Pediatr Cardiol. 2014;35(7):1232–8.

Ensing S, Kleinrouweler CE, Maas SM, Bilardo CM, Van der Horst CM, Pajkrt E. Influence of the 20-week anomaly scan on prenatal diagnosis and management of fetal facial clefts. Ultrasound Obstet Gynecol. 2014;44(2):154–9.

Ephraim PL, Dillingham TR, Sector M, Pezzin LE, Mackenzie EJ. Epidemiology of limb loss and congenital limb deficiency: a review of the literature. Arch Phys Med Rehabil. 2003;84(5): 747–61.

EUROCAT Guide 1.3 and reference documents. Instructions for the Registration and Surveillance of Congenital Anomalies 2005. http://www.eurocat-network.eu/content/EUROCAT-Guide-1.3.pdf. Accessed 1 July, 2011.

Fratelli N, Papageorghiou AT, Bhide A, Sharma A, Okoye B, Thilaganathan B. Outcome of antenatally diagnosed abdominal wall defects. Ultrasound Obstet Gynecol. 2007;30(3):266–70.

Gaglioti P, Danelon D, Bontempo S, Mombrò M, Cardaropoli S, Todros T. Fetal cerebral ventriculomegaly: outcome in 176 cases. Ultrasound Obstet Gynecol. 2005;25:372–7.

Gagnon A, Wilson RD, Allen VM, Audibert F, Blight C, Brock JA, et al. Society of Obstetricians and Gynaecologists of Canada. Evaluation of prenatally diagnosed structural congenital anomalies. J Obstet Gynaecol Can. 2009;31(9):875–81. 9.

Garne E, Haeusler M, Barisic I, Gjergja R, Stool C, Clemete M, EUROSCAN Study Group. Congenital diaphragmatic hernia: evaluation of prenatal diagnosis in 20 European regions. Ultrasound Obstet Gynecol. 2002;19:329–33.

Garne E, Loane M, Addor MC, Boyd PA, Barisic I, Dolk H. Congenital hydrocephalus–prevalence, prenatal diagnosis and outcome of pregnancy in four European regions. Eur J Paediatr Neurol. 2010;14(2):150–5.

Garne E, Loane M, Dolk H, De Vigan C, Scarano G, Tucker D, et al. Prenatal diagnosis of severe structural congenital malformations in Europe. Ultrasound Obstet Gynecol. 2005;25:6–11.

Gascard-Battisti C, Dubois-Lebbe C, Chatelet-Cheront C, Ferrant L, Sales A, Houzé de l'Aulnoit D. Antenatal screening for congenital heart disease: a retrospective analysis of 20 years experience. J Gynecol Obstet Biol Reprod. 2006;35:472–6.

Gramellini D, Fieni S, Vadora E. Prenatal diagnosis of isolated limb defects: an updated review. Fetal Diagn Ther. 2005;20(2):96–101.

Grande M, Arigita M, Borobio V, Jimenez JM, Fernandez S, Borrell A. First-trimester detection of structural abnormalities and the role of aneuploidy markers. Ultrasound Obstet Gynecol. 2012;39(2):157–63.

Grandjean H, Larroque D, Levi S. The performance of routine ultrasonographic screening of pregnancies in the Eurofetus Study. Am J Obstet Gynecol. 1999;181:446–54.

Hanikeri M, Savundra J, Gillett D, Walters M, McBain W. Transabdominal ultrasound detection of cleft lip and palate in Western Australia from 1996-2003. Cleft Palate Craniofac J. 2006;43: 61–6.

Hannon T, Tennant PW, Rankin J, Robson SC. Epidemiology, natural history, progression, and postnatal outcome of severe fetal ventriculomegaly. Obstet Gynecol. 2012;120(6):1345–53.

Hendler I, Blackwell SC, Bujold E, Treadwell MC, Mittal P, Sokol RJ, et al. Suboptimal second-trimester ultrasonographic visualization of the fetal heart in obese woman: should we repeat the examination? J Ultrasound Med. 2005;24:1205–9.

Hern WM. Fetal diagnostic indications for second and third trimester outpatient pregnancy termination. Prenat Diagn. 2014;34(5):438–44.

Hillman SC, McMullan DJ, Hall G, Togneri FS, James N, Maher EJ, et al. Use of prenatal chromosomal microarray: prospective cohort study and systematic review and meta-analysis. Ultrasound Obstet Gynecol. 2013;41:610–20.

Hillman SC, Willams D, Carss KJ, Mcmullan DJ, Hurles ME, Kilby MD. Prenatal genetic diagnosis for fetuses with structural abnormalities, the next step. Ultrasound Obstet Gynecol. 2015;45:4. doi:10.1002/uog.14653.

Holder-Espinasse M, Devisme L, Thomas D, Boute O, Vaast P, Fron D, et al. Pre- and postnatal diagnosis of limb anomalies: a series of 107 cases. Am J Med Genet A. 2004;124A(4): 417–22.

Hui L, Bianchi DW. Prenatal pharmacotherapy for fetal anomalies: a 2011 update. Prenat Diagn. 2011;31:735–43.

International Society of Ultrasound in Obstetrics & Gynecology Education Committee. Sonographic examination of the fetal central nervous system: guidelines for performing the 'basic examination' and the 'fetal neurosonogram'. Ultrasound Obstet Gynecol. 2007;29(1): 109–16.

International Society of Ultrasound in Obstetrics and Gynecology, Carvalho JS, Allan LD, Chaoui R, Copel JA, DeVore GR, Hecher K, et al. ISUOG Practice Guidelines (updated): sonographic screening examination of the fetal heart. Ultrasound Obstet Gynecol. 2013;41(3):348–59.

Jaeggi ET, Carvalhho JS, De Groot E, Api O, Clur SA, Rammeloo L, et al. Comparison of transplacental treatment of fetal supraventricular tachyarrhythmias with digoxin, flecainide, and sotalol: results of a nonrandomized multicenter study. Circulation. 2011;124(16):1747–54.

Jaeggi ET, Sholler GF, Jones OD, Cooper SG. Comparative analysis of pattern, management and outcome of pre- versus postnatally diagnosed major congenital heart disease: a population-based study. Ultrasound Obstet Gynecol. 2001;17(5):380–5.

Johnson CY, Honein MA, Dana Flanders W, Howards PP, Oakley Jr GP, Rasmussen SA. Pregnancy termination following prenatal diagnosis of anencephaly or spina bifida: a systematic review of the literature. Birth Defects Res A Clin Mol Teratol. 2012;94(11):857–63.

Jones KL, Jones MC, Del Campo M, editors. Smith's recognizable patterns of human malformation. 7th ed. Philadelphia, PA: Saunders-Elsevier; 2013.

Khoury MJ, Moore CA, Evans JA. On the use of the term "syndrome" in clinical genetics and birth defects epidemiology. Am J Med Genet. 1994;49:26–8.

Lepigeon K, Van Mieghem T, Vasseur Maurer S, Giannoni E, Baud D. Gastroschisis – what should be told to parents? Prenat Diagn. 2014;34(4):316–26.

Levi S. Ultrasound in prenatal diagnosis: polemics around routine ultrasound screening for second trimester fetal malformations. Prenat Diagn. 2002;22(4):285–95.

Lubinsky M. Vater and other associations: historical perspectives and modern interpretations. Am J Med Genet Suppl. 1986;2:9–16.

Manning FA. Imaging in the diagnosis of fetal anomalies. In: Creasy RK, Resnik R, Iams JD, editors. Creasy and Resnik's maternal-fetal medicine: principles and practice. 6th ed. Philadelphia, PA: Saunders Elsevier; 2009.

Martínez-Frías ML. The primary developmental field I: clinical and epidemiological characteristics. Am J Med Genet. 1995;56:374–81.

Martinez-Zamora MA, Borrell A, Borobio V, Gonce A, Perez M, Botet F, et al. False positives in the prenatal ultrasound screening of fetal structural anomalies. Prenat Diagn. 2007;27:18–22.

National Institute for Clinical Excellence. Antenatal Care: Routine Care for the Healthy Pregnant Woman. Clinical Guideline CG62. London: NICE; 2008. http://guidance.nice.org.uk/CG62

Nell S, Wijngaarde CA, Pistorius LR, Slieker M, ter Heide H, Manten GT, et al. Fetal heart disease: severity, associated anomalies and parental decision. Fetal Diagn Ther. 2013;33(4):235–40.

NHS Commissioning Board. NHS Fetal Anomaly Screening Programme. November 2012. http://fetalanomaly.screening.nhs.uk/standardsandpolicies

Nicolaides KH, Brizot ML, Snidjers RJM. Fetal nuchal translucency: ultrasound screening for fetal trisomy in the first trimester of pregnancy. Br J Obstet Gynaecol. 1994;101:782–6.

Novelli A, Grati FR, Ballarati L, Bernardini L, Bizzoco D, Camurri L, et al. Microarray application in prenatal diagnosis: a position statement from the cytogenetics working group of the Italian Society of Human Genetics. Ultrasound Obstet Gynecol. 2012;39(4):384–8.

Opitz JM. The developmental field concept. Am J Med Genet. 1985;21:1–11.

Oster ME, Kim CH, Kusano AS, Cragan JD, Dressler P, Hales AR, et al. A population-based study of the association of prenatal diagnosis with survival rate for infants with congenital heart defects. Am J Cardiol. 2014;113(6):1036–40.

Pagani G, Thilaganathan B, Prefumo F. Neurodevelopmental outcome in isolated mild fetal ventriculomegaly: systematic review and meta-analysis. Ultrasound Obstet Gynecol. 2014;44(3): 254–60.

Pereira S, Ganapathy R, Syngelaki A, Maiz N, Nicolaides KH. Contribution of fetal tricuspid regurgitation in first-trimester screening for major cardiac defects. Obstet Gynecol. 2011; 117(6):1384–91.

RANZCOG College Statement: C-Obs 35. The Royal Australian and New Zealand College of Obstetricians and Gynaecologists. March 2013. https://www.ranzcog.edu.au/college-statements-guidelines.html

RCOG, The Royal College of Obstetricians and Gynaecologists. Termination of Pregnancy for Fetal Abnormalities in England Scotland and Wales. Report of a Working Party, May 2010.

RCOG, The Royal College of Obstetricians and Gynaecologists. Ultrasound Screening Supplement to *Ultrasound Screening for Fetal Abnormalities*. 2013. http://www.rcog.org.uk/womens-health/clinical-guidance/ultrasound-screening

Ruano R, Yoshisaki CT, da Silva MM, Ceccon ME, Grasi MS, Tannuri U, et al. A randomized controlled trial of fetal endoscopic tracheal occlusion versus postnatal management of severe isolated congenital diaphragmatic hernia. Ultrasound Obstet Gynecol. 2012;39(1):20–7.

Salomon LJ, Alfirevic Z, Berghella V, Bilardo C, Hernandez-Andrade E, Johnsen SL, et al. ISUOG Clinical Standards Committee. Practice guidelines for performance of the routine mid-trimester fetal ultrasound scan. Ultrasound Obstet Gynecol. 2011;37(1):116–26.

Salomon LJ, Alfirevic Z, Bilardo CM, Chalouhi GE, Ghi T, Kagan KO, et al. ISUOG Practice Guidelines: performance of first-trimester fetal ultrasound scan. Ultrasound Obstet Gynecol. 2013;41:102–13.

Saltvedt S, Almstrom H, Kublickas M, Valentin L, Grunewald C. Detection of malformations in chromosomally normal fetuses by routine ultrasound at 12 or 18 weeks of gestation – a randomised controlled trial in 39,572 pregnancies. BJOG. 2006;113:664–74.

Siebert JR, Kapur RP. Diagnosing congenital malformations in the fetus. Society for Pediatric Pathology Workshops, Seattle, WA. 2001; 3–34.

SOGC Committee Opinion. (Society of Obstetricians and Gynaecologists of Canada). Evaluation of prenatally diagnosed structural congenital anomalies. No 234, September 2009. J Obstet Gynaecol Can. 2009;31(9):875–81.

Souka AP, Pilalis A, Kavalakis I, et al. Screening for major structural anomalies at the 11-14 week ultrasound scan. Am J Obstet Gynecol. 2006;194:393–6.

Spranger J, Benirschke K, Hall JG, Lenz W, Lowry RB, Opitz JM, et al. Errors of morphogenesis: concepts and terms. Recommendations of an international working group. J Pediatr. 1982;100:160–5.

Springett A, Draper ES, Rankin J, Rounding C, Tucker D, Stoianova S, et al. Birth prevalence and survival of exomphalos in England and Wales: 2005 to 2011. Birth Defects Res A Clin Mol Teratol. 2014;100:721. doi:10.1002/bdra.23301.

Stoll C, Wiesel A, Queisser-Luft A, Froster U, Bianca S, Clementi M. Evaluation of the prenatal diagnosis of limb reduction deficiencies. EUROSCAN Study Group. Prenat Diagn. 2000; 20(10):811–8.

Syngelaki A, Chelemen T, Dagklis T, Allan L, Nicolaides KH. Challenges in the diagnosis of fetal non-chromosomal abnormalities at 11–13 weeks. Prenat Diagn. 2011;31:90–102.

Tararbit K, Bui TT, Lelong N, Thieulin AC, Goffinet F, Khoshnood B. Clinical and socioeconomic predictors of pregnancy termination for fetuses with congenital heart defects: a population-based evaluation. Prenat Diagn. 2013;33(2):179–86.

Tower C, Ong SS, Ewer AK, Khan K, Kilby MD. Prognosis in isolated gastroschisis with bowel dilatation: a systematic review. Arch Dis Child Fetal Neonatal Ed. 2009;94(4):F268–74.

Wapner RJ, Martin CL, Levy B, Ballif BC, Eng CM, Zachary JM, et al. Chromosomal microarray versus karyotyping for prenatal diagnosis. N Engl J Med. 2012;367:2175–84.

Watkins ML, Rasmussen SA, Honein MA, Botto LD, Moore CA. Maternal obesity and risk for birth defects. Pediatrics. 2003;111(5 Pt 2):1152–8.

Wiesel A, Queisser-Luft A, Clementi M, Bianca S, Stoll C, EUROSCAN Study Group. Prenatal detection of congenital renal malformations by fetal ultrasonographic examination: an analysis of 709,030 births in 12 European countries. Eur J Med Genet. 2005;48(2):131–44.

Witlox RS, Lopriore E, Oepkes D. Prenatal interventions for fetal lung lesions. Prenat Diagn. 2011;31:628–36.

Yang J, Cummings EA, O'Connell C, Jangaard K. Fetal and neonatal outcomes in diabetic pregnancies. Obstet Gynecol. 2006;108(3 Pt 1):644–50.

Chapter 5
Medical Reasons for Pregnancy Interruption: Fetal Reduction

Mark I. Evans, Stephanie Andriole, Shara M. Evans, and David W. Britt

History

Pregnancy management via fetal reduction (FR) has evolved dramatically since we first published on the subject in the 1980s (Evans et al. 1988). FR started out as a desperate management strategy in high order multiple pregnancies that carried extreme risks to both mother and fetuses due to the presence of multiple embryos. Selective termination (as it was then called) of some of the embryos was performed to (1) increase the viability of the remaining ones and (2) reduce the risk of morbidity and mortality for the mother. FR has followed the pattern of numerous other technological advances, i.e., new technologies begin with matters of life and death but as they eventually become accepted indications graduate from crisis "life and death" into issues of quality of life (Cohen and Hanft 2004; Evans and Hanft 1997).

More than 2,000,000 in vitro fertilization (IVF) babies have been born since the birth of Louise Brown in 1978. A demonstrable, common, side effect of infertility treatments has been a skyrocketing incidence of multiple gestations. In the USA, twins now represent nearly 3 % of all births—a tripling of the rate prior to the widespread use of infertility treatments (Centers for Disease Control 2013; Martin et al. 2013).

M.I. Evans, M.D. (✉)
Department of Obstetrics & Gynecology, Mt. Sinai School of Medicine,
131 E. 65th St., New York, NY 10065, USA
e-mail: evans@compregen.com

S. Andriole, M.S., C.G.C. • S.M. Evans, M.P.H., M.Sc.
Comprehensive Genetics, PLLC, 131 E. 65th St., New York, NY 10065, USA

D.W. Britt, Ph.D.
FMFA, 131 E. 65th St., New York, NY 10065, USA
e-mail: dwbrit01@me.com

J.P. Galst, M.S. Verp (eds.), *Prenatal and Preimplantation Diagnosis*,
DOI 10.1007/978-3-319-18911-6_5

Table 5.1 Longitudinal trends in multiples in the USA (Martin et al. 2013)

Year	Twins	Triplets	Quads	Quints+
2012	131,024	4598	276	45
2011	131,269	5137	239	41
2010	132,562	5153	313	37
2008	138,660	5877	345	46
2006	137,085	6118	355	67
2003	128,615	7110	468	85
2001	121,246	6885	501	85
1996	100,750	5298	560	81
1989	90,118	2529	229	40
% Increase 1989–2012	45.39 %	81.81 %	20.52 %	12.5 %

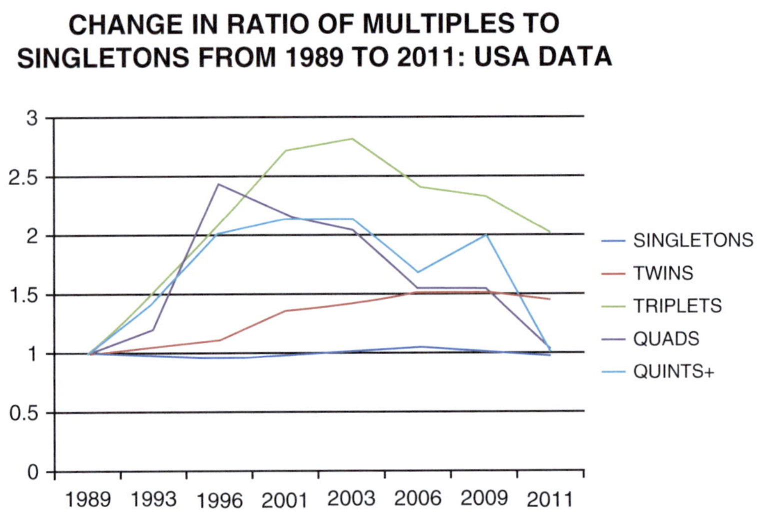

Fig. 5.1 Using 1989 data set as baseline (1), ratio incidence of cases for the years listed on the *X* axis

While higher-order multiples (triplets and above) have plateaued to an extent, IVF programs create as many multiple gestations as singletons (Centers for Disease Control 2013; Martin et al. 2013). Fortunately, the incidence of very high order pregnancies has dramatically fallen over the past several years, but twins and triplets remain very common. The US Society for Assisted Reproductive Technology (SART) reported 32,305 singleton and 13,655 multiple pregnancies producing 60,190 infants in 2009. Nearly half the babies born from IVF in the USA are part of multiple pregnancies (Martin et al. 2013) (Table 5.1, Fig. 5.1).

In addition to changing from the use of gonadotropins only to the greater control conferred by IVF, another key development allowing control of the number of embryos implanting has been the development of norms and expectations regarding

Table 5.2 IVF Management: maternal age and transfer numbers (Lawlor and Nelson 2012)

SART		<35	35–39	40+
Mean transfer	2009	2.1	2.5	3.0
	2012	1.9	2.2	2.6
SET (%)	2009	7.0	3.0	0.5
	2012	14.8	4.5	1.0

SART = Society for Assisted Reproductive Technologies, SET = single embryo transfer

single-embryo transfers (Martin et al. 2013; Society of Assisted Reproductive Technologies 2011; MMWR: Assisted Reproductive Technology Surveillance—USA 2009). Single embryo transfer (SET) has many medical advantages; however, the economics of IVF in the USA make it highly unlikely that SET will ever be predominant. As an illustration, SART guidelines state that only two embryos should be transferred in women under age 35. However, the average number is actually 2.4, according to Centers for Disease Control and SART data (Martin et al. 2013; Society of Assisted Reproductive Technologies 2011; MMWR: Assisted Reproductive Technology Surveillance—USA 2009). High costs for every cycle (commonly $15,000 or more with variable insurance coverage) result in substantial economic pressures. Both patient and IVF provider—have significant incentive to achieve a very high pregnancy rate with each cycle. Even with any health care "reform" that may ultimately be operative in the USA, this is unlikely to change. For example, 2009 SART data showed that only 7 % of US cases in women under 35 were SET, and the numbers were much lower in older women (Table 5.2) (Martin et al. 2013; Society of Assisted Reproductive Technologies 2011; MMWR: Assisted Reproductive Technology Surveillance—USA 2009).

Lawlor and Nelson in 2012 showed that the success rate for live born babies was higher by about 7 % when transferring two embryos in one cycle rather than one each for two cycles (Lawlor and Nelson 2012). Regardless, the percentage of live births per transfer—both for fresh and frozen cycles—clearly diminishes with advancing maternal age. Therefore, the desire to be more aggressive in transfers is understandable, but also correlates with increased risks of multiples. Egg donors tend to be younger so statistically they resemble the <35-year-old cohort (Tables 5.3 and 5.4) (Martin et al. 2013; Society of Assisted Reproductive Technologies 2011; MMWR: Assisted Reproductive Technology Surveillance—USA 2009; Lawlor and Nelson 2012).

Loss of the pregnancy is not the only potential negative outcome of a multiple gestation. Decades of data have correlated the incidence of prematurity and related sequelae with fetal number (Fig. 5.2) (Martin et al. 2013; Society of Assisted Reproductive Technologies 2011; MMWR: Assisted Reproductive Technology Surveillance—USA 2009; Lawlor and Nelson 2012). Additionally, about one-fifth of babies born at less than 750 g develop cerebral palsy (Task Force of American College of Obstetricians and Gynecologists 2003). Peterson et al. (in West Australia) showed that the rate of cerebral palsy was 4.6 times higher for twins than for singletons per live birth, but 8.3 times higher when calculated per pregnancy (Petterson

Table 5.3 Centers for disease control 2010 data

Non donor eggs	Age	# Fresh	# Trans	% LB/ tran	% Mult	# Frozen	# Trans	% LB/ tran	% Mult
	<35	41,744	2.0	47.6	34.0	12,631	2.0	38.4	?
	35–37	21,369	2.2	38.3	28.7	6195	1.9	34.7	?
	38–40	21,741	2.6	28.1	23.3	4682	2.1	28.4	?
	41–42	10,122	3.0	16.7	18.0	1591	2.2	21.5	?
	43–44	4501	3.2	7.4	10.2	710	2.2	16.8	?
	45+	1347	2.7	1.8	(2/14)	432	2.0	13.0	?
Donor eggs		9866	2.0	55.8	?	6665	2.0	34.9	?

Table 5.4 Number of embryos transferred nondonor eggs

Year	<35	35–37	38–40	41–42	43–44	45+
1998	3.4	3.6	3.7	3.9		
2001	2.8	3.1	3.4	3.7		
2004	2.5	2.7	3.0	3.3		
2007	2.2	2.5	2.8	3.1	3.2	
2010	2.0	2.2	2.6	3.0	3.2	2.7
2012	1.9	2.0	2.4	2.9	2.9	

US Centers for Disease Control: Assisted Reproductive Technology Reports

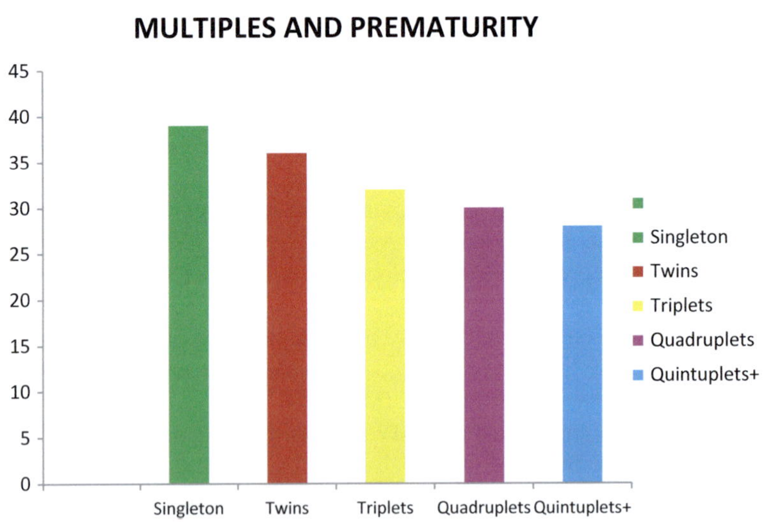

Fig. 5.2 Average gestational age at delivery axis is gestational weeks at delivery

et al. 1993). Pharoah and Cooke calculated cerebral palsy rates per 1000 first year survivors at 2.3 for singletons, 12.6 for twins, and 44.8 for triplets (Pharoah and Cooke 1996; Dimitiiou et al. 2004). We have witnessed a growing sensitivity to these risks among older patients and a corresponding increase in the use of prenatal diagnosis and FR. More recent data have shown improvements; a Dutch study suggested an 8.5 % risk of cerebral palsy in babies born before 27 weeks (Tronnes et al. 2014).

Over $10 billion was spent in the USA on the 12.3 % of babies born preterm in 2003 (Cuevas et al. 2005). Data from 2005 show that there is considerably higher neurologic and developmental disability in 6-year-olds who survived birth at 26 weeks or less (Marlow et al. 2005; Rosenbaum et al. 2007). Significant cerebral palsy was present in 12 % (Rosenbaum et al. 2007). The rates of severe, moderate, and mild disability were 22 %, 24 %, and 34 % respectively. Hack et al. showed that, the rate of cerebral palsy was 14 %, as opposed to 0 % for controls, in babies born at less than 1000 g. Asthma, poor vision, IQ <85 and poor motor skills were all also substantially higher (Hack et al. 2005). Neonatal care advancements have had significant impact on reducing mortality, in particular, at early gestational ages with the resultant increase in compromised, surviving infants (Stoll et al. 2010). We would expect changes in insurance coverage and the shaping of practice in IVF clinics, as well as a continued increase in sensitivity to these issues, especially among at-risk patients who are aware of escalating costs.

Development of Fetal Reduction Techniques

FR was developed as a clinical procedure in the 1980s by a small number of clinicians in the USA and Europe who attempted to reduce the usual and frequent adverse sequelae of multifetal pregnancies by selectively terminating or reducing the number of fetuses to a safer number. The first European reports by Dumez and Oury (1986), and the first American report by Evans, et al. (1988), followed by a further report by Berkowitz, et al. (1988), and later Wapner, et al. (1990), described a surgical approach to improve the outcome in such cases.

A needle was inserted transabdominally and maneuvered into the fetal thorax. The most common method has been injection of potassium chloride (KCl). Mechanical disruption of the fetus, air embolization, and electrocautery have also been used. Initially, transcervical aspirations were also tried, but with minimal success. Transvaginal mechanical disruption or KCl was also used in some centers, but data suggested a significantly higher loss rate than with the transabdominal route (Timor-Tritsch et al. 1993). Today, virtually all experienced operators perform the procedure by inserting a needle transabdominally under ultrasound guidance into the thorax, but intraabdominal and intracranial injections are also used when intrathoracic injections are not feasible (Li et al. 2013). Of concern, published and unpublished data suggest that some centers continue to use transvaginal reduction procedures despite loss rates 5–10× that of the abdominal approach.

Table 5.5 Risks of multiple pregnancies and improvements with FR

Starting number	Spontaneous loss rates (%)	Finishing number	Reduction of risk of loss (%)
6+	90–99	2	90–10
5	75	2	50–7
4	25	2	25–4
		1	25–7
3	15	2	15–3.5
		1	15–4
2	8	1	8–2.5

Data are extrapolations of multiple papers. When there are monozygotic twins as part of the multiple, the overall risk is increased as if there were 1 more as the starting number

Over time, as with other surgical procedures, data have shown improvements in understanding the nature of the clinical situation, the risks and benefits of the different approaches, and how these services should best be presented to patients and executed by clinicians. In the early 1990s several centers with the world's largest experience began collaborating to leverage their data. In 1993 our first collaborative report showed a 16 % pregnancy loss rate through 24 completed weeks (Evans et al. 1993). These numbers represented a major improvement for higher order multiple pregnancies. Subsequent collaborative papers showed dramatic improvements in the overall outcomes of such pregnancies (Table 5.5, Fig. 5.3). Twenty-five years ago, the first question asked was: "at how many fetuses was it reasonable to offer FR"? Generally, the answer varied between triplets and quadruplets, with wide differences in perception of risks by specialty and religious beliefs (Evans et al. 1991). In the 1990s, multiple papers demonstrated that there was clear improvement in outcomes by reducing to twins from triplets or more. Yaron et al. (1999) compared triplets-to-twins and unreduced triplet data with two large cohorts of twins. Reduced twins showed substantial improvement as compared to triplets. Pregnancy outcomes for cases starting at triplets or even quadruplets reduced to twins at about 12 weeks do as well as pregnancies starting as twins, as suggested by the 2001 collaborative series, and others. Antsaklis et al. showed a decrease of losses from 15.41 to 4.76 % for twins and diminishment of low birth weight from 28 to 11 % (Antsaklis et al. 2004)

These data supported guarded aggressiveness in infertility treatment in challenging clinical scenarios. However, good outcomes clearly diminished when higher number pregnancies occurred. Luke et al. suggested that FR increased the risk for birth at <30 weeks and for very low birth weight, and slowed mid-gestational growth in twin pregnancies initiated with assisted reproduction (ART) (Luke et al. 2004). This analysis, however, ignored the starting conditions. i.e., what would be the outcome of unreduced quadruplets? Kozinsky et al. demonstrated that the perinatal outcomes of singleton and twin pregnancies following ARTs were comparable to matched pregnancies that were spontaneously conceived (Kozinsky et al. 2003). In a meta-analysis, McDonald et al. showed that even when matched to spontane-

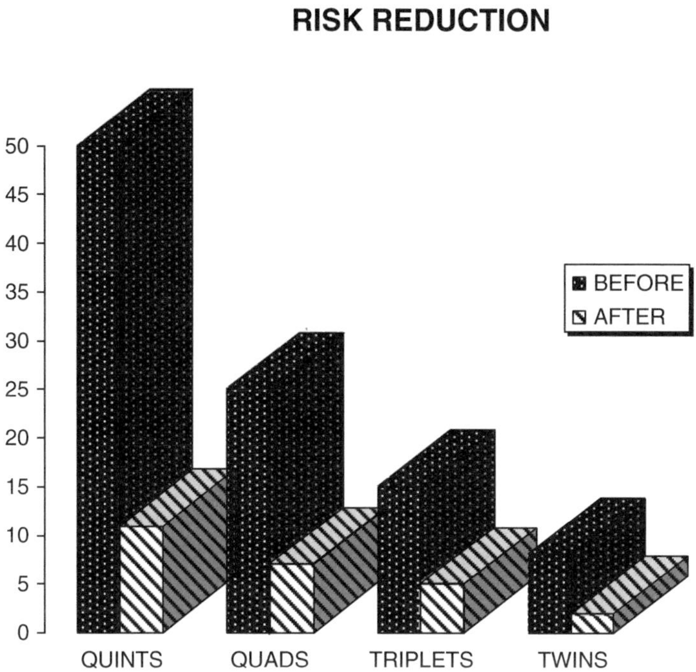

Fig. 5.3 Reduction of pregnancy loss with FR. *Y* Axis is % loss before 24 weeks

ously conceived twins, twins from IVF had a higher risk for preterm birth, but no significant differences in low birth weight, perinatal death, or congenital malformations (McDonald et al. 2005). Over the last decade, several other papers have also demonstrated higher risks for "unreduced" triplets than for reduced cases (Leondires et al. 1999; Lipitz et al. 2001; Sepulveda et al. 2003; Francois et al. 2001). In his large database Blickstein reported that triplets did worse than reduced twins in every perinatal category (Blickstein 2004). It is clear that one must use extreme caution in choosing comparison groups.

The 2001 collaborative data using late first trimester procedures similarly demonstrated clearly that outcomes of triplets reduced to twins, and quadruplets reduced to twins, were essentially as if they began as twins (Evans et al. 2001). Pregnancy loss rates substantially decreased, and so did the rate of very early prematurity. Both outcomes continued to be correlated with the starting and finishing numbers. Continued improvements in management and overall outcomes have been shown at experienced centers in more recent data (Table 5.5).

Changes in infertility management and evolving experience have also lead to novel situations. The number and proportion of monozygotic twins has increased significantly in the last decade, parallel to changes in IVF laboratory techniques and increasing use of blastocyst transfers (MMWR: Assisted Reproductive Technology Surveillance—USA 2009; Evans and Britt 2011; Rosner et al. 2013).

Approximately 7 % of our triplets + cases include a monochorionic–diamniotic twin pair (Rosner et al. 2013). Provided the "singleton" seems healthy (by CVS and ultrasound), our experience shows that the best outcomes are achieved by reduction of the MZ twins. If the singleton does not appear healthy, then keeping the twins is the best choice; however, not every center has shown comparable improvement in outcomes (Chaveeva et al. 2013).

In the 2001 collaborative report, the subset of patients who reduced from 2 to 1 suggested a loss rate comparable to that of patients who reduced from 3 to 2, however, about one third of the 2 to 1 cases had an additional complicating medical indication for the procedure—e.g., prior twin pregnancy with severe prematurity, or uterine abnormality, or maternal cardiac disease, thereby raising the overall risks (Blickstein 2004). However, demographics have changed in recent years, and the vast majority of such cases now are less medically complicated but often involve women in their 40s, or even their 50s, some of whom are using donor eggs. Many of these women only want a singleton pregnancy, for both medical and social reasons (Evans et al. 2004; Templeton 2004; Kalra et al. 2003). Our data suggest that twins reduced to a singleton do better than continuing as twins (Evans et al. 2004; Templeton 2004). Consistent with the above, more women are requesting to reduce to a singleton. In a series of triplets from the late 1990s, we found that the average age of our patients reducing to twins was 37 years and to a singleton 41 years (Yaron et al. 1999). While the reduction in risk of pregnancy loss for triplets to singleton was not as much as triplets to twins in the 90s (15–7 % and 15–5 %, respectively), the gestational age at delivery for the resulting singleton was higher, and the incidence of births <1500 g was 10× higher for twins than singletons. As reducing to a singleton has become more mainstream, more recent data show the age difference between those reducing to twins and those to a singleton has disappeared (Rosner et al. 2013). These data have made counseling patients far more complex. Accordingly, it is not surprising that there are often differences between members of the couple as to the desirability of twins or a singleton, or even as to the total number of fetuses desired, which sometimes is more than two for one member of the couple (Kalra et al. 2003). As a result of all of the above and the changing demographics of who is having infertility treatment and desiring reductions, we believe that reduction of twins to a singleton is reasonable and will continue to increase.

Changing Perspectives

Over the last 25 years we have observed changes in both issues and outcomes. Outcomes have steadily improved (Evans et al. 2004; Templeton 2004; Kalra et al. 2003; Evans and Britt 2009, 2010). Overall statistics on reductions have improved noticeably (Rosner et al. 2013; Balasch and Gratacós 2011, 2012). In the early 1990s when half the cases were quadruplets or more, loss rates (up to 24 weeks) were 13 %. Early premature (<28 weeks) deliveries were an additional 10 %. Now, with decreased starting numbers, better ultrasound, better understanding of zygosity, and a limited number of practitioners with extensive experience accounting for a high percentage of reductions, they are down to about 4 %. Counseling should be tailored to specific starting and finishing numbers (Table 5.5, Fig. 5.2). Currently, we still do most FR procedures in one session, but have seen that when reducing from higher orders (5+) to a singleton, we break it up into two sessions separated by about a week which we believe can produce better outcomes.

The pattern of patients seeking FR has evolved over the last 10 years in response to predictable demographic and cultural shifts (Centers for Disease Control 2013; Martin et al. 2013). There has been a strong trend—common throughout the developed world—of increasing age at which women give birth to their first child. The increase is actually a function of two parallel but independent trends: fewer deliveries (and terminations) in lower and middle class teenagers, and more women, regardless of income, postponing child bearing for a wide range of personal or professional reasons from their 20s to their 30s and 40s. The latter is, of course, the group that is most relevant to our discussion here (Martin et al. 2013). As the risks of delayed childbearing have become more widely known (Marlow et al. 2005; Balasch and Gratacós 2011), there has been a corresponding increase in the demand for donor eggs as a means of moderating the risks for older women (Balasch and Gratacós 2012).

The number of "older women" seeking FR has increased dramatically with the rapid expansion of the availability of donor eggs, and the increasing sensitivity and specificity of diagnostic testing offered. In our experience, more than 10 % of our patients seeking FR are now over 40 years of age, and almost half of them are using donor eggs (Rosner et al. 2013). It would appear that as medical advances in achieving pregnancies and moderating risks for older women have developed, more women are electing to do so.

As a consequence of the shift to older patients, there is an increased desire by these patients to have only one (or one more) child. Many of our patients already had previous relationships and children. There is still a very limited number of experienced centers willing to reduce from twins to singleton, but we believe that it can be justified in most circumstances, based upon improvement of outcomes. Twin pregnancies currently constitute about 25 % of the patients we see (Rosner et al. 2013).

For patients who are "older," particularly those using their own eggs, genetic diagnosis has also become a more salient issue. In 2009, about 60 % of patients in the USA having ART cycles were over age 35. Using the criteria of risk for a chromosome abnormality comparable to that of a 35-year-old, about 90 % of IVF patients are at increased chromosomal aneuploidy risk (Evans et al. 1988) (Table 5.6).

Most FR practitioners make their decisions as to which fetuses to keep or reduce by ultrasound evaluation only. In the 1980s most of our procedures were performed between 9 and 10 weeks, and our decisions were based principally on basic ultrasound and fetal position (Evans et al. 1988). For those patients for whom genetic assessment was appropriate, we asked them to undergo amniocentesis several weeks later at their home center (McLean et al. 1998). We subsequently changed our practice

Table 5.6 Risk for chromosome abnormality in fetus of IVF pregnancy

Factor	Risk	% of IVF pregnancies with factor
AMA	>0.5 %	60
TWINS+	Age 30 with two fetuses risk = that at age 35	34
ICSI	1 %	66
PGD	1 % error	4

AMA = advanced maternal age, ICSI = intracytoplasmic sperm injection, PGD = preimplantation diagnosis

to doing CVS a week after reduction to twins. In the mid 90s a small but increasing percentage of patients were reducing to a singleton; it seemed prudent to assess the viability of the one embryo we were keeping, before committing to a particular embryo. However, waiting for a full karyotype was problematic both because of the time interval to get results, and the fact that others reported a 1 % error rate as to which embryo was which at the time of the reduction (Wapner et al. 1993; Brambati et al. 1995). As fluorescent in situ hybridization (FISH) technology became reliable, we began to do procedures on two consecutive days (CVS with FISH on the first, FR on the second) on a routine basis (Evans and Britt 2010; Balasch and Gratacós 2012). Over the last two decades, the percentage of patients having CVS before FR has risen from about 20 % in 2000 to about 85 % of our patients (Rosner et al. 2013).

While there have been many publications on the risks of prenatal diagnosis (Tabor and Alfirevic 2010), we believe that in multiples—in the most experienced hands—risks incurred by diagnostic procedures are offset by not inadvertently failing to reduce a fetus with a serious problem that is more likely to be spontaneously lost than is a healthy fetus (Rosner et al. 2013).

Another distinct cohort of patients are those who consider a reduction procedure in a multiple pregnancy because of a diagnosed abnormality in one of the fetuses, rather than because of the inherent risk of carrying a multiple pregnancy (Evans and Britt 2009, 2010). The literature uses the term fetal reduction (FR) for reductions performed for fetal number, predominantly in the first trimester. The term selective termination (ST) is used for cases done for a diagnosed anomaly, predominantly in the second trimester. Occasionally, diagnosed abnormalities are discovered even in the third trimester posing medical, ethical, and legal issues (Hern 2004). We and others have published large series over the past decades that have described the similarities and differences when there is a confirmed abnormality (Evans et al. 1999; Eddleman et al. 2002). The majority of this literature focuses on twins—particularly on twin to twin transfusion syndrome (TTTS), in which laser therapy has become the mainstay of therapy, but ST is still sometimes necessary in other situations (Lu et al. 2013). A complete discussion of these issues is beyond the scope of this paper.

Modern Management

Ideally, we believe that a rigorous evaluation of the fetal status should be a part of the decision process prior to reduction, a process which includes more than just a nuchal translucency ultrasound and determination of the position of the fetuses. As noted above, we typically perform a 2 day procedure on most patients at about 12 weeks: CVS on the first day with FISH analyses overnight for chromosomes 13, 18, 21, X, and Y (Rosner et al. 2013) (Fig. 5.4). The results come back the next afternoon, at which time we do the reduction. By definition, FISH for five chromosomes cannot detect all chromosomal abnormalities; however, modeling and our experience suggest only about a 1/400 residual risk of an abnormal karyotype (Rosner et al. 2013) We believe this to be a lower risk than that of sending the patient home, to return nearly 2 weeks later, with the attendant risk of interval loss associated with higher order multiples, and the potential confusion as to which embryo/fetus was which on the ultrasound (Wapner et al. 1993; Brambati et al. 1995).

Over recent years, about 85 % of our patients have combined CVS and FR procedures. With an increasing proportion of older patients; new data suggesting higher risks of chromosomal and other anomalies in patients conceiving by IVF, especially with intracytoplasmic sperm injection (ICSI); and the inaccuracy rate of PGD (3–6 %), we anticipate the utilization of CVS prior to reduction will increase even further (Rosner et al. 2013; Evans and Britt 2010; Balasch and Gratacós 2012) We

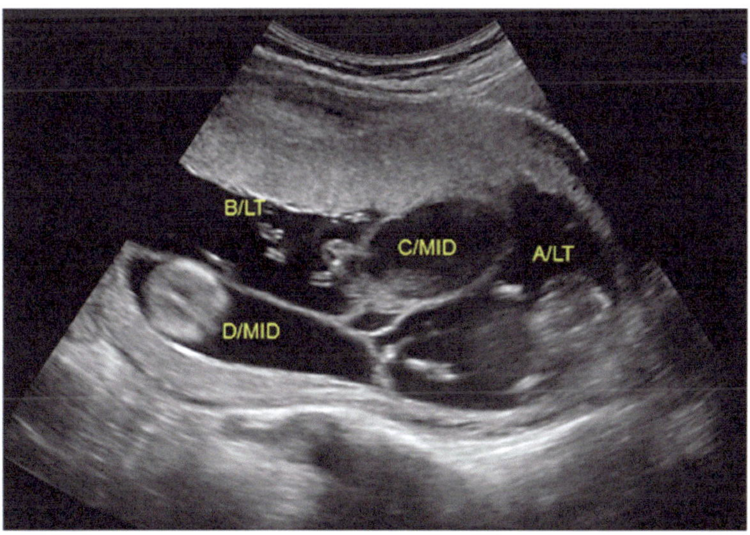

Fig. 5.4 Evaluating and documenting fetal positions in sextuplet pregnancy. Fetal positions of A, B, C, and D on longitudinal scan

have also found that many couples in their 40s or 50s who are using donor eggs still want CVS prior to FR, even though the chromosomal risk is the age of the egg donor, because their "tolerance" for having a child with special needs is more akin to that of those their actual ages, not the egg donor's.

Our recent data show that our protocol of CVS followed by overnight FISH analysis with FR the next day substantially improves outcomes. In pregnancies with normal-appearing fetuses on ultrasound prior to first trimester FR, 3.1 % of women had a fetus with an abnormal karyotype, 90 % of which FISH detected (Rosner et al. 2013). Virtually all of the remaining 10 % were confined placental mosaicisms for unstudied chromosomes or culture artifacts. Of 350 patients with normal-appearing first trimester fetuses, 9 had abnormal CVS by either karyotype or FISH. Those abnormal FISH and ultrasound results guided decisions at the time of the reduction procedure. Ultimately, 90 % of those abnormal FISH results were confirmed on final karyotype. Of false negatives, most were for chromosomes for which there weren't FISH probes used, and most of them were actually confined placental mosaicisms. Ultimately, only 1 of the 350 cases (0.3 %) had a clinically relevant false negative (sex chromosome mosaicism). On balance, we believe that the risk of a false negative is lower than the risks entailed in waiting between procedures, which increases loss rates because of the higher fetal number and the risk of making a mistake as to which fetus is which when returning for the FR procedure.

While it has worked best for us to use FISH for rapid diagnoses, other methods have been and will be available in the near future. Earlier methods included direct preparation CVS, which was used frequently in the 1980s but was largely abandoned because of high rates of mosaicism and aneuploidies that did not reflect the actual fetal status (Pergament et al. 1992). Qualitative fluorescence-polymerase chain reaction (QF-PCR) can also be used for rapid preparation and evaluation of chromosome number (Nicolini et al. 2004). Microarrays can provide greater detail than whole chromosome studies, but currently are expensive (particularly with multiple pregnancies) and time consuming. We routinely offer microarrays in all singleton pregnancies but not yet in multiples because the waiting time to get microarray results in such pregnancies would significantly postpone the reduction and increase the chance of loss before reduction. However, as microarrays decrease in price and turn around speed improves, molecular sub-chromosomal techniques will certainly move into the mainstream of multiple pregnancy evaluation prior to reduction (Wapner et al. 2012).

As utilization of pre-implantation genetic diagnosis (PGD) as part of the IVF process increases, many patients have questioned if traditional CVS still has a role in reduction decisions (Dreesen et al. 2014). Our experience over the past 5 years has shown a 2–3 % discordancy between PGD results and those we have seen on CVS—with chromosomal discordancies being greater than Mendelian (Rosner et al. 2013). As new PGD microarray-like methods are incorporated, the discordancy rate is likely to fall. We speculate that in the long run, the rate will be roughly 1 %. Similarly, with the advent of noninvasive prenatal screening (NIPS) techniques, the same questions arise (Lo 2013). Our perspective is that both PGD and NIPS are excellent screening tests, but they are not diagnostic: we have observed a number of instances in which errors have occurred, resulting in babies born affected by the disorders for which screening was performed. Also in multiples, NIPS and PGD cannot distinguish between individual fetuses; if an abnormality is detected, diagnostic techniques will still be required to determine the affected fetus.

An increasingly more common scenario is a pregnancy with a set of monozygotic twins plus one or more singletons (Pantos et al. 2009). Changes in IVF culture techniques, including growing use of blastocyst transfers have significantly increased the incidence of monozygotic twinning. Our data suggest that dichorionic, triamniotic triplets, for example, have far higher rates of pregnancy loss, TTTS, and complications of prematurity than tri–tri pregnancies (Peeters et al. 2014).

In the vast majority of cases, the primary genetic risk factor in determining which fetuses to keep or reduce is chromosomal risk. However, the same principles can be applied to Mendelian risks. For example, we assessed a couple, both of whom were cystic fibrosis carriers, with a triplet pregnancy. Using appropriate probes, we were able to ascertain that two of the fetuses were carriers, and one was affected, which was later reduced.

As part of the FISH panel, we also learn gender. Historically, we perceived a significant bias among those patients who were interested and whom mostly expressed a preference for boys (Kalra et al. 2003; Evans and Britt 2009). These requests disproportionately came from patients of cultural backgrounds that classically valued males over females. Due to such bias, we categorically refused to allow gender influence decisions, with the rare exception of genetic diseases with known gender discordancy. Ironically, in X-linked disorders, it is the males at risk, making females the safer option. However, over the past 15 years, we noticed a change to requests coming from all ethnic groups and a seeming equalization of gender preferences. In the early 2000s, our ethics consultant, John Fletcher, Ph.D., pushed us to reevaluate.

Overall, decisions about which fetuses to keep or reduce have progressed over the years from a relatively simplistic ultrasound assessment of abnormalities and position to now a detailed evaluation of fetal status.

We prioritize FR decisions by:

1. Did we find a “problem?”
2. Are we “suspicious” about something, such as increased nuchal translucency (>2 mm), smaller fetal size (e.g., >½ week than expected by gestational age), smaller gestational sac size, or placental concern?
3. If none of the above apply, then and only then, we will consider gender preference.

Patients are told that we will have a “poker faced” discussion with them when we get the chromosome results, in which gender is not disclosed. They will then choose which of four categories concerning gender they prefer. The groups are:

1. Those patients who want to know “everything,”
2. Those who want to know “nothing,”
3. Those who have no preference but want to know what they’ve kept (but not the reduced), and

Table 5.7 Fetal gender options and patient's choices

	Gender option (*N*, %)	Chose all M[a]	Chose all F[b]	Chose MF[c] twins	*p*
Triplets to twins	79 (51 %)	1 (1 %)	7 (9 %)	71 (90 %)	<0.001
Triplets to singletons	20 (25 %)	10 (50 %)	10 (50 %)	NA	NS
Twins to singletons	44 (27 %)	20 (45 %)	24 (55 %)	NA	NS

NA not applicable, *NS* not significant
[a]Male
[b]Female
[c]Male and female

4. Those who, considering all other factors, do have a preference (but don't want to know the reduced fetus' or fetuses' genders) (Evans et al. 2013a).

Recently, we published data that show that such requests now come from patients of all ethnic backgrounds and cultures (Evans et al. 2013a). When patients do have a gender preference, they are equally likely to prefer a female as a male. For patients reducing to twins, the vast majority prefer one of each; for those reducing to a singleton, it is almost a 50/50 split (Table 5.7) (Evans et al. 2013a).

Recently, we have also been able to use technology to extend services to a previously underserved group of patients. In the past few years we have seen several gay male couples, using surrogate carriers with egg donation, both partners having fertilized the eggs. The couples desired FR for the typical clinical reasons, but they requested if possible to be left with twins—one fathered by each of them. We elected to consider this request using the same protocol as we did for gender preference: i.e., if—and only if—there are no higher clinical priorities. In multiple cases we have been able to assess the pregnancies with CVS and ultrasound, document normal genetic results, perform paternity testing, and find that one man fathered one and the other the remaining two of a triplet gestation. In such cases we then reduced one of the two embryos fathered by the same man (Evans et al. 2013b).

Ethical Issues

Prima facie respect for the intrinsic value of human life is a common moral norm. Prima facie means that a norm is binding absent conflicting obligations. "Intrinsic" means to value something in and for itself, independent of its results for or our relations to us or other people. Convictions about intrinsically valuing human life are universal among the medical community. However, these convictions often conflict with responsibilities of other moral norms, e.g., to do justice, to benefit others, to respect and defend autonomous decisions, to prevent or minimize harm and suffering, to use proportionality when faced with inevitable risks, etc. (Beauchamp and

Childress 2001) Only moral compromise can "split the differences" between such diverse interpretations in policy and in practice (Benjamin 1990).

When such conflicts occur in reproductive choices currently our society does not generally interfere in parents' consultations with obstetricians, geneticists, or moral advisors. However, this has not stopped politicians from enacting legislation that seriously encroaches upon doctor-patient relationships, particularly in regard to issues of reproductive choice. The right to privacy, as originally interpreted by Roe v. Wade (1973), is certainly not absolute and has been scaled back several times in the four decades since the landmark US Supreme Court decision. The Court's opinion expects physicians to counsel patients about the reasons for their actions, and to be responsible in providing terminations. The value of respect for human life lies behind this concern. Society also defends a clinician's conscientious refusal to participate in abortions or reductions, constrained by their obligation to refer patients to competent sources for assistance.

Compromise is often the best path, as all moral judgments are fallible and their interpretations change as circumstances evolve. Ultimately, no matter how well-considered, predictions of consequences are restricted by our inability to know the future. Political and social interests cannot be eliminated from moral assessment. Both sides must remember that integrity and advocacy does not disappear in an authentic compromise. We acknowledge moral uncertainty about unknown effects of twin reduction, and reductions more generally, for individuals, families, and society. But we can see in retrospect how some of the issues have changed over time.

Increasing use of ART, coupled with improved outcomes, have led to an evolution in the ethical questions being discussed. Nearly 30 years ago, FR seemed acceptable only in life and death situations. As has been seen in numerous innovative technologies, once concepts are supported by data, the focus and application can shift from "life and death" to "quality of life." Such has been the case here, but because of the context of the abortion debate, FR will always be controversial. In our experience opinions on FR have never followed the classic "pro-choice/pro-life" dichotomy (Evans et al. 1991; Evans and Britt 2010; Balasch and Gratacós 2012).

It is essentially impossible to separate ethical debates from the situation in which they occur—especially the presenting number of embryos with which patients enter an FR clinic. The number of couples presenting with quadruplets and quintuplets has declined dramatically. The focus of care rightfully continues to be on fertilization strategies that offer greater control over the incidence of high multiples.

Triplets are still plentiful. Even with the improved control of embryo-transfer, the economics of IVF favor a modest risk of multiples, particularly among women with constrained resources (for whom the cost of IVF cycles is a significant burden) and those who are over 35 (for whom the risks of larger transfer numbers are proportionate to their greater difficulty in getting pregnant). The significant debate is no longer about whether it is appropriate to offer FR for triplets, but about whether or not it is appropriate to offer FR routinely for twins (Templeton 2004).

Our data show that reduction of twins to a singleton improves the overall outcome of the remaining fetus (Evans and Britt 2009, 2010; Balasch and Gratacós 2012). Despite the data, no consensus on appropriateness of routine $2 \rightarrow 1$ reduction is ever likely to emerge, because of the sharp ethical divide over women's reproductive rights the issue poses. We speculate that the total number of women with twins reducing to singletons will remain small. However, the overall proportion of such patients reducing will steadily increase over the next several years, and we believe this option should be presented to all patients.

With a continuing decrease in starting numbers, the emphasis has shifted to prevention of serious morbidities, i.e., cerebral palsy from prematurity. Many studies have suggested that the rate of cerebral palsy for singletons is approximately 1/700; twins 1/100; and triplets 1/25–30 (Petterson et al. 1993; Pharoah and Cooke 1996; Dimitiiou et al. 2004). If the definition of success is a healthy mother and healthy family, for both morbidity and mortality, the data conclusively show that with multiples, fewer is always better.

Unsurprisingly, there are frequently differences in opinion between members of the couple as to the desirability of twins or singleton (Evans and Britt 2009). We believe that reduction of twins to a singleton is likely to increase over the next several years, as a result of all of the above and the changing demographics of infertility and desire for a reduction. In our patients, the proportion of those with twins who request a reduction is now 25 % and may rise as high as 50 % (Rosner et al. 2013). Many couples or single mothers would not reduce twins to a singleton for social or economic reasons. However, if it is right for a pluralistic society to curb a state's interference with the choice of abortion or other reproductive options, how could it be wrong for society to respect and protect the freedom of couples to choose to have one rather than two infants? This so-called "negative right," i.e., to non-interference, differs from a "positive right" to society's encouragement and aid in the action (Wenar 2011).

Other parental decisions also deserve protection and respect from interference. Some couples with few assets want to keep twins, knowing that one or both have a genetic condition requiring lifelong care. Society does not and should not interfere with this choice nor deny its resources to care for children with disabilities.

We have previously developed the concept of "frames"; lenses through which patients incorporate and interpret information (Britt and Evans 2007a). For some, the escalation of mortality and morbidity risks is so definite that even those patients who rely on a "conceptional frame" (a frame that defines conception as the beginning of life, rather than viability) will follow a proportionality rule, in which they try to balance the mounting risks and the ethical hazards of reduction by reducing only to triplets versus twins or a singleton. Reduction to twins or a singleton is less challenging for those with a "medical frame" (one that focuses on maximizing the chances of having a successful birth(s)) or a "lifestyle frame" (one that emphasizes the balancing of career and family interests, in whatever proportions the patient chooses). As technology advances, utilization is expanding to groups such as gay and lesbian couples who previously often could not take advantage of advances in "family building".

Thus, we view framing as an ongoing and evolving process in society, with highly different perceptions of reality being embraced by highly different couples. All wish to overcome the difficulties of having children and living some semblance of a "normal" family life. "Family" is not a concept limited to heterosexual couples, but "normal" is an attribution that may be slow in coming in some conservative communities, if at all. We see evidence of these trends in how all couples share their experience of FR as a pregnancy-management strategy, supported by knowledge of same-sex couples who have gone through (with or without a surrogate) fertility therapy and ended up choosing FR as a pregnancy-management strategy.

We have described four sharing strategies that differed among FR patients in how selectively they shared information (Britt and Evans 2007b). Strategies for sharing varied in terms of selectivity from a *defended-relationship* approach in which only the partner and patient were aware of the problems faced by the patient and the decision to reduce, up through a *qualified family and friends* strategy, in which information is shared only with those whom the patient believes to be trustworthy in terms of their responses. Our analysis also highlighted two other less selective strategies. In the first, *both sets of parents* are privy to what the couple is going through, and finally, there is an extended, *open network* strategy of family, friends and colleagues being in the loop (Britt and Evans 2007a, b).

No sharing strategy is entirely free of the risk of facing judgment. However, the odds of encountering hostility are significantly greater with the more open, less selective strategies. In our experience, the less selective, more open strategies are more prevalent in cosmopolitan surroundings, with the more limited sharing strategies typical of more conservative settings. As our population shifts toward urbanization, one might expect an increasing proportion of open strategies over time.

Legal Issues

Legal concerns about IVF have been considered for over 30 years including a paper we wrote in 1981 envisaging a range of problems likely to be encountered, almost all of which eventually occurred, including problems with surrogate mothers (Evans and Dixler 1981). In contrast, while there has been widespread civil and criminal litigation concerning abortion, and limitations imposed on its use, there has been so far a scarcity of direct legal cases relating to the legality of FR. Most jurisdictions in the USA have kept silent on the subject, although Michigan, for example, specifically requires the same 24 h waiting period between counseling and procedure as it applies to abortions, per se. There have been some malpractice litigation cases, but these have conformed to the expected scenarios such as reduction of the wrong fetus in situations with anomalies, alleged failures to provide informed consent as to procedure risks, and for various poor outcomes.

Despite distinct differences, most practitioners of fetal reduction have followed the guidelines applying to abortions, e.g., performing the procedures only at gestational ages that would be permissible for abortion, and conforming to legally mandated informed consent procedures for abortion.

Summary

Over the past 25 years, data from around the world have demonstrated that pregnancy outcomes are significantly improved by reducing the number of fetuses in multiples. All but the most conservative of critics have long since accepted the efficacy and safety of reduction of triplets or higher order pregnancies. The medical data now also demonstrate that reduction of twins to a singleton improves outcomes. The FR debate then shifts to an ethical one on which there will never be universal agreement, but we argue that from an autonomy and public health perspective, FR must be seen as a necessary but hopefully increasingly rare procedure.

Acknowledgement The authors wish to acknowledge the contributions to our thinking on this subject of John C. Fletcher, Ph.D., who, before his death several years ago, laid the foundation for the ethical analysis of this subject.

References

Antsaklis A, Souka AP, Daskalakis G, et al. Embryo reduction versus expectant management in triplet pregnancies. J Matern Fetal Neonatal Med. 2004;16:219–22.

Balasch J, Gratacós E. Delayed childbearing: effects on fertility and the outcome of pregnancy. Fetal Diagn Ther. 2011;29:263–73. doi:10.1159/000323142.

Balasch J, Gratacós E. Delayed childbearing: effects on fertility and the outcome of pregnancy. Curr Opin Obstet Gynecol. 2012;24(3):187–93.

Beauchamp TL, Childress JC. Principles of biomedical ethics. 5th ed. New York, NY: Oxford University Press; 2001. p. 358–9.

Benjamin M. Splitting the difference. Compromise and integrity in ethics and politics. Lawrence, KA: University Press of Kansas; 1990. p. 72–4.

Berkowitz RL, Lynch L, Chitkara U, et al. Selective reduction of multiple pregnancies in the first trimester. N Engl J Med. 1988;318:1043.

Blickstein I. How and why are triplets disadvantaged compared to twins. Best Pract Res Clin Obstet Gynecol. 2004;18:631–44.

Brambati B, Tului L, Baldi M, Guercilena S. Genetic analysis prior to selective fetal reduction in multiple pregnancy: technical aspects and clinical outcome. Hum Reprod. 1995;10:818–25.

Britt DW, Evans MI. Sometimes doing the right thing sucks: frame combinations and multifetal pregnancy reduction decision difficulty. Soc Sci Med. 2007a;65:2342–56.

Britt DW, Evans MI. Information sharing among couples considering multifetal pregnancy reduction. Fertil Steril. 2007b;87:490–5.

Chaveeva P, Kosinski P, Puglia D, Poon LC, Nicolaides KH. Trichorionic and dichorionic triplet pregnancies at 10–14 weeks: outcome after embryo reduction compared to expectant management. Fetal Diagn Ther. 2013;34:199–205.

Cohen AB, Hanft RS. Technology in American health care: policy direction for effective evaluation and management. Ann Arbor, MI: Univ Michigan Press; 2004.

Cuevas KD, Silver DR, Brooten D, et al. The cost of prematurity: hospital charges at birth and frequency of rehospitalizations and acute care visits over the first year of life: a comparison by gestational age and birth weight. Am J Nurs. 2005;105:56–64.

Dimitiiou G, Pharoah PO, Nicolaides KH, et al. Cerebral Palsy in triplet pregnancies with and without iatrogenic reduction. Eur J Pediatr. 2004;163:449–51.

Dreesen J, Destouni A, Kourlaba G, Degn B, Mette WC, Carvalho F, et al. Evaluation of PCR-based preimplantation genetic diagnosis applied to monogenic disease: a collaborative ESHRE PGD consortium study. Eur J Hum Genet. 2014;22:1012. doi:10.1038/ejhg.2013.277.

Dumez Y, Oury JF. Method for first trimester selective abortion in multiple pregnancy. Contrib Gynecol Obstet. 1986;15:50.

Eddleman KA, Stone JL, Lynch L, Berkowitz RL. Selective termination of anomalous fetuses in multiple pregnancies: two hundred cases at a single center. Am J Obstet Gynecol. 2002;187: 1168–72.

Evans MI, Britt DW. Selective reduction in multifetal pregnancies. In: Paul M, Grimes D, Stubblefield P, Borgatta L, Lichfield S, Creinin M, editors. Management of unintended and abnormal pregnancy. London: Blackwell-Wiley Publishing Co; 2009. p. 312–8.

Evans MI, Britt DW. Fetal reduction: ethical and societal issues. In Sauer M (ed). Sem Reprod Med. 2010;28:295–302.

Evans MI, Britt DW. Medical, ethical, and legal aspects of fetal reduction. In: Schenker JL, editor. Ethical and legal aspects of ART. New York, NY: Walter De Gruyter GmbH & Co.; 2011. p. 121–30.

Evans MI, Dixler AO. In vitro fertilization: some legal issues. JAMA. 1981;245:2324–7.

Evans MI, Hanft RS. The introduction of new technologies. ACOG Clin Semin. 1997;2(5):1–3.

Evans MI, Fletcher JC, Zador IE, Newton BW, Struyk CK, Quigg MH. Selective first trimester termination in octuplet and quadruplet pregnancies: clinical and ethical issues. Obstet Gynecol. 1988;71:289–96.

Evans MI, Drugan A, Fletcher JC, Platt LD, Rodeck CA, Hansmann M, Bottoms SF. Attitudes on the ethics of abortion, sex selection & selective termination among health care professionals, ethicists & clergy likely to encounter such situations. Am J Obstet Gynecol. 1991;164: 1092–9.

Evans MI, Dommergues M, Wapner RJ, Lynch L, Dumez Y, Goldberg JD, Zador IE, Nicolaides KH, Johnson MP, Golbus MS, Boulot P, Berkowitz RL. Efficacy of transabdominal multifetal pregnancy reduction: collaborative experience among the world's largest centers. Obstet Gynecol. 1993;82:61–7.

Evans MI, Goldberg J, Horenstein J, Wapner R, Ayoub MA, Stone J, Lipitz S, Achiron R, Holzgreve W, Brambati B, Johnson A, Johnson MP, Berkowitz R. Selective termination (ST) for structural (STR), chromosomal (CHR), and Mendelian (MEN) anomalies: international experience. Am J Obstet Gynecol. 1999;181:893–7.

Evans MI, Berkowitz R, Wapner R, Carpenter R, Goldberg J, Ayoub MA, Horenstein J, Dommergues M, Brambati B, Nicolaides K, Holzgreve W, Timor-Tritsch IE. Improvement in outcomes of multifetal pregnancy reduction with increased experience. Am J Obstet Gynecol. 2001;184(2):97–103.

Evans MI, Kaufman MI, Urban AJ, Krivchenia EL, Britt DW, Wapner RJ. Fetal reduction from twins to a singleton: a reasonable consideration. Obstet Gynecol. 2004;104:102–9.

Evans MI, Rosner M, Andriole S, Alkalay A, Gebb J, Britt DW. Evolution of gender preferences in multiple pregnancies. Prenat Diagn. 2013a;33:935–9. doi:10.1002/pd.4167.

Evans MI, Andriole S, Pergament E, Curtis J, Britt DW. Paternity balancing. Fetal Diagn Ther. 2013b;34:135. doi:10.1159/000351857.

Francois K, SEARS C, Wilson R, Elliot J. Twelve year experience of triplet pregnancies at a single institution. Am J Obstet Gynecol. 2001;185:S112.

Hack M, Taylor HG, Drotar D, et al. Chronic conditions, functional limitations, and special health care needs of school-aged children born with extremely low birth weights in the 1990s. JAMA. 2005;94:318–25.

Hern WM. Selective termination for fetal anomaly/genetic disorder in twin pregnancy at 32+ menstrual weeks. Report of four cases. Fetal Diagn Ther. 2004;19:292–5.

Kalra SK, Milad MP, Klock SC, Grobman WA. Infertility patients and their partners: differences in the desire for twin gestations. Obstet Gynecol. 2003;102:152–5.

Kozinsky Z, Zadori J, Ovros H, et al. Obstetric and neonatal risk of pregnancies after assisted reproductive technology: a matched control study. Acta Obstet Gynecol Scand. 2003; 82:850–6.

Lawlor DA, Nelson SM. Effect of age on decisions about the number of embryos to transfer in assisted conception: a prospective study. Lancet. 2012;379:521–7.

Leondires MP, Ernst SD, Miller BT, et al. Triplets: outcomes of expectant management versus multifetal reduction for 127 pregnancies. Am J Obstet Gynecol. 1999;72:257–60.

Li R, Yang R, Chen X, Yang S, Ma C, Liu P, Qiao J. Intracranial KCl injection – an alternative method for multifetal pregnancy reduction in the early second trimester. Fetal Diagn Ther. 2013;34:26–30.

Lipitz S, Shulman A, Achiron R, et al. A comparative study of multifetal pregnancy reduction from triplets to twins in the first versus early second trimesters after detailed fetal screening. Ultrasound Obstet Gynecol. 2001;18:35–8.

Lo YM. Non-invasive prenatal testing using massively parallel sequencing of maternal plasma DNA: from molecular karyotyping to fetal whole genome sequencing. Reprod Biomed Online. 2013;37:593. doi:10.1016/j.rbmo.2013.08.008. pii: S1472-6483(13)00466-5.

Lu J, Ting YH, Law KM, Lau TK, Leung TY. Radiofrequency ablation for selective reduction in complicated monochorionic multiple pregnancies. Fetal Diagn Ther. 2013;34:211.

Luke B, Brown MD, Nugent C, et al. Risk factors for adverse outcomes in spontaneous versus assisted conception in twin pregnancies. Fertil Steril. 2004;81:315–9.

Marlow N, Wolke D, Bracewell MA, et al. Neurologic and developmental disability at six years of age after extremely preterm birth. N Engl J Med. 2005;352:9–19.

Martin JA, Hamilton BE, Osterman MHS, Curtin SC, Matthews TJ. Births: final data for 2011. National Vital Statistics Reports. 62#9. Hyattsville, MD: National Center for Health Statistics; 2013.

McDonald S, Murphy K, Beyene J, et al. Perinatal outcomes of in vitro fertilization twins: a systematic review and meta analysis. Am J Obstet Gynecol. 2005;193:141–52.

McLean LK, Evans MI, Carpenter RJ, Johnson MP, Goldberg JD. Genetic amniocentesis (AMN) following multifetal pregnancy reduction (MFPR) does not increase the risk of pregnancy loss. Prenat Diagn. 1998;18(2):186–8.

MMWR: Assisted Reproductive Technology Surveillance – United States, 2009. Centers for Disease control and prevention. 2012;61#7

National Survey of Family Growth. Centers for Disease Control 2013 http://www.cdc.gov/nchs/nsfg/abc_list_i.htm#infertilityservices

Nicolini U, Lalatta F, Natacci F, Curcio C, Bui TH. The introduction of QF-PCR in prenatal diagnosis of fetal aneuploidies: time for reconsideration. Hum Reprod Update. 2004;10(6):541–8.

Pantos K, Kokkali G, Petroutsou K, Lekka K, Malligiannis P, Koratzis A. Monochorionic triplet and monoamniotic twins gestation after intracytoplasmic sperm injection and laser-assisted hatching. Fetal Diagn Ther. 2009;25:144–7.

Peeters SH, Evans MI, Slaghekke F, Klumper FJ, Middeldorp JM, Lopriore E, Oepkes D. Pregnancy complications for di-chorionic, tri-amniotic triplets: markedly increased over trichorionic and reduced cases. Am J Obstet Gynecol. 2014;210:S288.

Pergament E, Schulman JD, Copeland K, Fine B, Black SH, Ginsberg NA, Frederiksen MC, Carpenter RJ. The risk and efficacy of chorionic villus sampling in multiple gestations. Prenat Diagn. 1992;12:377–84.

Petterson B, Nelson K, Watson L, et al. Twins, triplets, and cerebral palsy in births in Western Australia in the 1980s. BMJ. 1993;307:1239–43.

Pharoah PO, Cooke T. Cerebral Palsy and multiple births. Arch Dis Child Fetal Neonatal Ed. 1996;75:F174–7.

Roe v. Wade, 410 US 113 1973:at 153

Rosenbaum P, Paneth N, Leviton A, Goldstein M, Bax M, Damiano D, Dan B, Jacobson B. A report: the definition and classification of cerebral palsy April 2006. Dev Med Child Neurol. 2007;49:8–14. doi:10.1111/j.1469-8749.2007.tb12610.x. Corrected in Rosenbaum, P; Paneth, N; Leviton, A; Goldstein, M; Bax, M; Damiano, D; Dan, B; Jacobsson, B (2007). "A report:

The definition and classification of cerebral palsy April 2006". *Developmental medicine and child neurology. Supplement* **109**: 8–14. doi:10.1111/j.1469-8749.2007.tb12610.x.

Rosner M, Pergament E, Andriole S, Gebb J, Dar P, Evans MI. Detection of genetic abnormalities using CVS and FISH prior to fetal reduction in sonographically normal appearing fetuses. Prenat Diagn. 2013;33:940–4. doi:10.1002/pd.4213.

Sepulveda W, Munoz H, Alcalde JL. Conjoined twins in a triplet pregnancy: early prenatal diagnosis with three-dimensional ultrasound and review of the literature. Ultrasound Obstet Gynecol. 2003;22:199–204.

Society of Assisted Reproductive Technologies 2011 Statistics. https://www.sartcorsonline.com/rptCSR_PublicMultYear.aspx?ClinicPKID=0

Stoll BJ, Hansen NI, Bell EF, Shankaran S, Laptook AR, Walsh MC, et al. Neonatal outcomes of extremely preterm infants from the NICHD Neonatal Research Network. Pediatrics. 2010;126:443–56. doi:10.1542/peds.2009-2959.

Tabor A, Alfirevic Z. Update on procedure-related risks for prenatal diagnosis techniques. Fetal Diagn Ther. 2010;27:1–7.

Task Force of American College of Obstetricians and Gynecologists. Neonatal Encephalopathy and Cerebral Palsy: defining the pathogenesis and pathophysiology. Washington, DC: ACOG; 2003.

Templeton A. The multiple gestation epidemic: the role of the assisted reproductive technologies. Am J Obstet Gynecol. 2004;190:894–8.

Timor-Tritsch IE, Peisner DB, Monteagudo A, Lerner JP, Sharma S. Multifetal pregnancy reduction by transvaginal puncture: evaluation of the technique used in 134 cases. Am J Obstet Gynecol. 1993;168:799–804.

Tronnes H, Wilcox AJ, Lie R, Markestad T, Moster D. Risk of cerebral palsy in relation to pregnancy disorders and preterm birth: a national cohort study. Dev Med Child Neurol. 2014;56:779. doi:10.1111/dmcn.12430.

Wapner RJ, Davis GH, Johnson A. Selective reduction of multifetal pregnancies. Lancet. 1990;335:90–3.

Wapner RJ, Johnson A, Davis G, Urban A, Morgan P, Jackson L. Prenatal diagnosis in twin gestations: a comparison between second-trimester amniocentesis and first-trimester chorionic villus sampling. Obstet Gynecol. 1993;82:49–56.

Wapner RJ, Martin CL, Levy B, Ballif BC, Eng CM, Zachary JM, et al. Chromosomal microarray versus karyotyping for prenatal diagnosis. N Engl J Med. 2012;367:2175–84.

Wenar L. Rights. The Stanford encyclopedia of philosophy, Fall 2011 Edition, Edward N. Zalta (ed.). http://plato.stanford.edu/archives/fall2011/entries/rights/

Yaron Y, Bryant-Greenwood PK, Dave N, et al. Multifetal pregnancy reduction (MFPR) of triplets to twins: comparison with non-reduced triplets and twins. Am J Obstet Gynecol. 1999;180:1268–71.

Chapter 6
Fetal Pain

Stuart W.G. Derbyshire

Introduction

Discussion regarding the possibility of fetal pain began in earnest after it was discovered that the fetus will mount a hormonal stress response during invasive procedures (Giannakoulopoulos et al. 1994). The release of cortisol and β-endorphin following fetal tissue damage raised concern that the fetus may feel pain and generated considerable scientific and public debate. Scientific debate has largely focused on understanding the critical periods of change during fetal development that may bear on the experience of pain (Lee et al. 2005). Public debate has largely focused on the implications for abortion and the possibility (now a reality in large parts of America) that abortion should be restricted or regulated to prevent fetal pain (Brugger 2012).

In line with the dominant scientific debate, this review first focuses on the critical neurodevelopmental moments that are thought to be necessary for fetal pain experience. Serious limitations of this approach, however, will also be raised to explain why a neuroscientific answer to the issue of fetal pain remains inaccessible. Finally, it will be argued that fetal pain is an immensely provocative and thought-provoking issue that cannot be usefully used to guide clinical practice or policy.

S.W.G. Derbyshire, Ph.D. (✉)
Psychology and A*STAR-NUS Centre for Clinical Imaging, Faculty of Arts and Sciences, National University of Singapore, Singapore 117570, Singapore
e-mail: stuart.derbyshire@nus.edu.sg

J.P. Galst, M.S. Verp (eds.), *Prenatal and Preimplantation Diagnosis*,
DOI 10.1007/978-3-319-18911-6_6

Approaches from Neuroscience

Probably the most audacious, and brilliant, attempt to end the fetal pain debate comes from the work of Mellor (2005). In 2005, Mellor published a comprehensive review documenting many decades of highly detailed observations of, mostly, fetal lambs. Those observations indicated that the fetal lamb rarely shows any behavioral signs of waking or alertness during gestation. In addition, the EEG pattern of fetal lambs indicates continuous sleep and that sleep pattern is not broken by hypoxic stress. Indeed, the EEG pattern shifts to a more quiescent state during periods of hypoxic stress (Hunter et al. 2003).

Based on observation and deduction, Mellor argued that the fetus is in a constant state of sedation or sleep throughout the whole of pregnancy, and never awakens. The environment of the womb is dark, quiet, warm, and buoyant, which places an emphasis on sleep. In addition, there is no avenue of escape or possibility of rescue from the womb, so there is nothing to be gained by expending energy on activity when under threat. Finally, the placenta provides a chemical environment, involving the release of adenosine, which maintains or enhances sleep.

The Mellor argument potentially ends the discussion about fetal pain because, regardless of any arguments about the neural or psychological readiness of the fetus, it is broadly accepted that feeling pain during sleep is not possible (Nofzinger and Derbyshire 2007; Wang et al. 2004). There are, however, important problems with Mellor's argument and, ultimately, the argument has failed to end the fetal pain debate. The failure is, however, highly interesting, and has important implications for all attempts to resolve the question of fetal pain using neuroscientific observations.

Problems begin with the interpretation of fetal EEG as "sleep" and "quiescence." When hypoxic stress is induced, the fetal lamb EEG shows a clear transition from a heightened state of activity to a reduced state of activity that can be viewed as a relative quiescence (Hunter et al. 2003). Within that relative quiescence, however, are various bursts and spikes of activity that are clearly not indicative of silence. The meaning of those bursts and spikes is uncertain, but they are not easily explained as "sleep." Furthermore, the normal EEG pattern of the fetus is not easily recognizable as a typical "sleep" pattern. In adult mammals, sleep is accompanied by characteristic stages of EEG wave patterns that are used to define the type of sleep that is occurring, such as dream sleep or deep sleep (Hobson 2005). These stages, however, are not apparent in the newborn neonate, which has essentially the same EEG pattern during waking and sleep (Weerd and Bossche 2003). Thus, it is not surprising that the EEG patterns observed in the fetus cannot be easily mapped onto the EEG patterns observed during sleep in the mature mammal. Although it is plausible that the fetus transitions from one state of sleep to a deeper state of sleep during stress, as Mellor argues, it is possibly more reasonable to state that the fetus transitions from one uncertain state of being to another uncertain state of being. The terms "sleep," "wakefulness," and so on imply a state of subjective existence that is not directly apparent in any of the EEG or other technical measures that might be made during gestation.

There is a difficulty in using terms that are, at least partially, subjective, such as "sleep," in association with technical measurements, such as EEG. Technical measurements, such as EEG waveforms, are inherently precise and provide units that deliver exact information. In contrast, subjective states, such as wakefulness, are less precise. There is a tendency to read the technical precision into the subjective state, as if the technical measure *were* the subjective state or as if the subjective state has the same precision as the technical measurement. This problem is evident for all attempts to resolve the question of fetal pain with neuroscience as will now be explored in more detail.

Neurodevelopmental Stages Relevant to Pain

Several distinct stages in development have been identified as important for pain. The earliest gestational moment at which pain has been suggested is 7–8 weeks when the first reflex responses to touch appear (Humphrey 1964). At this point, there is evidence of free nerve endings in the periphery (skin) that are necessary for detecting stimuli in the noxious range. Reflex responses to touch demonstrate that there are connections from the periphery to the spinal cord and there is also evidence of further projections into the thalamus (Fitzgerald 1987).

Reflex responses mediated by the spinal cord, however, are not considered sufficient to support conscious pain experience. Indeed, spinal reflexes occur in mature adults and precede conscious experience; rapid withdrawal from an unexpected noxious stimulus occurs automatically, without conscious intervention (Petkó and Antal 2000). Although further projection from the spinal cord to the thalamus provides an additional neural basis for conscious experience, it should be noted that at 7–8-week gestation, the thalamus is profoundly immature. At this gestation, the thalamus lacks all evidence of the cellular structure associated with the more mature thalamus (Hevner 2000; Larroche 1981). Neuroscientists are yet to fully understand the precise relationship between structure and function; however, it is evident that some relationship exists. The stark immaturity of the thalamus at 7–8 weeks casts doubt on the likelihood of the thalamus delivering a mature function, such as would be necessary to generate an experience of pain.

In addition, however, at 7–8-week gestation the cortex is almost entirely absent and there are no thalamocortical projections. Although contentious, as discussed later, most neuroscientists view the cortex as necessary for pain experience (reviewed in RCOG 2010).

The next gestational moment that has been identified as important for pain occurs at 12–18 weeks when the subplate begins to form (Ulfig et al. 2000). The subplate is a developmental structure that forms underneath the cortical plate proper from 12-week gestation. Neurons destined for the cortical plate first migrate into the subplate where they wait until the cortical plate above is sufficiently mature, and then the neurons migrate to their mature position in the cortex. At 18-week gestation, there are the first projections from the thalamus into the cortical subplate. As the neurons migrate, the subplate withers away and becomes the underlying white matter connecting cortical regions. This migration begins around 24-week gestation (Kostovic and Judas 2010).

There is evidence that the connections from the thalamus to the subplate are functional, and some have interpreted this functionality as sufficient for an experience of pain (Bhutta and Anand 2002). Similar to the immature thalamus, however, the subplate is not a mature structure. Typically, the subplate is understood as a developmental structure that is necessary for mature development (Ulfig et al. 2000). In itself, however, the subplate is not a mature structure capable of mature function such as the delivery of pain experience.

At 18-week gestation, it has been demonstrated that the fetus mounts a hormonal stress response (release of cortisol and β-endorphin) in response to noxious stimulation (Giannakoulopoulos et al. 1994). As mentioned earlier, this report largely began the current debate about fetal pain because the authors stated that "[the hormonal stress response of the fetus raises] the possibility that the human fetus feels pain in utero." That statement, however, somewhat overstated what can be inferred from a hormonal stress response. While certainly consistent with an experience of pain, increases in cortisol and β-endorphin also occur when someone is anxious, exercising, or undergoing surgery with a general anesthetic (Mellor et al. 2005). Thus, the stress response cannot be equated with pain and is better understood as a generalized response mediated by brainstem circuits.

The next gestational moment that has been identified as important for pain occurs at 24–28-week gestation. By 24-week gestation, the cortical plate proper shows clear signs of maturity (including a laminar structure), and receives direct projections from the thalamus (Kostovic and Judas 2002). In addition, experiments with very premature infants at an equivalent age of around 24-week gestation show a clear cortical response following a standard heel lance procedure (Slater et al. 2006). Thus, by around 24-week gestation, there is good evidence of a complete connection from the periphery, through the spinal cord, into the thalamus and into the cortex. And there is also good reason to consider that connection functional and able to deliver nociceptive signals. Many have interpreted this moment as the point at which fetal pain is at least possible and, more typically, probable (Lee et al. 2005; RCOG 2010). If there is any consensus on the question of fetal pain, it is that fetal pain is unlikely before 24-week gestation, but increasingly likely afterwards. A committee of clinicians, academics, and medical professionals reporting on the possibility of fetal awareness for the British Royal College of Gynecologists (RCOG) summarized this consensus position:

> In reviewing the neuroanatomical and physiological evidence in the fetus, it was apparent that connections from the periphery to the cortex are not intact before 24 weeks of gestation and, as most neuroscientists believe that the cortex is necessary for pain perception, it can be concluded that the fetus cannot experience pain in any sense prior to this gestation. (RCOG 2010).

Challenging the Neurodevelopmental Evidence

While a general consensus has emerged that fetal pain is not possible before 24-week gestation, a number of clinicians and investigators forcefully argue that fetal pain is possible well before 24 weeks (Anand 2007; Lowery et al. 2007; Merker 2007). There appear to be two dominant arguments within this position of dissent. The first is that the cortex is not necessary for pain experience and that pain can, instead, be supported by subcortical structures. The second is that observations of fetal behavior and facial expressions are sufficient to directly infer, or intuit, conscious states such as pain.

These arguments often run together. For example, Merker has reported that anencephalic infants, who survive with no, or highly minimal, cortex, go on to become infants with a clear emotional and conscious existence (Merker 2007). Merker bases his conclusion on observations of anencephalic infants who clearly laugh, show signs of upset, and generally display evidence of affective behavior. More anecdotally, obstetrician/gynecologist Stuart Campbell (personal communication) has observed the facial expressions of fetuses under 20 weeks with 4D ultrasound and claimed that the images indicate evidence of smiling and grimacing. More controlled examinations of 4D ultrasound images have provided similar, albeit more nuanced, interpretations (Reissland et al. 2011, 2013).

From these observations of apparent emotional responses, it is argued that the available underlying neural circuitry must be sufficient to support fetal experience, including fetal pain. The logic of the argument is compelling. Fetuses respond to a noxious event with a withdrawal, which at least demonstrates some capacity to detect damaging stimuli. The detection and withdrawal are dependent upon coherent activity within a signaling system, which is typically taken to be thalamic-brainstem-spinal circuitry. Although the consensus position is that the cortex is necessary for pain, there is no adequate explanation for how the cortex might directly give rise to pain. Consequently, it is difficult to explain why coherent activity within other parts of the nervous system cannot also give rise to pain. The argument is especially compelling because observation of the fetus gives a direct impression of pain; it just seems intuitively right that something akin to pain is being experienced.

The Argument from Intuition

In 1764, Voltaire issued a direct challenge to those, such as Descartes, who claimed that animals could not feel pain:

> Answer me, machinist, has nature arranged all the springs of sentiment in this animal that he should not feel? Has he nerves, and is he incapable of suffering?

Here Voltaire argues from what appears to be intuitively correct. If the animal has a nervous system and responds as if it feels, how could it be that the animal does not feel? The position Voltaire adopts is one that many spontaneously feel is self-evidently correct. A similar position is adopted by many who argue that the fetus feels pain as soon as there is evidence of a behavioral reaction, which is before 10-week gestation.

Although this argument from intuition has some purchase, there are important limitations to an argument that relies on what "feels" right. The most important limitation is precisely that assumptions made based on observation and intuition can be incorrect. Cartoon characters can be observed to "emote" and "experience" but we know that the inference is incorrect and directly manipulated by the makers of the cartoon. Formal study has demonstrated that the inference of intention and feeling can be induced for colored shapes using relatively minor animations (Hamlin et al. 2007). If such an inference can be made with fairly crude images, then it is unsurprising that exquisite 4D ultrasound images have created quite powerful inferences about the experiences of the fetus.

To answer Voltaire, the cartoonist, for sure, has precisely "arranged all the springs of sentiment" without the cartoon feeling anything. The spontaneous feeling that objects and moving images are feeling is not accepted as indicating the true feelings of objects and moving images. Interestingly, prenatal health professionals also spontaneously ascribe feelings and thoughts to their fetal patients but when directly asked about the nature of those feelings and thoughts, the intuitions about fetal experience can diminish. Consider this comment from a midwife who was asked if the fetus could feel pain:

> … it's most bizarre, now that you've asked me that question [can the fetus feel pain?], I kind of can't make the leap. (Williams 2005).

What this comment represents is a real tension between pain as a direct response to injury, which is apparently self-evident, and pain as a conscious experience, which is much less self-evident. Injury and behavior can be directly observed but experience cannot be. For older adults and infants, language is used to directly communicate experience. When used honestly, language provides an accurate portrayal of personal experience. In the absence of language, experience has to be inferred, and the process of inference is fraught with difficulty.

To summarize, direct empirical observation and intuition, either apart or combined, fail to adequately resolve whether the fetus feels pain. In light of these failings, the next section offers an alternate approach.

The Argument from "Reason"

A problem with both a pure empirical approach and an approach from intuition is the lack of any clear statement or investigation of the pain experience itself. The construct of pain is not examined and is, instead, presented as something already known and understood. The problem with such an approach is that pain can be understood as something extremely complex or something relatively straightforward. The International Association for the Study of Pain (IASP), for example, defines pain as "an unpleasant sensory and emotional experience associated with actual or potential tissue damage, or described in terms of such damage" (Merskey 1991). The definition goes on to explain that "pain is always subjective. Each individual learns the application of the word through experiences related to injury in early life." Thus the IASP definition describes pain as multidimensional and subjective. The definition also implies that pain cannot be experienced before developmental processes that occur after birth.

In contrast, Anand and Craig (1996) have criticized the IASP definition as involving more complexity than necessary for an experience of pain that might be relevant to the fetus. Thus, the fetus may have a first-order, direct and immediate, painful experience without second-order reflection and knowledge of being in pain. A fetus gripped by forceps might just be "in pain" without an explicit recognition of being in pain or knowing that "I am in pain" (Tallis 2005).

The distinction between "being that" and "knowing that" might be useful in separating the IASP definition of pain from the definition provided by Anand and Craig (1996). Being in pain implies a direct apprehension of a stimulus without any comprehension. Direct apprehension might be something attributable to a fetus but not comprehension, which would involve knowledge such as the body part being threatened, identification of the sensation (crushing or stinging, for example), and reflection on the broader implications (fear of injury or death). Direct apprehension avoids attributing a level of knowledge that is implausible for the fetus. For a fetus to experience a crushing sensation in his or her leg, for example, the fetus would need some knowledge of what it is to be crushed—the difference between compression and torque—and knowledge of separate bodily appendages. These conceptual items of knowledge, however, will not be available to the fetus and so the IASP definition of pain cannot be easily mapped onto "fetal pain."

From the above discussion, if the fetus does feel pain then it is a pain without the fear and sensory identity that is typical of pain experiences known to mature human beings. A pain without explicit localization, sensory components, and fear will, at least, lack some of the paradigmatic components of a typical pain experience (Corns 2014). Some of the negativity of pain is bound up in the threat to bodily integrity that is known to the injured subject and which cannot be easily reduced to measures of physical damage (Pustilinik, 2012). Human beings experience pain partly *through* the unpleasantness and anxiety that come from associating the outcome (a crushed limb) with concern for greater, more unpleasant outcomes (free movement, infection, death) (Derbyshire and Raja 2011).

In addition to the above limitations, it is unclear whether an "experience" of pain that is a pure immediacy and without comprehension is possible, or could ever constitute something deserving the term "experience." At any given moment, many sensory neurons will be firing in response to different pressures, lights, sounds, smells, and so forth. Think right now of the many sensory neurons firing as you hold and manipulate this book. The sensory receptors in your hands, for example, will fire as you adjust and relocate the book in your field of view. In general, however, you will not be aware of sensations associated with holding and manipulating the book. Your focus of attention, understanding, and experience will be dominated by the flow of understanding as you take in the words. Being aware of every sensation would drown out your ability to read and understand, because the cacophony of sensations would deliver a totality of being to your consciousness. You would, however, not be able to experience that totality because conscious beings experience specifics and not a totality. Human beings are "self-located" within experience. Viewing a Rothko canvas that includes 32 m of red, for example, may fill the viewer with an experience of red, but he or she will not become the experience red; they will remain self-located within the experience of red.

Some sort of conceptual apparatus is necessary to divide up the sensory world into that which fits together and requires attention, and that which can be ignored. A conceptual system that holds sensations together, *and* keeps sensations apart, seems necessary even for raw and immediate sensory experience. Such a conceptual apparatus is generally not considered to be available until sometime after birth (Hobson 2002; Vygotsky 1978).

Conclusion

Most discussion of fetal pain summarizes evidence from neuroscience. This approach is compelling and, to a point, highly persuasive. To the author's knowledge, every commentary on fetal pain accepts that a minimum nervous system is necessary for pain (Anand and Hickey 1987; Brusseau 2008; Derbyshire 2006; Lee et al. 2005; Mellor et al. 2005; Vanhatalo and van Nieuwenhuizen 2000; Van Scheltema et al. 2008). That minimum nervous system includes peripheral nerve fibers that can detect noxious stimuli, and a central nervous system that can receive input from peripheral nerve fibers. The earliest that such a system is available in the human fetus is between 8- and 12-week gestation. Consequently, it is essentially agreed that pain is not possible until the latter part of the first trimester.

After 12 weeks, however, there is an intact peripheral and central nervous system that can, at least, process noxious stimulation in some fashion. Consensus over what experience might follow from this processing becomes much less clear. The majority of neuroscientists argue that the cortex is necessary for pain and, as the cortex is not a "functional unit" and is not connected to the periphery via the thalamus before 24-week gestation, pain is not possible until the third trimester (RCOG 2010). A significant minority of neuroscientists and clinicians, however, argue that subcortical circuitry, possibly combined with activity in the cortical subplate, is sufficient for fetal pain (Anand 2007; Lowery et al. 2007; Merker 2007). Thus, these authors suggest the possibility of fetal pain from 12-week gestation with increasing certainty from 18 weeks when the first thalamocortical fibers reach the subplate (Ulfig et al. 2000).

Rejecting this minority position on neuroscientific grounds alone is difficult. There is, currently, no comprehensive account of how neural activity gives rise to pain experience or to any other experience. It remains highly uncertain exactly what neural activity means in terms of experience. Efforts to reject fetal pain on the grounds that the fetal EEG indicates "sleep" fail because it is not clear what "sleep" means for a fetus. Sleep can be described in terms of relative behavioral inactivity, reductions in electromyogram activity, changes in EEG activity, and changes in sensory and cognitive awareness (Hobson 2005). Physiological measurements of the fetus are generally consistent with the fetus being asleep but there are inconsistencies, including mobility in response to noxious stimuli, and EEG patterns that are not precisely consistent with known sleep stages (Hunter et al. 2003; Williams 2005). Most importantly, however, the very notion of "sleep" is a construction that arises largely from the subjective experience of a nightly fading consciousness combined with a loss of volitional control. All physiological measures are interpreted with reference to that construction of sleep but they do not bind or constitute sleep. Consequently, physiological recordings from the fetus cannot resolve whether the fetus is in a state of sleep or wakefulness. Fetal EEG recordings, for example, might not display patterns that are equivalent to mature states of wakefulness, but that does not mean the fetus lacks the capacity for some sort of wakefulness and, with it, some form of conscious experience, including pain (Van Scheltema et al. 2008). In essence, without a comprehensive understanding of how conscious states fall out of neural states, we have no principled position from which any fetal experience might be accepted or refuted.

Given this difficulty, some investigators and commentators have claimed that fetal experience can be accepted on intuitive grounds: there is a minimal nervous system present for the processing of noxious stimuli from at least 18-week gestation and, at the same gestation, the fetus will flinch, move away from a noxious stimulus, and show evidence of facial grimacing during noxious procedures (Reissland et al. 2011, 2013; Savell 2007; Williams 2005). When this evidence is taken together, it seems right to accept fetal pain.

The argument from intuition, however, fails for the same reason that it succeeds. When asked to rate the pain and distress of neonates under medical care, parents and health professionals can rate neonates as being "in pain" but not "in distress" (Elias et al. 2014). It is difficult to understand how a being might be in pain but not distressed. It is possible that healthcare teams make a distinction between pain in the sense of tissue damage, and pain in the sense of experience (Corns 2014). When pressed to describe pain in terms of experience, even those who work with fetuses and neonates in need of clinical care have difficulty in accepting the notion of fetal pain (Williams 2005). Thus, there may be a spontaneous intuition that fetal pain is possible but a more reflective intuition that the experience of pain imparts too much conceptual structure onto the fetus.

The lack of definitive answers from neuroscience and intuition suggests that the concerned putative parent and clinician must turn elsewhere to understand whether fetal pain is possible. Pain scientists long ago adopted a definition and understanding of pain as a multidimensional and subjective state that would appear to, *prima facie*, rule out the possibility of fetal pain (Merskey 1991). If pain is a highly abstract, conceptual, subjective experience, then fetal pain is not possible; it is implausible to attribute so much conceptual and subjective experience to the fetus.

Opposition to this understanding of pain has led to suggestions that pain experience, for the fetus and neonate, might be more immediate, raw, and relevant to the needs and processing capacity of the more immature nervous system (Anand and Craig 1996). Thus, the fetus might experience something akin to pain without the self-reflective, explicit knowledge of *being in* pain (Derbyshire and Raja 2011).

While this distinction between a raw and more knowledge-based experience of pain looks like it may be useful and true, there remain considerable difficulties in explaining how the non-conceptual mind of a fetus might grab hold of any single experience amongst the cacophony of other possible experiences. The nervous system continuously receives an abundance of sensory input that could generate any number of experiences together. Consciousness experiences a singular stream of awareness, not a totality.

On balance, it is reasonable to conclude that the fetus cannot experience pain, at least not in any equivalent way to how mature infants and adults experience pain. An immediate, fleeting, experience, even if possible, will lack the precision and associated fear and dread of a more mature pain experience.

The above conclusion may provide sufficient reassurance for many clinicians and women seeking fetal procedures that fetal pain is not something for concern. It is, however, not possible to use fetal pain to provide a definitive guide for clinical practice or legal policy regarding the fetus. The fetal patient undergoing therapeutic surgery is not the same as a more mature infant who will self-explicitly report their feelings, distinguish the experience from other experiences, and remember the events of surgery. In the absence of a subjectivity to engage and without the possibility of a subjectivity that will be retained, the clinician can focus on other, measurable and objective, indicators of well-being. Rates of surgical complication, morbidity and mortality, unlike speculation about fetal pain, can provide a definitive guide to surgical practice (Anand et al. 1987). The later good that will accrue to the fetus from the minimizing of negative surgical outcomes provides sufficient moral justification for the followed procedures.

In the case of a woman seeking a pregnancy termination, there is no life to lead after the procedure and so there is no later good that will accrue to the fetus. The pregnant woman is precisely choosing to end her pregnancy, and while she may have concerns about the well-being of her fetus, that concern is obviously bounded by the greater decision to end the life of the fetus. Currently, the law in most countries recognizes that the definite subjectivity and personhood of the woman take precedence over the highly uncertain subjectivity, and not-yet personhood, of the fetus. Arguments about whether such laws are right or wrong cannot be resolved via the discussion of fetal pain (Derbyshire 2006).

In summary, assessing the evidence for and against fetal pain is not straightforward, and cannot be resolved with neuroscience or intuition. Whether the fetus can feel pain critically depends on what is meant by "pain." For the older infant and adult, pain is a multidimensional, subjective state that cannot be plausibly experienced by the fetus. By that account, fetal pain is impossible at any stage of gestation.

The younger infant and fetus, however, may experience a rawer, more immediate, "pain" that gradually matures into the multidimensional, subjective experience of older infants and adults. Even this experience, however, is not obviously plausible without a conceptual apparatus that can, at least, isolate one sensory state from another. The need for some psychological development to experience even the most basic of states seems necessary, and rules out fetal pain at any stage of gestation.

The vexed nature of the argument about fetal pain renders it an unsuitable grounding for deciding clinical practice or policy. Instead, therapeutic surgery for the fetus can be guided by objective measures of outcomes decided in clinical trials. Policy towards termination can be guided by democratic discussion of when society thinks it is acceptable for a woman to decide that she will not continue to be pregnant.

Acknowledgments The author is grateful to Dr. Nina Powell for comments and edits of an earlier draft of this chapter.

References

Anand KJS. Consciousness, cortical function, and pain perception in non-verbal humans. Behav Brain Sci. 2007;30:82–3.

Anand KJS, Craig KD. New perspectives on the definition of pain. Pain. 1996;67:3–6.

Anand KJS, Hickey PR. Pain and its effects in the human neonate and fetus. N Engl J Med. 1987;317:1321–9.

Anand KJS, Sippel WG, Aynsley-Green A. Randomised trial of fentanyl anesthesia in preterm babies undergoing surgery: effects on the stress response. Lancet. 1987;1:243–8.

Bhutta AT, Anand KJS. Vulnerability of the developing brain: neuronal mechanisms. Clin Perinatol. 2002;29:357–72.

Brugger EC. The problem of fetal pain and abortion: towards an ethical consensus for appropriate behavior. Kennedy Inst Ethics J. 2012;3:263–87.

Brusseau R. Developmental perspectives: is the fetus conscious? Int Anesthesiol Clin. 2008; 46:11–23.

Corns J. The inadequacy of unitary characterizations of pain. Philos Stud. 2014;169:355–78.

Derbyshire SWG. Can fetuses feel pain? Br Med J. 2006;332:909–12.

Derbyshire SWG, Raja A. On the development of painful experience. J Conscious Stud. 2011;18:233–56.

Elias LSDT, Santos AMN, Guinsburg R. Perception of pain and distress in intubated and mechanically ventilated newborn infants by parents and health professionals. BMC Pediatr. 2014;14:44.

Fitzgerald M. The prenatal growth of fine diameter afferents into the rat spinal cord - a transganglionic study. J Comp Neurol. 1987;261:98–104.

Giannakoulopoulos X, Sepulveda W, Kourtis P, Glover V, Fisk NM. Fetal plasma cortisol and β-endorphin response to intrauterine needling. Lancet. 1994;344:77–81.

Hamlin JK, Wynn K, Bloom P. Social evaluation by preverbal infants. Nature. 2007;450:557–60.

Hevner RF. Development of connections in the human visual system during fetal mid-gestation: a DiI-tracing study. J Neuropathol Exp Neurol. 2000;59:385–92.

Hobson JA. Sleep is of the brain, by the brain and for the brain. Nature. 2005;437:1254–6.

Hobson P. The cradle of thought: exploring the origins of thinking. London: Macmillan; 2002.

Humphrey T. Some correlations between the appearance of human fetal reflexes and the development of the nervous system. Prog Brain Res. 1964;4:93–135.

Hunter CJ, Bennet L, Power GG, Roelfsema V, Blood AB, Quaedackers JS, et al. Key neuroprotective role for endogenous adenosine A1 receptor activation during asphyxia in the fetal sheep. Stroke. 2003;34:2240–5.
Kostovic I, Judas M. Correlation between the sequential ingrowth of afferents and transient patterns of cortical lamination in preterm infants. Anat Rec. 2002;267:1–6.
Kostovic I, Judas M. The development of the subplate and thalamocortical connections in the human foetal brain. Acta Paeditrica. 2010;99:1119–27.
Larroche JC. The marginal layer in the neocortex of a 7 week-old human embryo: a light and electron microscopic study. Anat Embryol.1981;162:301–12.
Lee SJ, Ralston HJP, Drey EA, Partridge JC, Rosen MA. Fetal pain: a systematic multidisciplinary review of the evidence. JAMA. 2005;294:947–54.
Lowery CL, Hardman MP, Manning N, Hall RW, Anand KJS. Neurodevelopmental changes of fetal pain. Semin Perinatol. 2007;31:275–82.
Mellor DJ, Diesch TJ, Gunn AJ, Bennet L. The importance of 'awareness' for understanding fetal pain. Brain Res Rev. 2005;49:455–71.
Merker B. Consciousness without a cerebral cortex: a challenge for neuroscience and medicine. Behav Brain Sci. 2007;30:63–81.
Merskey H. The definition of pain. Eur Psychiatry. 1991;6:153–9.
Nofzinger EA, Derbyshire SWG. Pain imaging in relation to sleep. In: Lavigne G, Sessle BJ, Choiniere M, Soja PJ, editors. Sleep and pain. Seattle, WA: IASP Press; 2007. p. 153–73.
Petkó M, Antal M. Propriospinal afferent and efferent connections of the lateral and medial subdivisions of the dorsal horn (laminae I-IV) in the rat lumbar spinal cord. J Comp Neurol. 2000;422:312–25.
Pustilnik AC. Pain as fact and heuristic: how pain neuroimaging illuminates moral dimensions of law. Cornell L Rev. 2012;97:801–47.
Reissland N, Francis B, Mason J, Lincoln K. Do facial expressions develop before birth? PLoS One. 2011;6:e24081.
Reissland N, Francis B, Mason J. Can healthy fetuses show facial expressions of "pain" or "distress"? PLoS One. 2013;8:e65530.
Royal College of Obstetricians and Gynaecologists (RCOG). Fetal awareness review of research and recommendations for practice: report of a working party. London: RCOG Press; 2010.
Savell K. Life and death before birth: 4D ultrasound and the shifting frontiers of the abortion debate. J Lipid Mediat. 2007;15:103–16.
Slater R, Cantarella A, Gallella S, Worley A, Boyd S, Meek J, Fitzgerald M. Cortical pain responses in human infants. J Neurosci. 2006;26:3662–6.
Tallis R. The knowing animal: a philosophical inquiry into knowledge and truth. Edinburgh: Edinburgh University Press; 2005.
Ulfig N, Neudorfer F, Bohl J. Transient structures of the human fetal brain: subplate, thalamic reticular complex, ganglionic eminence. Histol Histopathol. 2000;15:771–90.
Wang X, Inui K, Qiu Y, Kakigi R. Cortical responses to noxious stimuli during sleep. Neuroscience. 2004;128:177–86.
Weerd AW, Bossche AS. The development of sleep during the first few months of life. Sleep Med Rev. 2003;7:179–91.
Williams C. Framing the fetus in medical work: rituals and practices. Soc Sci Med. 2005; 60:2085–95.
Vanhatalo S, van Nieuwenhuizen O. Fetal pain? Brain Dev. 2000;22:145–50.
Van Scheltema PNA, Bakker S, Vandenbussche FPHA, Oepkes D. Fetal pain. Fetal Maternal Med Rev. 2008;19:311–24.
Vygotsky LS. Mind in society: the development of higher psychological processes. Cambridge, MA: Harvard University Press; 1978.

Chapter 7
Giving Bad and Ambiguous News

Joan G. Lalor

Introduction

This chapter is a fusion of knowledge gained from my lengthy experience as a clinical midwife, sonographer and subsequently as a researcher. During the 20 years of these interconnected activities I have often imparted the news to parents that there is a problem with their fetus. I have witnessed the psychological impact and aftermath of the traumatic loss that results from a prenatal diagnosis of a fetal abnormality. Initially, when I began my work in obstetric and gynecological ultrasound, my chief concern was the accuracy of the diagnosis, and my main fear was that I might miss something. However, it soon became apparent that the impact of *what* I was saying, and *how* I was saying it, should have primacy. Although the evidence I present in this chapter is based on extensive research with women and their male partners following a diagnosis of fetal abnormality, my understanding of parental reactions is influenced by the work of eminent scholars such as (but not limited to) Barbara Katz Rothman, Rayna Rapp, Faye Ginsburg, Monica Casper, Lynn Morgan and Meredith Wilson Michaels, Gail Landsman, Richard Lazarus and Susan Folkman, Ronnie Janoff-Bulman, Bob Neimeyer, and Colin Murray-Parkes.

My early research focussed on whether women were fully and accurately informed regarding the capability and limitations of second-trimester ultrasound (Lalor and Devane 2007). More than 460 women at a tertiary referral site were surveyed. The findings demonstrated that women received little information regarding the limitations of ultrasound, and that their expectations exceeded the capability of the examination. However, each of the women who responded indicated that they were concerned with fetal health and that from their perspective a reassuring

J.G. Lalor, Ph.D. (✉)
Trinity College Dublin, School of Nursing and Midwifery,
24 D'Olier Street, Dublin 2, Ireland
e-mail: j.lalor@tcd.ie

J.P. Galst, M.S. Verp (eds.), *Prenatal and Preimplantation Diagnosis*,
DOI 10.1007/978-3-319-18911-6_7

ultrasound result equated with confirmation of fetal normality (Lalor and Devane 2007). Although women were aware that a fetal anomaly could be uncovered, none expected to be the recipient of such devastating news.

In order to develop an understanding of the emotional impact of an adverse diagnosis and the process of adaptation, I began a longitudinal study of women's experiences of carrying a fetus with an abnormality from diagnosis up to and beyond the birth (Lalor et al. 2009). This research was designed to determine the best practices in caring for women after diagnosis, irrespective of the type of anomaly detected, likely prognosis, or outcome of the pregnancy. The suggestions I offer here are based on the empirical findings from that study and my ongoing work in this area.

The Technological Determination of Fetal Normality or Abnormality

Because some women participating in routine ultrasound screening programs will inevitably be faced with an adverse finding, it has been recommended by many that detailed information regarding ultrasound should be given to women before examination (Rapp 1999). Research has demonstrated that the provision of both written and verbal information in relation to routine ultrasound in pregnancy is limited, yet uptake rates for ultrasound screening programs are almost 100 % (Campbell and Smith 1983; Katz Rothman 1988; Lalor and Begley 2006; Lalor et al. 2006, 2007). Women who are offered routine ultrasound frequently see the examination as non-threatening and may perceive it as a social event (Proud 1985). By understanding why this is the case we, as practitioners, can learn how to impart bad or ambiguous news sensitively and responsively.

The last 25 years have witnessed significant advances in prenatal screening, yet much of this progress has occurred in the area of technology. The concept of the fetal "patient" has emerged as in utero interventions and fetal surgical techniques have developed and continue to develop, while the boundaries of fetal survival at earlier gestations are pushed back through advances in neonatal intensive care. In comparison, how women and couples react to and cope with the diagnosis of fetal abnormality has received relatively little attention. In order to appreciate the impact of our words and actions as we convey the diagnosis to parents, we must understand why parents are shocked and how they cope with the repercussions for the pregnancy and for their dreams of their future family.

The Assumption of Normality

The importance of providing information to women before they are scanned has been debated (Kolker 1989), and the evidence demonstrates that in spite of variations in the level of pre-ultrasound information, women still remain unprepared for the diagnosis of an abnormality. This is in stark contrast to experiences with other forms of screening (mammography, MRI, CT scanning) where concerns regarding the test are associated with the probability of an adverse outcome. Routine ultrasound screening in pregnancy represents an example of the newer paradigm of surveillance medicine whereby normal populations are screened for an illness that has not manifested itself in the identification of risk factors (Statham et al. 1997). This blurring of traditional boundaries between health and illness is evident in women's experiences, as ultrasound has been "normalized" in pregnancy to just another aspect of routine antenatal care. The feminist argument that routine scanning promoted medical over maternal expertise (Hyde 1986; Lalor and Devane 2007; Statham et al. 1997) that was evident in women's accounts of their attitudes to scanning 20 years ago (Eurenius et al. 1997) is no longer a dominant feature. Screening has become an integral part of women's experience of pregnancy and ultrasound is now seen as a necessary source of reassurance. As almost all pregnant women currently experience the procedure, the anxiety that is associated with ultrasound has moved from that related to participation in screening into the possibility of non-reassuring results. Women without a family history of birth defects anticipate that their fetus will be healthy and do not perceive themselves to be at risk for a fetal anomaly. When ultrasound is mentioned to couples by friends or family it is in a positive context. Proud parents commonly exhibit ultrasound photos with pride (Baillie and Hewison 1999), and this is reflective of the social aspect that routine ultrasound has acquired (Larsen et al. 2000). The influence of ultrasound on parental emotional well-being is strong (Lalor 2000) and many parents have stated that their pre-ultrasound discussion in the waiting room was dominated more often by a debate as to whether to learn the fetal gender rather than by a heightened concern for fetal well-being. Why do couples hold such a firm belief that the scan will be reassuring?

Colin Murray Parkes (1971, 1988) developed the construct of the "assumptive world," and suggests that this construct is the ordering principle for the psychological and psychosocial construction of the human world. He defines it in terms of "the only world we know and it includes everything we know or think we know. It includes our interpretation of the past and our own expectation of the future, our plans and our prejudices" (Parkes 1971, p. 102). Parents experience natural excitement and anticipation at seeing their baby on screen (Ekelin et al. 2004; Eurenius et al. 1997; Lalor 2000), which frequently overrides any concerns raised by explicit pre-scan information on what *might* go wrong. Over the last 20 years I have heard repeatedly women's constructions of the normative constancy, experience of, and belief that pregnancy almost always culminates in the birth of a healthy baby (Lalor et al. 2009). A diagnosis of fetal anomaly is an unexpected event for the majority, shattering the couples' hopes and expectations of pregnancy and parenthood (Janoff-Bulman 1992). How clinicians communicate with women when conveying and confirming the diagnosis is critical to this process, as the repercussions of a negative encounter extend beyond the diagnosis or even beyond the death of the fetus or neonate. This form of ambiguous loss is complex, at times irrevocable and without closure, as the dream of a perfect child is lost. From the moment the sonographer detects an abnormal finding, interactions between caregivers and parents are intensified, and *what* is said and *how* it is said become central as couples attempt to cope and adapt to an unforeseen and frequently unpredictable future.

There are several key differences between giving bad or ambiguous news as a consequence of a routine prenatal ultrasound examination compared with such news in other health care settings. Firstly and most importantly, parents expect a normal result. As the anomaly is visualized while the examination is in progress, there is little time for the sonographer (a stranger to the parents) to prepare to deliver this devastating news. It is not unusual for multiparous women who have previously had a normal outcome to attend the examination either unaccompanied by their partner or with a young child. This adds to the challenge of preparing parents for hearing that all is not as expected.

Shocking News and Shattered Assumptions

The social role of obstetric ultrasound and parental reactions to the images obtained are often more complex than foreseen. As image quality improves, the technologically mediated representation of the fetus gives parents an impression of fetal maturity incongruent with gestational age, raising expectations of the treatment possibilities available and reinforcing the image of the *child* to be (RCOG 1997).

> *If you had seen the baby it was like she was ready to be born … turning around and scratching her neck, God how could anything be wrong with this child?*

It is precisely because ultrasound is a technology of visualization that couples may recognize either that the image on the screen is abnormal or that the ultrasonographer is focused particularly on one fetal part. The sense of alarm may be heightened by subtle changes in the ultrasonographer's behavior:

> *Me and my husband went in all excited and the midwife was pointing out all the bits, but she started to focus on the head. She was getting more serious, she was measuring and measuring, she measured the same thing a number of times. Then she brought in another midwife and they were printing pictures, the head looked a bit big, they didn't like the look of it but they couldn't tell us anymore than that, I knew it was all going wrong.*

Once a deviation from normal is identified, the process of breaking the news to parents begins.

> *They* [*radiographers*] *told us absolutely nothing … it left us a little bit more frightened, you know not knowing, saying nothing and standing scanning, looking very worried. I mean, you're there and you're thinking what is it, what's wrong? You're looking at someone's face and I remember looking at her and she looked so worried.*

It is at this point in the care pathway that a sense of trust or mistrust in the clinical team can be sealed. In order to maximize the development of a trusting relationship it is critical that clinicians recognize and understand different coping styles. Recognizing cues in parents' initial reactions can guide clinicians to tailor information in a way that will improve couples' experiences of their interactions with caregivers, and reduce occurrences of suboptimal care. Consequently, as the picture of the abnormality is emerging it may be useful to consider the following issues before delivering the news:

- *Is the diagnosis clear-cut? Is the anomaly isolated or are there multiple anomalies?*
- *Is it likely that further testing such as amniocentesis will be required?*
- *Do I have access to a fetal medicine specialist immediately, and if not, when might a second opinion be arranged?*
- *What words should I use?*
- *What is this woman's coping style and information preference?*

The Importance of Recognizing Coping Styles When Informing Couples of an Adverse Finding

Both clinicians and members of the public may be ignorant of the diversity of meaning that individuals attribute to the loss of a "normal" child and the extent to which the threat of such a loss can be simultaneously paralyzing, chaotic, and emotionally overwhelming. In order to best respond to parents trying to come to terms with what is a very traumatic experience, it is necessary to consider how individuals process information during times of distress. Horowitz (1992, p. 92) has suggested that when experiencing a traumatic event, there is a need to "*match new information with inner models based on older information and the revision of both until they agree*." At times this reconciliation can be so excruciating as to interrupt information processing temporarily (information avoidance), while for others there is an attempt to reduce the threat and control their fear through seeking information to clarify the situation or solve the problem.

Miller and Mangan (Miller 1980; Miller and Mangan 1983) have described two primary approaches undertaken by people facing stressful health-related situations. "*Monitors*" are those that seek out information, monitor the threat, and require a high level of detail as they seek to understand the implications of the news while simultaneously trying to evaluate the level of the threat. In contrast, "*Blunters*" have a low preference for information and may appear to avoid engagement with the issues until confirmation of the anomaly is received from the fetal medicine specialist or obstetrician/gynecologist.

Once a concern is raised, *monitors* frequently ask a series of rapidly fired questions as they endeavor to find a solution to the problem. Women and men who exhibit monitoring-type behavior need to have control over the situation in order to cope with what they are being told, and see information as the key to regaining that control. This behavior may also re-emerge later in the pregnancy if a new variable is introduced into the situation such as a change in the fetal condition or the discovery of an additional anomaly or variant, regardless of the impact that this new variable might have on the predicted outcome. This need for control in a stressful situation has been previously described as a problem-focused approach to coping, where the focus is to manage the problem and minimize the distress (Lazarus and Launier 1978).

How to Recognize and Respond to Parents Using Problem-Focused Coping Strategies (Monitors)

In most cases parents are utterly unprepared for bad news and irrespective of their coping strategy may take a few moments to process that the information you are giving actually relates to their baby:

> *I just would not have expected it to happen to me. It happens to someone else and you feel just so awful for them but it doesn't happen to me. I think you know, up to this point in my life I have been quite, quite lucky. Nothing really bad has happened to me … so you just think that is someone else's life, not mine.*

Honesty in the context of uncertainty is critical. Monitors will often ask questions such as: *What is it*? *Why me*? *Did I do anything to cause it*? *Could I have prevented it*? *What will happen to the baby in the womb*? *What will happen to the baby during the birth*? *What can you do to fix this*? *What is the treatment*? *Will I need a caesarean section*? Couples with a high preference for information frequently find it particularly difficult to cope when the diagnosis is uncertain. They may even perceive, albeit erroneously, that information is being withheld, leading to a sense of mistrust in the treating clinician. Consequently, these couples are less likely to develop a sense of mistrust when they are informed that further testing is required to reach a "certain" diagnosis. However, there are times when the diagnosis is unequivocal, such as anencephaly. In such situations and when parents are exhibiting monitoring behavior, revealing the diagnosis in full and without delay is the most appropriate approach. At other times, ultrasound alone is not sufficient for a definitive diagnosis; for example, on many occasions a structural anomaly may be associated with a chromosomal disorder. In situations such as this, parents exhibiting a preference for high levels of information still prefer the clinician to reveal what is known:

> *This is not good news …. They were quite clear, which was a good thing; they booked an appointment for the consultant later that day. I said* [*looking at the screen*] *that doesn't look right … she* [*midwife*] *told us there was a hole in the heart … we needed to have an amniocentesis to confirm if there was something else or worse wrong but at least we knew.*

Having spoken to many colleagues over the years, some have expressed concern that while waiting for confirmation there is a hesitance to commit to a diagnosis. For women and men who adopt a problem-solving approach to coping, honesty in uncertainty is critical. If the anomaly is complex or ambiguous and the prognosis is not clear this should be clearly explained to the parents. Being honest in the context of uncertainty is not the same as withholding information. Although withholding information may not be a deliberate act, it may be perceived as such if, before the clinician is ready to reveal the news, the woman has noticed a change in the clinician's body language and facial expression, or that the examination seems particularly focused on one fetal part. Although a staged approach to revealing information to parents exhibiting information avoidance behaviors may be appropriate, any perceived difficulty in accessing information quickly can add to a *monitor's* distress.

> *She told us it was bad … things were not what she was expecting … but I would need more facts* [*than that*] *…I was trying to find out what about the other organs, was there something else* [*affected*]*, where was this coming from, where was it originating from, but she* [*the midwife*] *couldn't answer all the questions … now I wasn't leaving there that day without seeing* [*the consultant*]*. I was asking her loads of questions. But straight away my reaction was 'right, tell me what is going on'.*

Failing to respond to requests for information leads to further distress as it is incongruent with a problem-focused coping strategy. As *monitors* require a high and detailed level of disclosure, difficulties experienced accessing information from clinicians can lead to mistrust and anxiety. Statham et al. (2003) have previously cautioned against making the assumption that parental reactions will vary in accordance with the relative severity of the anomaly.

> *I suppose you are a bit taken aback when you are not expecting anything. Then I suppose if it's something you are familiar with, the language is very difficult isn't it? She said like a club foot but we said what is a club foot? But she didn't have any more information in leaflet or oral form to give me on it. I didn't feel that she was definitely able to tell me. I felt she should have been able to explain to me what it was so that I knew what I was dealing with. We did ask I think we asked several questions and we got a bit of information but not much. I think we felt we would just go and find out ourselves. I think if I had been able to ask the questions and get the information, it's just not knowing, that's the worst … I just felt if you are going to tell people, I know there are a lot of different things that could be wrong but they should have leaflets available to explain to you*

Needless to say there are risks associated with concluding the consultation when parents still feel that they are not fully informed. Many will turn to the Internet to try and fill the information deficit but, unfortunately, many of the sites accessed are not subjected to critical appraisal by health professionals.

> *If I had been told even in passing don't be alarmed by what you read on it. I have seen some horrific stuff on the internet I actually feel now that the information should be available quicker. The internet is a very dangerous tool. The diagnosis of polycystic was absolutely horrific on the net, it was like more or less death and you know, even though we had been told the other kidney looked okay.*

From my many years of experience in the field, I would suggest that parents need to be given written information that points them towards reliable websites, and they should be forewarned that what may be an isolated anomaly (such as talipes) can also be associated with more serious outcomes, such as trisomy 18. Parents need to be made aware in no uncertain terms if the more serious anomaly is being considered in their case.

Although couples with a high need for information often find it difficult to cope with uncertainty, not all women will confront the problem when suspicions of an abnormality are first raised.

How to Recognize and Respond to Parents Using Emotion-Focused Coping Strategies (Blunters)

In contrast to a problem-solving approach, "*Blunters*" avoid information that may result in increasing anxiety. Women who adopt blunting strategies continue to avoid seeking information regarding the fetal condition, particularly when it is of a negative nature. This coping process has been described as emotion focused (Folkman and Lazarus 1980), and the authors suggest that this behavior manifests more often in circumstances that are appraised as unchangeable. Although outright cognitive avoidance of the reality that a problem could be present is unlikely, some will defer engagement with the problem until it has been confirmed by a second party. This strategy is likely employed to protect oneself from overwhelming emotions (Landsman 2002).

> *We could see everything, which is why we were so shocked; we were in there for an awful long time … And she [radiographer] was there just like checking everything, and mm … you still don't think that she is going to say to you that something is there, I just thought they were being extra thorough. And then she just said to me eh …. she saw a little abnormality with the heart and she asked me would I ring the hospital at 8.30 in the morning to get an appointment with [FMS]. But she didn't go into much detail either she just said she could see abnormalities … so I said to myself whatever the problem is he is obviously moving around in there so he is not too bad. She [radiographer] didn't really say what was wrong, I thought I would get to the fetal medicine expert and they would say it's all a mistake, after all they have better machines … they can see more.*

Couples exhibiting *blunting* strategies have the potential to become overwhelmed in the face of distressing information. These parents often don't ask any questions in response to hearing that a problem has been detected, or may ask in spite of what is said if everything will be all right. It is not unusual for a woman using this coping strategy to climb off the examination table hurriedly and even seek to end the consultation abruptly. Some will become very distressed, crying uncontrollably, whereas others may become almost frozen in fear, seemingly unable to hear anything else that is said. This does not imply that they have not understood what is conveyed but rather that once they have been told that all is not well, there is a limit to the amount of negative information that can be processed at that moment. Women who adopt blunting strategies may continue to avoid information regarding the fetal condition, particularly when it is of a negative nature.

Women exhibiting this coping process require more positive information about the fetus, such as pointing out what is normal about the baby, or highlighting fetal growth or movement even when the fetal condition and prognosis remain grave. One's approach to information processing can be viewed in terms of the pace at which one attempts to adjust to negative information and the extent to which one tries to regain control over events. Some clinicians struggle with the notion of offering positive comments about fetal well-being when the situation is dire. I have had conversations with colleagues who have expressed concern that when women seek positive information about the fetus, it may indicate that the woman has failed to understand or accept that fetal mortality is probable. However, when women are using information avoidance strategies as a coping mechanism, a continued focus exclusively on the negative will result in added distress. The imperative to ensure that patients are fully informed may have emerged from ethical obligations related to full disclosure and patient autonomy. However, if patient autonomy requires full disclosure in all circumstances, other principles such as beneficence and non-maleficence are ignored. Cognizance of the relative certainties and uncertainties of prenatal diagnoses requires discretion, as much harm can be done by delivering bad news in a manner perceived as cold and factual and in a way that fails to acknowledge the impact of the news. Breaking bad news in a prenatal context requires compassion, sensitivity, emotional intelligence, and a commitment to support the couple after the diagnosis has been revealed.

Referral for an Expert Opinion: Expectations of the Consultation

Waiting for important news is not an easy experience, and waiting for information on fetal well-being presents added challenges due to the potentially life-changing implications of the diagnostic, prognostic, or risk information about to be revealed. Irrespective of the information preference exhibited, it is critically important that follow-up with a fetal medicine specialist or equivalent (e.g., obstetrician-geneticist, neonatologist) is arranged speedily. It is my experience that "*monitors*" in particular value the second consultation as soon as possible and preferably the same day. However, irrespective of the information preference demonstrated, all couples prefer for that follow-up to be arranged within 24 h. Given that a same-day appointment with a fetal medicine specialist cannot always be provided, women were asked if there were any alternative strategies that might provide support during this particularly difficult time of uncertainty.

> *Give us written information on the problem, it would sort out things, rather than have us looking at websites, … just to be able to take it away would help.*

Some have suggested that clinic policies ought to ensure that, in so far as is practicable, women should be given a name and description of the diagnosis before leaving the unit (Mitchell 2004). Empirical evidence from previous studies (Lalor et al. 2007, 2008, 2009) indicates that having a name for the condition assists those using "*monitoring*" strategies to search for information in a more targeted way that is less likely to reveal incorrect diagnoses. Many using "*blunting*" strategies suggested that having written information would have afforded them the opportunity to review at their own pace what they had been told during the examination. Information from the initial scan may assist in formulating relevant questions for the fetal medicine specialist. This is critically important for those using emotion-focused coping strategies, as they risk becoming emotionally overwhelmed again as the diagnosis unfolds at the second consultation.

> *So it was just up to me to keep it together now, ask your questions, see what you can find out … nobody will talk to you if you're crying.*

Ambiguous Diagnosis: A Pandora's Box of Possibilities

Couples commonly express concern that the diagnosis of a treatable anomaly is not quite as definitive as clinicians first believe and may in fact resemble Pandora's box. Women using a problem-focused approach to coping have stated that opening this box with the diagnosis of one treatable abnormality could herald the discovery of increasingly serious anomalies at future ultrasound examinations, obliterating the hope of a healthy or "near" healthy child.

> *It's not just the condition … it's is there anything else or is it worse than they think it is.*

Women with a preference for information avoidance may prefer "*to cross that bridge when they come to it*." Understanding parental fear of the disclosure of further anomalies can assist clinicians in understanding what seems like an overreaction to the diagnosis of a seemingly minor or treatable anomaly.

The Five Horsemen of Trusting Relationships: How Environments Can Foster Trust or Mistrust

The initial interaction with the specialist shapes the development of the relationship between the woman and her caregivers for the remainder of the pregnancy and beyond.

Honesty and sensitivity are key components in the development of a trusting relationship.

> *I wanted to know what was the bottom line, but when they [fetal medicine team] told me … there was all kinds of pain, they were really good, good bedside manners, they had been very direct about the whole thing.*

> *We just wanted the facts and exactly what the problem was. He [FMS] went quite quiet and you know his hand kind of went up to his mouth while he was looking. We were very, we were anxious, nervous. I think I was being hopeful that everything was okay. We saw him focusing on the hands and feet; we had read that if it's a chromosome abnormality it will affect the development of the limbs. He was saying he thought he saw a hand kind of folded up like this [make a clenched fist with her hand]. I thought the feet looked funny even though he didn't say anything. But he had got a picture of the feet and I thought why they are pointing in like that although nothing was said about it and I didn't ask. So we said what do you think it is? and he said I think it's chromosomal. At that point I got very upset and he was very kind to us.*

> *I can remember it was pretty devastating. Mm I was in a room in [fetal medicine unit] and I called him [partner to give him the news] and he [FMS] had just gave me some privacy to make the call. By the time he got back the water works had started and everything, and you know he was very nice and he asked me was I okay and everything else. But mm he asked me how I was getting home.*

Couples are particularly appreciative of acknowledgement of the human tragedy that is an adverse prenatal diagnosis.

> *I felt they cared- I wasn't just another interesting science project, they said we know this is very disappointing for us- focusing in on the emotional.*

> *It was extremely difficult for him to tell us this news … clearly bad results happen fairly often and doctors have to give bad news, but I think it was nice, after all we were losing our baby.*

However, institutional procedures that limit sonographers' interaction with the patient or individual sonographers' personal lack of confidence in breaking bad news is problematic for couples, and can lead to a sense of mistrust that may start at the initial scan (Mitchell 2004). Partial disclosure (seen by couples as antithetical to honesty) during the examination leaves couples feeling frustrated; many have described the worry of *not knowing* as worse than the truth.

> *So then she scanned me* [radiographer]*, and then a doctor* [radiologist] *came in and he just basically pointed out the problem to her and then he walked back out again, there was no talking. I said is there something wrong? She said I can't read it … I think if I had been able to ask the questions and get the information, it's just not knowing what you are thinking about and that's the worst.*

When couples ask questions during the examination and clinicians fail to respond, parents are left feeling that the clinician is insensitive to their need for information. The sonographer's discomfort at breaking bad news may be reflected in a falsely optimistic prognosis. If couples feel that they have been misled, regardless of the intention, it can foster feelings of mistrust, complicating future interactions with staff.

> *She said* [radiographer] *here is a bit of fluid around the brain … you see kids with hydrocephalus and a lot of them have been coming back to us and the child is perfect. I'm going down to the doctor just to check, she just walked out. She* [the obstetrician] *didn't even come up to look at it, just yeah there's water on the brain and I'm sending you to the fetal medicine expert.*

If *partial disclosure* is inevitable based on local unit policies, then same-day referral to an expert becomes even more critical as the wait for further information can be unbearable.

> *I lost my child for about four days* [until I met the fetal medicine specialist] *and it was like a big black cloud and you wake up in the morning and you think I can't get out of this.*

Couples exhibit a range of emotional reactions in response to the shock such as crying, disbelief, and fear, as they attempt to come to terms with the apparent randomness of this traumatic event. Any tendency to delay appointments with the fetal medicine specialist on the basis that couples are too shocked to process additional information is to be discouraged. Couples have high expectations of the consultation with the specialist in terms of certainty of diagnosis. This may be particularly problematic when the diagnosis remains uncertain. When couples are given the name of a particular specialist often referred to as the "expert," they expect to meet him/her rather than a substitute clinician at the consultation. The need to meet the named person is likely to represent an attempt at maintaining some level of control in an otherwise uncertain context. The anxiety associated with seeking confirmation by the diagnosis and understanding the significance of the abnormality is influenced by level of disclosure/confusion associated with the initial scan, time waiting for the consultation, access to information prior to the appointment, and level of pre-consultation professional support from the referring clinician (midwife/obstetrician/radiographer).

Acknowledgement of the human tragedy that is the loss of a healthy baby is of paramount importance from the point at which suspicions are raised, as clinician sensitivity is highly valued by couples. It is not uncommon for women to try to control their emotional reaction to the loss in order to access information regarding the diagnosis. Specialist fetal medicine units are also training sites for residents and fellows in fetal medicine, and consequently, it is likely that a trainee will attend the high-risk clinic. In some units it may be customary for the trainee to perform an initial assessment/diagnosis, which is subsequently confirmed with a follow-up examination by the specialist. One woman describes how having waited 24 h for her appointment, the urgency to access information regarding the fetal outcome became so acute that she couldn't cope with this process.

> *He* [*FMS*] *said I am going to let* [*SPR*] *have a look first, do a scan. I am going to go away and then I will come back and I will have a look and we will talk to each other and see if we see the same things because I want to be objective and that was fine, you know. We had no problem with that. I just started crying and* [*fellow in fetal medicine*] *said what is wrong and I just said I don't know what I am going to hear today. I just, I knew things were going to be bad. I didn't know what they were going to tell me next, I really didn't. It was panic and fear I think. So actually the midwife went and said look we will get him back in now because I think I had waited long enough, we had a bad night, I just couldn't wait any longer, you know. She* [*fellow*] *was trying to say things mightn't be as bad, but we knew there wasn't going to be a positive outcome. Then* [*FMS*] *came in and gave it to us between the eyes … blunt, that is what you want straight talking, we were here to get the truth.*

When asked how she felt about the initial reassurance she replied:

> *A bit resentful, yeah we are not here for that, we are here to get the truth, you know. We are here to be told exactly what you as a professional think about this and not pat my hand.*

It goes without saying that the training needs of the fellow in fetal medicine should not be prioritized above the needs of the couple to get a diagnosis and prognosis about the pregnancy. Unfortunately I have spoken with women who have reported feeling that they had been treated like a "science project" when the trainee focused on the disease process associated with the fetal condition, rather than on the tragedy associated with the loss of a healthy baby.

> *Is it going to die? Is it going to have lifelong problems? … I found it difficult to get information from her* [*trainee*] *she was there to get her own information; I felt I was intruding on what she was doing, I felt like a science experiment, something of interest.*

Although one would hope that experiences similar to the one outlined above are rare, women do acknowledge the need for training. The trainee will be accepted as part of the team once properly introduced. Women in general have no difficulty with providing trainees with an opportunity to learn, but prefer to meet them at subsequent examinations, not at the first meeting with the specialist.

Straight Talking: With Carefully Chosen Words

As with many aspects of health care, the terminology used is frequently not that which is commonly used in everyday conversation, and many women comment on the inaccessibility of technical language or medical jargon.

10% mortality, it didn't register with me, now a 1 in 10 chance your baby could die is high … you need to know to prepare.

Survival in the long-term may mean something to a medical practitioner, it doesn't mean anything to me … in accounting terms it's more than five years.

Women have described how, in the first hours after the initial scan, they became preoccupied with working through an endless list of worst-case scenarios. Consequently, at the time of the first meeting with the fetal medicine specialist, critical information regarding the anomaly and the outcome needs to be clear, using language common in everyday conversation. Even when medical terminology is avoided, many women have indicated that further explanation through the use of a combination of fetal ultrasound images, percentile charts, and diagrams can help them to grasp a basic understanding of what seems incomprehensible (Drugen et al. 1990).

They [fetal medicine team] showed us the back of the baby's head, the skull hadn't formed right and we could see it on the screen.

I had never heard of it [Triploidy] … they sat me at the computer [showed me the measurements], it made things quite clear.

He drew a diagram and showed me the valve, drew a diagram with a regular valve and showed me that this valve wasn't free flowing.

It is also important that couples are afforded the time to ask questions while acknowledging that many of their queries often emerge after they leave the hospital. This time with the fetal medicine team is very precious to parents, and, ideally, clinicians should ensure that they are not disturbed by cell phones or pagers. Assimilating information when under enormous stress is challenging, and couples may not retain all that they have heard. In addition, they may not have time to ask all the questions that they intended to; consequently, it is important that access to a named contact person between scheduled appointments is arranged.

Look you are going to have some questions when you go home, you can ring me or the midwife tomorrow and he [FMS] circled his number and said that is no problem to contact him … Come in anytime, the amount of times I was handed paper with the number on it, it was great. I've always felt the doors are wide open.

As fetal medicine consultants are not always available, the nurse/midwife may in fact be best placed to offer ongoing support between appointments.

After that scan the midwife, the midwife I must say was very nice and she, the fact that she was caring and understanding made a hell of a difference like, she was worried about what she was telling me like, you could see that in her face like, she didn't just say that's it and away you go like, no she was very nice and she gave us her name and her number and she told us to ring her, you know after, to, ring her with any other questions.

Receiving contact from members of the fetal medicine team between clinic appointments was viewed by women as an acknowledgement of the awfulness of the news they had just been given, and this contact made women feel as though they weren't forgotten as soon as they had left the unit.

A relationship had built up, they knew where we were at, it wasn't that we had to tell our story to strangers each time.

Being with the one person just gives you a lot of confidence in them, you feel there is more support going to one person and you know its such a big hospital and so many midwives, it has been very good that she [midwife] has been there when we come in because if we had to go to different ones it would be really hard.

For couples that cope as a "unit" (Morgan et al. 2005) inclusion of the partner in the conversation is essential. These couples present themselves as a unit, representing both the collectiveness and individuality of how they reacted to this loss. This process of merging strengths has been identified as a coping strategy used by couples in other traumatic health care situations (Morgan et al. 2005).

Speaking to both of us, both of us are dealing with this … there was one midwife who didn't include him [husband] at all, which added to the upset.

Situations exist, however, where couples are dissatisfied with the consultation with the fetal medicine specialist.

The fetal medicine specialist said it was a multi cystic kidney and then threw in an association with a chromosome disorder … but he wasn't facing me. Edward's disease and it would be fatal, they could do an amniocentesis if we wanted. Now that whole conversation went very fast and he never looked at me face to face.

Couples may also express dissatisfaction with the perceived insensitivity of the specialist delivering the news. This can be exacerbated if they also receive insufficient detail regarding the prognosis or treatment available as quickly as they would have wished. Consequently, in the short time available the clinician also needs to try and identify if there is a high or low preference for information. Asking simple questions such as the following can assist the clinician in this determination:

- *When faced with making a decision, do you focus on every little detail or just focus on the main point*?

- *If you were undergoing a medical procedure, would you want to know if it was going to hurt in advance?*
- *If your doctor ordered a medical procedure, would you question if it is the best test for you or if there is an alternative?*
- *When you hear something upsetting, do you seek further detail, or prefer to think about pleasant things to distract yourself or try to find a way to end the conversation?*

Although much of the focus on how to communicate an adverse diagnosis is centered on serious or lethal conditions, women with ambiguous diagnoses or treatable anomalies also express acute distress and grief at the initial consultation, which may seem out of proportion to the clinician. These parents also need the attention and reassurance of the health care team and the care provider should attempt to understand how the woman has processed and understood the information she was given.

> *He [FMS] just said to us that there was a problem, there is fluid on the brain, and we said right what does that mean? and he went on to talk about chromosomes em, it could mean putting a shunt into the baby you know, it's brain. Or the baby might not survive the pregnancy if the fluid on the baby had expanded its head and then, you know, loads of different things … He went through everything in a matter of 10 minutes … I just broke down in the middle of it and then he left the room.*

Although clinic staffs are responding to time pressures, the consequences for women who feel rushed in this situation are significant.

> *We were booked in for 10.15 and we were told [by the secretary] we had to leave by 10.30, you need more time than that to open up.*

> *We were out the door before we realised, before we understood what was going on.*

Women who are dissatisfied with the initial encounter with the fetal medicine specialist or clinic staff have a tendency to feel antagonistic towards the specialist for the remainder of the pregnancy, placing a strain on the relationship, and limiting access to the information and support required to make sense of the situation. Negative encounters are generally characterized by a fear that queries will only be partially resolved and often hinder the search for answers to the question "*why did this happen to me*?" One of the reasons couples struggle to come to terms with an adverse diagnosis is because it is a commonly held belief that what happens to us is a consequence of our actions (Rotter 1966). However, when the traumatic event does not fit with this assumption, one can become an "innocent victim" and may be overwhelmed by the objectively uncontrollable nature of the crisis.

Pregnancy is unique as the "patient" with the abnormality is not actually the woman receiving care, and access to that "patient" is through the mother. Many women have spoken about how the focus on the fetal patient to the exclusion of the woman is unwelcome, and fosters a sense of being of clinical interest purely for scientific reasons. Receiving an adverse diagnosis can influence the mother's relationship with her unborn baby, and ambivalent feelings may become manifest to the clinician in the form of whether a woman looks at the screen during ultrasound examinations. Some women find it difficult to become attached and even try intentionally not to become attached. Not surprisingly, this is due to fear that developing a bond would intensify the emotional pain felt if the baby subsequently dies (Stainton et al. 1992).

> *I don't look at the scan, I can't get attached to it … I hoped it was going to die.*

This response may be more common in women who are considering terminating the pregnancy (Drugen et al. 1990).

Telling Family and Friends

When the diagnosis is made during a routine second-trimester ultrasound, it is likely that many couples will have already told friends and family of their ultrasound appointment. Once the possibility of an abnormality is raised couples start to wonder how they will break the news to others.

> *How do I explain this to the family, to my mother when I'm not certain what it is?*

In the space of 24 h women lose the assumption of fetal health and begin trying to come to terms with this devastating news. However, due to the positive context in which ultrasound is envisioned, most will have informed at least some family members or friends of the date of the ultrasound examination. Consequently, women frequently receive queries from friends within hours of receiving the diagnosis, and sharing the news to some extent is almost inevitable.

> *Oh God yeah, that was the unfortunate thing that I told a lot of people. I had a lot of people to explain it to afterwards. I regret that now. There are some obscure people that you just go God if I hadn't told them, they didn't need to know but you are just so excited you have to.*

> *There's only so much information you can take in. I don't even know if I slept that well that night, I can't remember if I got up the next day … I'm thinking God how am I going to deal with this … what am I going to tell people?*

Some women felt that they have no option but to inform relatives before they fully understand the situation themselves. This is often because others have been involved in taking care of their other children while they attended the examination.

> *I had to go straight up to my mother's;* [*my son*] *was up there so I had to tell them, because they all knew that there was something happening. They knew I was going for the scan. So mm and I was supposed to be dropping* [*my son*] *back there, and then I was supposed to go back to work.*

It appears that when the search for meaning is complex and there was difficulty in answering "why me?" there was an increased reluctance to discuss the diagnosis with others.

> *It's the worst thing about pregnancy, you can see it, I am a stranger in the street and you can see that I am pregnant, it's not a private thing, everybody knows. People are congratulating me and saying isn't it great? … but I just don't want to tell everyone. Then people*

who were delighted for me they are starting to notice they haven't seen me for a few weeks .... I don't want to talk about it. We asked our parents to tell them [*other family members*]. *They are a great support, but like tomorrow when we go in to* [*fetal medicine unit*] *there will be 6 or 7 phone calls made afterwards to tell our family how it went, or they will be ringing us ... a lot of repetition as well so it's difficult to get away from it.*

Parents are unprepared for this and the couple may have to relay painful information over and over again. Many women suggest that staff should forewarn parents of this possibility and advise them to nominate one family member who would notify all relevant others. Some couples will have family members who experience difficulty in acknowledging that not all babies are born healthy, and the clinical team should offer advice and strategies to communicate with the extended family.

Ultrasound is both a screening and a diagnostic tool; consequently, for some women carrying fetuses with structural abnormalities (e.g., anencephaly), certainty regarding the diagnosis can be achieved based on ultrasound findings alone. However, other defects (e.g., certain cardiac and gastrointestinal anomalies) can occur in isolation or in conjunction with a chromosomal defect. Clinicians may wonder why women would equivocate as to whether they should accept further testing (e.g., amniocentesis) to clarify the diagnosis. Having certainty is a relief for some (*monitors*), but it destroys hope for others (*blunters*).

[*Husband*] *asked him straight out, you know is this going to happen again? and he said he didn't think so, it just was one of those once off situations probably happened at the moment of conception, it was that unusual ..., you know he was talking about chromosomes and of course everybody thinks when they think chromosome they think Downs Syndrome. I had the amnio to try to deal with it ... I was delighted just to get a diagnosis ... there was a great sense of relief just knowing.*

We cried our eyes out, you know, what can you do like, you see you're expecting so much like [*prospective life with a healthy child*], *and we were coping you know, hoping that it won't be bad news and knowing deep down it will be. So I said it to* [*husband*] *should we go for it?* [*amniocentesis*], *I think we should because, it's better than not knowing ... but I suppose deep down you always cling onto the little bit of hope that there might be good news.*

The fetal karyotype result may be pivotal in the decision to continue or terminate the pregnancy. However, some women may choose not to have an amniocentesis (information avoidance) on the basis that there is little value to be gained from the information the test would reveal and the risk of a procedure-related loss is too high a price to pay.

I always thought there was something else underlying .... I didn't believe it was as simple as a multicystic kidney, now hopefully it will have been, I do believe now it will be that simple and that's it but no on that day, I was very matter of fact that day and he said the amniocentesis and I said no, what am I going to do? I'm not going to go [*to UK for TOP* [*termination of pregnancy*]], *so what's the point in knowing? If I lost the baby having an amniocentesis, you know and had the baby* [*prematurely*] *how would I cope, that would be a bigger problem ...* [*if*] *they couldn't medically do anything for this baby there was no point in having the test.*

Women also recommended four key elements (when, who, how, gender) that should be incorporated into the process of informing parents of test results: WHEN will the result be available, WHO will give it to me (named person), and HOW will I be informed, i.e., by phone or appointment in the unit. Staffs also need to be aware of whether the woman wishes to know the GENDER or not, as once it has been revealed it cannot be withdrawn.

Conclusion

The Miller and Mangan (Miller 1980; Miller and Mangan 1983) model of styles of information seeking is very useful in explaining the interaction between information need and coping style. The relationship between the woman and her caregivers forms a vital support structure in this stressful situation, as access to information is a key component in coping with this traumatic event. "*Monitor*"- and "*blunter*"-type behaviors are readily recognizable to the observer; therefore, responding appropriately to the information preference exhibited can be utilized to improve the effectiveness of the relationship between the woman and her caregivers.

> *I wanted information but not so much that it would freak me out. It's great to be prepared but you can get information overload.*

When women with a low preference for information receive more information than they can assimilate, the consequence is often increased anxiety and distress. Once a satisfactory level of factual knowledge relating to a definitive diagnosis is obtained, the need for ongoing information diminishes. However, if an additional variable or problem manifests during the pregnancy, the high need for information regarding the new variable will return for those using a problem-focused approach to coping. It is of importance to note that women who know that there is a real possibility the fetal condition might deteriorate yet neonatal intervention remains a possibility may struggle to cope with the constant demand of assimilating additional information, and require extra support during the pregnancy. For women who adopt blunting strategies, and where neonatal survival is predicted to be low but mortality is not a certainty, hearing something positive at the fetal medicine visit is important.

> *I haven't asked anymore about the problems. I don't ask too many questions it's just my way. If they* [the twins] *could have a bit more weight on them they might have a chance, a bit of positivity.*

The information preference that is exhibited throughout the pregnancy, in general, remains consistent up to the birth. Those using monitoring strategies prefer to have detailed information as the fear of not knowing what to expect is greater than knowing, whereas blunters often prefer to take a wait-and-see approach, and to assimilate information at their own pace. Women value continuity of care as it increases their sense of security while they are at their most vulnerable; the potential for a difficult relationship with caregivers exists if continuity is not provided.

Ameliorating stress for women learning of a fetal abnormality requires health care professionals to observe the coping strategies used by women and to respond appropriately. Miller and Mangan's (Miller 1980; Miller and Mangan 1983) model of informational coping styles provides a framework for allowing clinicians to match information need with information demand. Cognizance of information preferences has practical application in the care for these women.

Summary of Good Practice Points

The Initial Scan

- *Make introductions and ensure that you know the relationship of the companion to the woman before you begin.*
- *Try and avoid detectable changes in your facial expression and body language before you are ready to reveal the news.*
- *Take your time to complete the examination before you decide to inform the woman/parents that all is not as expected.*
- *Try to identify if there is a low or high preference for information:*
  - *Have the couple searched extensively for pre-scan information or relied on the information provided by the health care provider/friends/family,* etc.?
  - *Are they asking questions throughout the examination, hungry for detail, or are they focussing on the social aspects of the examination and the normalcy of pregnancy?*
  - *Are they seeking confirmation that all is normal or attentive to the possibility that it might not be or are they avoiding any questions regarding abnormality and focussing on the positive?*
- *Acknowledge this is a human tragedy and that you are very sorry to be giving such devastating news (or that the condition is treatable).*
- *Honesty is of paramount importance; if there is uncertainty then say so. If there is uncertainty or complexity outline clearly a plan to meet the fetal medicine specialist to achieve a diagnosis.*
- *Arrange a follow-up appointment with the fetal medicine specialist within 24 h if possible.*
- *Stop the scan to give the news—women with a preference for information avoidance may climb off the examination table, and women with a high need for information may wish the scan to continue to illustrate the areas of concern.*
- *Provide written information in whatever format is available,* e.g., *leaflets specific to the condition, a copy of the report, copies of fetal images, and hand-drawn diagrams.*
- *If a same-day appointment with the fetal medicine specialist is not possible, advise couples on the risk of searching the Internet and if possible give guidance*

on reputable websites. If the anomaly is associated with a more serious condition inform the couple if this is a concern in their case.

- *Give the couple time to ask questions before they leave the unit and ensure that they have someone available to bring them home.*
- *Advise them that family members will be concerned and recommend nominating one person to communicate with others on their behalf.*
- *Advise them to bring a list of questions to the fetal medicine clinic.*
- *Write the name of the consulting physician on the appointment card.*
- *Give your name and number so they can contact you between leaving the unit and the appointment the following day.*

The Fetal Medicine Clinic

- *Make introductions and ensure that you know the relationship of the companion to the woman before you begin.*
- *If there is a trainee in fetal medicine at the clinic do not prioritize training over the need to offer diagnostic certainty to the couple.*
- *Acknowledge this is a human tragedy and that you are very sorry to be giving such devastating news (or that the condition is treatable).*
- *Always give the diagnosis (certain or uncertain) with eye contact and after the examination has been completed.*
- *Try and identify if there is a low or high preference for information.*
- *Avoid medical jargon and don't soften the blow with overly reassuring comments:*
  - *There is a 1:10 chance your baby will die is more easily grasped than there is a 10% risk of mortality.*
  - *Avoid the phrase "incompatible with life"; parents prefer language like "your baby cannot survive outside the womb," or "the baby will die in the womb or soon after birth."*
  - *Provide written information in whatever format is available*, e.g., *leaflets specific to the condition, a copy of the report, copies of fetal images, hand-drawn diagrams, and relevant websites to guide further searching.*
  - *Ask the couple if they have a list of questions they would like to ask.*
  - *Outline the plan of care—further testing, seeking an opinion from another specialist, and options open to the couple regarding terminating the pregnancy.*
- *Give the couple time to ask questions before they leave the unit and ensure that they have a person to contact between visits to ask questions.*
- *Avoid being disturbed by pagers, cell phones,* etc.
- *Advise them that family members will be concerned and recommend nominating one person to communicate with others on their behalf.*
- *Give the couple a confirmed follow-up appointment before they leave.*
- *If the pregnancy is continuing ensure continuity of care.*

References

Baillie C, Hewison J. Should ultrasound scanning in pregnancy be routine? J Reprod Infant Psychol. 1999;17:149–57.

Campbell S, Smith P. Routine screening for congenital abnormalities by ultrasound. In: Rodeck CR, Nicolaides KN, editors. Proceedings of the 11th study group of The Royal College OF Obstetricians and Gynaecologists. London: RCOG; 1983.

Drugen A, Greb A, Johnson MP, Krivchenia EL, Uhlmann WR, et al. Determinants of parental decision to abort for chromosome abnormalities. Prenat Diagn. 1990;10:483–90.

Ekelin M, Crang-Svalenius E, Dykes A-K. A qualitative study of mothers' and fathers' experiences of routine ultrasound examination. Midwifery. 2004;20:335–44.

Eurenius K, Axelsson O, Gallstedt-Fransson I, Sjoden P-O. Perception of information, expectations and experiences among women and their partners attending a second-trimester routine ultrasound scan. Ultrasound Obstet Gynecol. 1997;9:86–90.

Folkman S, Lazarus R. An analysis of coping in a middle-age community sample. J Health Soc Behav. 1980;21:219–39.

Horowitz M. Stress response syndromes. Northvale, NJ: Jason Aronson Incorporated; 1992.

Hyde B. An interview study of pregnant women's attitudes to ultrasound scanning. Soc Sci Med. 1986;22:589–93.

Janoff-Bulman R. Shattered assumptions: towards a new psychology of trauma. New York, NY: The Free Press; 1992.

Katz Rothman B. The tentative pregnancy: prenatal diagnosis and the future of motherhood. London: Pandora Press; 1988.

Kolker A. Advances in prenatal diagnosis: social-psychological and policy issues. Int J Technol Assess Health Care. 1989;5:601–17.

Lalor JG. Routine antenatal ultrasound, reassuring or anxiety-provoking? A descriptive study. Unpublished M.Sc. Thesis. Trinity College, University Of Dublin, 2000.

Lalor J, Begley C. Fetal anomaly screening: what do women *want* to know? J Adv Nurs. 2006;55:11–9.

Lalor J, Begley C, Galavan E. A grounded theory study of information preference and coping styles following antenatal diagnosis of foetal abnormality. J Adv Nurs. 2008;64:185–94.

Lalor J, Begley C, Galavan E. Recasting hope: a process of adaptation following fetal anomaly diagnosis. Soc Sci Med. 2009;68:462–72.

Lalor JG, Devane D. Information, knowledge and expectations of the routine ultrasound scan. Midwifery. 2007;23:13–22.

Lalor J, Devane D, Begley C. Unexpected diagnosis of fetal abnormality: women's encounters with caregivers. Birth. 2007;34:80–8.

Lalor J, Devane D, McParland P. (2007) Ultrasound screening for fetal abnormality in Ireland: a national survey. Ir J Med Sci. 176(3):175–9

Lalor J, Devane D, Mc Parland P. Ultrasound screening in Ireland: how effective is the service? Ir Med J, 2006b; 99, 264–6.

Landsman I. Crises of meaning in trauma and loss. In: Kauffman J, editor. Loss of the assumptive world. A theory of traumatic loss. New York, NY: Brunner-Routledge; 2002.

Larsen T, Nguyen TH, Munk M, Svendsen L, Teisner L. Ultrasound screening in the 2nd trimester. The pregnant woman's background knowledge, expectations, experiences and acceptances. Ultrasound Obstet Gynecol. 2000;15:383–6.

Lazarus R, Launier R. Stress-related transactions between person and environment. In: Pervin L, Lewis M, editors. Perspectives in interactional psychology. New York, NY: Plenum; 1978.

Miller S. When is a little information a dangerous thing? Coping with stressful life-events by monitoring versus blunting. In: Levine S, Ursin H, editors. Coping and health. New York, NY: Plenum Press; 1980.

Miller S, Mangan C. Interacting effects of information and coping style in adapting to gynecologic stress: should the doctor tell all? J Pers Soc Psychol. 1983;45:223–36.

Mitchell LM. Women's experience of unexpected ultrasound findings. J Midwifery Womens Health. 2004;49:228–34.

Morgan PD, Fogel J, Rose L, Barnett K, Mock V, et al. African American couples merging strengths to successfully cope with breast cancer. Oncol Nurs Forum. 2005;32:979–87.

Parkes C. Psycho-social transition: a field of study. Soc Sci Med. 1971;5:101–15.

Parkes C. Bereavement as a psychosocial transition: processes of adaptation to change. J Soc Issues. 1988;44:53–65.

Proud J. Some problems encountered in obstetric ultrasound scanning. Midwives Chron. 1985; 98:289–90.

Rapp R. Testing women. Testing the fetus. New York: Routledge; 1999.

RCOG. Report of the RCOG Working Party on ultrasound screening for fetal abnormalities. London: RCOG Press; 1997.

Rotter J. Generalized expectancies for internal vs. external control of reinforcement. Psychol Monogr. 1966;80:1–28 (Whole Number 609).

Stainton M, Mcneil D, Harvey S. Maternal tasks of uncertain motherhood. Matern Child Nurs J. 1992;20:113–23.

Statham H, Green J, Kafetsios K. Who worries that something might be wrong with the baby? A prospective study of 1072 pregnant women. Birth. 1997;24:223–33.

Statham H, Solomou W, Green J. Continuing a pregnancy after the diagnosis of an anomaly: parents' experiences. In: Abramsky L, Chapple J, editors. Prenatal diagnosis: the human side. 2nd ed. Cheltenham: Nelson Thornes; 2003.

Part II
The Legal Landscape

Chapter 8
Legal Issues in Prenatal and Preimplantation Genetic Diagnosis

Valerie Gutmann Koch

Introduction

In considering the use of, access to, and regulation and oversight of preimplantation and prenatal genetic diagnosis, questions of law continuously arise. Legal claims generally fall under two areas of law: (1) constitutional law regarding privacy, autonomy, and the state's interest in protecting potential life, and (2) tort law, with a focus on provider liability. Preimplantation and prenatal genetic diagnosis implicates a diverse and varied set of legal questions and issues, including, but not limited to, the right to access reproductive technologies, the oversight and licensure of genetic tests and counselors, the right to terminate a pregnancy for fetal anomaly, considerations of disability and discrimination, provider liability for misdiagnosis, the right to use preimplantation genetic diagnosis in order to create "savior siblings," and the obligation to use these technologies for the medical benefit of future children.

This chapter focuses on four primary legal issues or areas associated with prenatal and preimplantation genetic diagnosis. The section entitled "Pregnancy Termination for Fetal Anomalies" addresses pregnancy termination for fetal anomalies discovered through prenatal genetic testing, both at the federal and state levels. The section entitled "Constitutional Law and Preimplantation Genetic Diagnosis" focuses on a constitutional analysis of access to preimplantation genetic diagnosis and the state's role in regulating the procedure. The next section, "Current Oversight

V.G. Koch, J.D. (✉)
IIT Chicago-Kent College of Law, 565 West Adams Street, Chicago, IL 60661, USA

MacLean Center for Clinical Medical Ethics, University of Chicago, Chicago, IL USA

New York State Task Force on Life and the Law, New York, NY, USA
e-mail: vgutmannkoch@kentlaw.iit.edu

J.P. Galst, M.S. Verp (eds.), *Prenatal and Preimplantation Diagnosis*,
DOI 10.1007/978-3-319-18911-6_8

of Preimplantation and Prenatal Genetic Diagnosis" discusses existing oversight of preimplantation and prenatal genetic diagnosis. Finally, the last section, "Tort Law/ Liability Considerations for Preimplantation and Prenatal Genetic Diagnosis", explores issues of tort liability in the use of preimplantation and prenatal genetic diagnosis. Importantly, this chapter addresses whether information gleaned through prenatal or preimplantation genetic diagnosis is actionable under current legal standards, rather than the ethical question of *whether* it *should* be actionable.

Pregnancy Termination for Fetal Anomalies

Federal Law

Legal questions surrounding the use of prenatal genetic diagnosis are inextricably connected to the ability to terminate a pregnancy for fetal anomalies. Thus, one of the central legal inquiries related to the use of prenatal genetic diagnosis is the extent to which an individual may seek an abortion based on the results of the intervention. As this Section will discuss, the right to terminate a pregnancy is anything but absolute. Supreme Court jurisprudence supports the government's authority to balance a woman's health against fetal life, thereby limiting a woman's access to abortion.

Importantly, and as will be explored throughout the rest of this Section, under current Supreme Court interpretation, the right to *seek* a legal abortion is a protected liberty interest that can be curtailed where the government has a legitimate state interest, as long as the regulation does not impose an undue burden on that protected liberty interest. In contrast, the ability to *obtain* an abortion has never been recognized as a constitutionally protected liberty interest, particularly if it requires subsidization by the state.

A brief history of key Supreme Court cases related to termination of pregnancy bears reviewing here. The oft-cited Supreme Court's seminal decision in *Roe v. Wade* stands for the (subsequently modified) proposition that a state can restrict and even regulate the fundamental right to seek an abortion only if the state's interest is compelling and the restrictive law was framed in the narrowest manner possible to achieve that compelling interest (410 U.S. 113 [1973]). A fundamental right is a right of personal liberty that the Bill of Rights explicitly prohibits the government from limiting or proscribing except where the action has a compelling purpose (the Fourteenth Amendment extends this limitation to the states as well). However, Supreme Court jurisprudence since 1973 has evolved, changing what was a fundamental right in *Roe v. Wade* into a protected liberty interest. A protected liberty interest is a claim of personal freedom that has been traditionally and historically protected but is not explicitly protected by the Bill of Rights. Such interests are constitutionally protected but may be limited by state action where the state action bears a reasonable relationship to a legitimate state purpose. In other words, state legislation that impinges upon a protected liberty interest is valid if it is rationally related to a legitimate state purpose.

Supreme Court decisions after *Roe v. Wade* shed light on this important shift in defining the right to seek an abortion from a fundamental right to a protected liberty interest. In the decades following the 1973 decision, abortion opponents have increasingly influenced state policy-makers to curb the practice of abortion. Thus, in the 1977 decision *Beal v. Doe*, the Supreme Court considered the Pennsylvania Medicaid statute that permitted reimbursement of only "medically necessary" (rather than "elective") abortions; the law singled out "medical evidence that an infant may be born with incapacitating physical deformity" as one of the five "medical necessit[ies]" permitting subsidized abortion (432 U.S. 438 [1977]). Although the Supreme Court reaffirmed abortion as a right, it allowed restriction of federal funding of abortion in the first trimester of pregnancy. It stated that the state has an interest in potential life throughout pregnancy even though such interest does not become compelling until viability.

By 1989, the Supreme Court modified the fundamental constitutional right to seek an abortion into a mere protected liberty interest (*Webster v. Reproductive Health Services*, 492 U.S. 490 [1989]). In *Webster*, the Court decided that it is permissible for a state to presume viability at 20 weeks of pregnancy based on the reasoning that the state can act to protect viable potential life. In other words, the holding in that case emphasized that the state's interest in protecting potential life could develop before fetal viability, thereby permitting states to regulate the abortion decision so as to protect potential life, regardless of maternal health consequences, after 20 weeks of gestation.

In replacing the trimester approach with a single cutoff—viability—after which regulation of abortion is permitted, the majority in the 1992 Supreme Court decision *Planned Parenthood of S.E. Pennsylvania v. Casey* adopted the reasoning in Justice Sandra Day O'Connor's concurring opinion in *Webster*: state legislation that regulates and limits the right to seek an abortion is legitimate unless it "unduly burdens" that right (505 U.S. 833 [1992]). Thus, the Court in *Casey* modified the previously established basis for the state's power, deciding that the state has a compelling interest in potential life from conception, but it cannot unduly burden the right of women to seek an abortion until at least potential viability. Consequently, the *Casey* decision permits state regulation of first *semester* abortions if the regulation has any sort of relationship to the legitimate state interests of protecting maternal health, encouraging childbirth, discouraging abortion, or protecting potential life, as long as the regulation does not impose an undue burden on the protected liberty interest of the woman seeking to terminate a pregnancy. This standard is not very instructive as to what sort of state action is constitutionally acceptable. Indeed, many argue that the *Casey* decision permits almost any abortion restrictions, based on the state's legitimate interest in protecting potential life (Mutcherson 2008).

Today, it is undisputed that the state may, at some point, exercise its power to intervene on behalf of the fetus. The Supreme Court has only addressed abortion a few times since its *Casey* decision, and therefore the limited Supreme Court case law on abortion provides little guidance about how to apply the *Casey* undue burden standard, particularly as new technologies proliferate.

In one of its few abortion-related decisions since 1992, the Supreme Court in *Gonzales v. Carhart* upheld the Partial-Birth Abortion Ban Act of 2003, which prohibited the procedure it referred to as "intact D&E" (otherwise termed "partial-birth abortions") (550 U.S. 124 [2007]). It held that despite the Act's blanket prohibition on a specific method of abortion, the ban was not unconstitutionally vague, overbroad, or an undue burden on the decision to obtain an abortion. In an often-quoted portion of the opinion, the Court stated,

> Where it has a rational basis to act, and it does not impose an undue burden, the State may use its regulatory power to bar certain procedures and substitute others, all in furtherance of *its legitimate interests in regulating the medical profession in order to promote respect for life*, including life of the unborn (emphasis added).

In its amicus brief in that case, the National Women's Law Center described the experiences of specific women who decided to end their pregnancies via intact D&E because prenatal testing revealed severe genetic disorders (in two cases, trisomy 13), and the procedure was both the safest and "most humane" option for the women and their families. Nevertheless, and despite the testimony of the American Congress of Obstetricians and Gynecologists (ACOG), the Court held that prohibiting access to this method was not unconstitutional, even though the alternative procedure may be less safe for the woman seeking to terminate a pregnancy. Thus, the Supreme Court has made it clear that the state has the authority to ban a particular procedure—even where it is the safest option for the woman and even if prohibiting the procedure does not "save" a fetal "life."

State Laws

As the state's interest in protecting potential life is increasingly recognized at the federal level, a woman's ability to terminate a pregnancy based on fetal anomaly discovered as a result of prenatal genetic diagnosis becomes more restricted. States have enacted legislation that results in diminished availability of abortions and are passing such laws at an increasing pace: 2011 saw more state-level "anti-abortion" legislation than any year since the 1973 Supreme Court decision in *Roe v. Wade* (Hill 2012), and 2013 saw the second highest number of abortion restrictions become law in a single year (22 states passed a total of 70 abortion restrictions) (National Women's Law Center 2013). Moreover, between 2011 and 2013, 205 abortion restrictions were enacted, surpassing the total number of restrictions—189—passed in the entire previous decade (Boonstra and Nash 2014). The proliferation of these legal restrictions has increasingly foreclosed abortion as an option that pregnant women can choose after learning of a fetal anomaly.

These laws and regulations run the gamut, focusing on banning abortion outright after a certain point during the pregnancy; reducing or forbidding state funding of abortion; requiring waiting periods before a woman may seek an abortion; mandating ultrasounds prior to terminating a pregnancy; requiring additional "informed consent" or counseling procedures before a woman may terminate a pregnancy; banning certain types of abortion procedures (like the "partial birth abortion" law at issue in *Gonzalez v. Carhart*); and imposing additional licensure requirements and regulation of abortion providers and facilities. This Section focuses specifically on the laws that are most likely to affect a woman's ability to terminate a pregnancy for fetal anomalies, rather than the panoply of laws regarding a woman's right to seek an abortion.

Wholesale prohibitions of abortion. As of 2014, forty-one states prohibit some abortions after a certain point in pregnancy (Guttmacher Institute, State policies on later abortions, 2014). A growing number of states have enacted laws that limit or prohibit abortion after viability. As of 2013, 39 states limit abortion after fetal viability, 21 of which prohibit abortion at viability and 3 of which prohibit abortion in the third trimester (Nash et al. 2013; Guttmacher Institute, State policies on later abortions, 2014).

Additionally, states are increasingly passing laws that prohibit abortion at or after 20 weeks after conception (before fetal viability). Often these laws are based on the (erroneous) premise that the fetus can feel pain after this point (Lee et al. 2005). In 2010, one state had such a law; by 2013, 12 states had passed measures that banned abortion at or before 20 weeks (Kliff 2013). In 2010 and 2011 alone, six states passed laws banning abortions before fetal viability (at 20 weeks post-fertilization), and in 2013, two states passed similar laws: North Dakota banned abortion procedures after approximately 6 weeks (after the detection of a fetal heartbeat) and Arkansas at 12 weeks (N.D. Century Code Chap. 14-02.1; Arkansas Human Heartbeat Protection Act, Ark. Code Ann. §§ 20-16-1301-1307). Both laws had few, if any, exceptions (National Women's Law Center 2013; Rebouché and Rothenberg 2012). In March 2014, the Alabama House passed a bill that would ban abortion after a fetal heartbeat is detected, with exceptions where the pregnancy would endanger the mother's life or physical health, and where the fetus has a "lethal anomaly," defined as a condition that will result in death within 3 months of birth (2014 Alabama House Bill No. 490).

Although many of these laws are not currently in effect due to pending legal challenges (in most cases, the lowest level federal courts blocked the laws because they conflicted with Supreme Court decisions such as *Roe v. Wade*), their initial passage is indicative of a national trend toward increased restriction of abortion (*McCormack v. Hiedeman*, 900 F. Supp. 2d 1128 [D. Idaho 2013]; *MKB Manag. Corp. v. Burdick*, 2014 WL 1653201 [D. N.D. 2014]; *Edwards v. Beck*, 2013 WL 2302323 [E.D. Ark. 2013]; *Edwards v. Beck*, 2014 WL 1245267 [E.D. Ark. 2014]).

Although only 1.3 % of abortions are performed after the 21st week of gestation (Pazol 2012), a majority of the abortions that occur in the second and third trimesters in the USA "are for reason of fetal condition" (Rebouché and Rothenberg 2012). Thus, these wholesale prohibitions on abortion—at least after a certain point during a woman's pregnancy—severely limit a woman's ability to terminate a pregnancy for fetal anomalies.

Exceptions or prohibition on abortions for sex selection and genetic abnormalities. Some states allow pregnancy termination for either lethal or serious fetal anomalies—often without clearly defining these terms. Four states—Georgia, Louisiana, Texas, and Utah—allow exemptions for abortions for only *lethal* genetic anomalies (Ga. Code Ann. § 31-9B-2; Vernon's Texas Statutes and Codes Annotated § 171.046; West's Utah Code Annotated § 76-7-302; West's Louisiana Statutes Annotated § 1299.30.1; Thomson-Deveaux 2014). In an interesting version of these laws, a proposed Alabama bill would require a woman seeking an abortion because of a lethal fetal anomaly to receive counseling on perinatal hospice services, ostensibly to influence the woman not to terminate the pregnancy (2014 Alabama House Bill No. 493). Moreover, several states explicitly allow abortion for *serious* (rather than lethal) genetic anomalies. Maryland's law, which has been in effect since 1968—5 years before the Supreme Court decided *Roe v. Wade*—states that "the State may not interfere with the decision of a woman to terminate a pregnancy … [a]t *any time during the woman's pregnancy*, if … the fetus is affected by genetic defect or serious deformity or abnormality." (Md. Code Ann., Health-Gen. § 20-209(b)(2)(ii), emphasis added). In April 2014, Mississippi enacted a measure banning abortions at 20 weeks post-conception, except in cases where the pregnancy would endanger the mother's life, the possibility of "substantial and irreversible physical impairment of a major bodily function," or "severe fetal abnormalities." (2014 MS H.B. 1400; Guttmacher Institute, Major developments, 2014). Arizona's law, which was similar to Mississippi's, was struck down based on the holding that the statute violated the right of women to make the ultimate decision to terminate a pregnancy prior to fetal viability, after the Supreme Court refused to hear a challenge that could have restored the ban (*Horne v. Isaacson*, 134 S. Ct. 905 [2014]; Ariz. Rev. Stat. § 36-2151 (Botkin 2003)). If the Mississippi law is challenged and upheld, the Supreme Court may have to decide the issue after all, in order to resolve a potential split between the different Circuit courts.

However, many laws that limit or prohibit abortion after viability do not include exceptions for fetal anomalies—even lethal abnormalities that would require a woman to carry a nonviable fetus to term (Thomson-Deveaux 2014; Corrigan 2013). Blanket post-viability prohibitions (or laws without an exception for fetal anomalies) impact a woman's ability to terminate a pregnancy based on fetal abnormalities, because a number of these anomalies, such as renal agenesis, limb-body wall complex, encephalocele, severe hydrocephaly, meningomyelocele, and lethal skeletal dysplasias, cannot be detected until at least the second trimester (Corrigan 2013). However, this may change with the increased availability of diagnostic methods that allow for the discovery of information at a much earlier point in the pregnancy "when the termination options may be more tolerable both physically [due to the availability of medical, rather than surgical, abortion] and emotionally" (King 2011).

Recently, states have begun to introduce (and in a few cases, enact) measures to ban abortion targeted toward specific information, such as sex and genetic abnormalities, like Down syndrome and trisomy 18. In 2013, seven states—Arizona, Illinois, Kansas, North Carolina, North Dakota, Oklahoma, and Pennsylvania—had laws on the books that banned sex selection abortions, none of which have been struck down in the courts (National Women's Law Center 2013). Oklahoma's law requires that the physician complete a form that states the reason the woman is seeking to terminate the pregnancy; "Mother wanted a child of a different sex" is one of the options on the required form (Okla. Stat. Ann. tit. 63, § 1-738k(F) (Ethics Committee of the American Society for Reproductive Medicine 2013)). Of those seven states, North Dakota's law is the only one that also prohibits abortion for genetic abnormality. It explicitly forbids the provision of an abortion if the provider knows the woman is obtaining the abortion for purposes of sex selection or because the fetus has been "diagnosed with either a genetic abnormality or a potential for a genetic abnormality" (N.D. Cent. Code Ann. § 14-02.1-04.1). The law defines "genetic abnormality" broadly.

In the first 5 months of 2014 alone, legislators in 12 states introduced abortion laws addressing sex, race, or genetic selection, and South Dakota became the most recent state to enact legislation that criminalizes the provision of an abortion if the provider knows the woman is obtaining the abortion for purposes of sex selection (2014 South Dakota House Bill No. 1162; Guttmacher Institute, Major developments, 2014). Almost every one of these laws bans abortion for sex selection at any point during the pregnancy.

Laws forbidding abortion for genetic abnormality or sex selection may still be challenged in the courts, and although the Supreme Court has held that the state may place limits on *when* a woman may seek an abortion (*Roe v. Wade, Planned Parenthood of S.E. Pennsylvania v. Casey*) and on certain abortion procedures (*Gonzalez v. Carhart*), it has not addressed the state's interest in controlling access to pre-viability abortion based on a woman's *reasons* for having the procedure (besides, of course, in cases of medical necessity). However, states' willingness to pass laws that prohibit abortion for sex selection or fetal anomaly may indicate an increase in regulation of the reasons for seeking abortion, including for medically significant information like that revealed via prenatal genetic testing.

State funding of abortion. When determining whether to allocate state funds for abortion services, 32 states and the District of Columbia follow the federal standards established by the Hyde Amendment, of which a version has been passed annually by Congress since 1976 and which has been upheld by the Supreme Court. The Hyde Amendment prohibits the expenditure of federal funds for abortion except in cases of rape, incest, or danger to the life of the pregnant woman. Seventeen other states allow the use of state funds for "medically necessary" abortions, often as a result of a court order to do so (Guttmacher Institute, State funding of abortion under medicaid, 2014).

Certain states that generally follow the federal standard forbidding the provision of government funds for abortion not only permit abortion for fetal anomalies, but also allow medicaid funding for such procedures. Specifically, Iowa, Mississippi, and Virginia provide state funds for abortion in cases of fetal impairment (Guttmacher Institute, State funding of abortion under medicaid, 2014). Thus, although a small handful of states provide funds for abortion for fetal anomalies, most states may control access to pregnancy termination for fetal anomalies by restricting government funds for such procedures.

Targeted regulation of abortion providers (TRAP). States are more and more frequently enacting laws that govern the licensure and credentialing of abortion providers, as well as the type and size of facilities in which abortions may be provided, effectively restricting the ability of women to access abortions. In 2013, eight states enacted new, targeted regulation of abortion providers (TRAP), including licensing requirements for abortion clinics and providers (Nash et al. 2013). As of 2014, eight states have laws requiring abortion providers to have hospital admitting privileges; five of these laws are currently in effect (Guttmacher Institute, An overview of abortion, 2014). Texas became the most recent state to pass a law that would restrict access to abortion providers based on such requirements (2013 Texas House Bill No. 57). The law would require that all abortion providers have admitting privileges at a nearby hospital and that all abortion clinics must become ambulatory surgical centers, which will (or already has) effectively shut down a majority of the state's clinics (Eckholm, Abortion providers in Texas sue over a restrictive rule that could close clinics, 2014). The law has been temporarily enjoined, and had faced a number of legal challenges (*Planned Parenthood of Greater Texas Surgical Health Services v. Abbott*, 748 F. 3d 583 [2014]; Eckholm, Court panel upholds Texas law on abortion, 2014). In the first months of 2014, at least two other states followed suit, introducing similar legislation requiring providers to have admitting privileges at a nearby hospital (Monthly state updates 2014). Although TRAP provisions are generally applicable to abortion providers, they may greatly impact a woman's ability to terminate a pregnancy for fetal anomalies.

Conscience clauses. In the health care setting, a "conscientious objection" is the refusal to perform a legal role or responsibility based on the provider's personal beliefs, often premised in moral or religious terms. A number of laws, including the federal health care provider conscience protection statutes and international policy statements such as the Declaration of Helsinki, protect health care providers' conscience rights or acknowledge a universal right to freedom of conscience. As a general rule, these laws forbid discrimination against health care providers who refuse to provide health care services on the basis of religious beliefs and conscientious convictions. At the federal level, the Church Amendments, Section 245 of the Public Health Service Act, and the Weldon Amendment are collectively known as the "federal health care provider conscience protection statutes," and were generally enacted to prohibit recipients of federal funds from discrimination based on their refusal to participate in certain health care services—in particular, abortion—that they find religiously or morally objectionable (U.S. Department of Health and Human Services).

At the state level, newly passed conscience clauses are targeting genetic counselors—those who are often the individuals who provide the results of and interpret preimplantation and prenatal genetic tests for patients. In 2014, Virginia enacted a law governing the licensure of genetic counselors, which contained a conscience clause that can presumably allow counselors to refuse to provide fetal test results for genetic abnormalities (including Down syndrome or Tay-Sachs Disease) if they believe it could cause a woman to terminate her pregnancy (2014 Virginia House Bill No. 612). Significantly, genetic counselors are tasked with screening pregnant women for exactly these types of fetal abnormalities. Virginia is not alone: as of 2014 two out of the 15 states that license genetic counselors have conscience clauses that allow them to refuse to provide information about abortion (Thomson-Deveaux 2014). Both Nebraska and Oklahoma's genetic counseling licensure acts state that nothing in the statutes may be construed to require any genetic counselor or other person to mention, counsel, or refer for abortion (Neb. Rev. St. § 38-3424; Okla. Stat. tit. 63, § 1-568). Moreover, Missouri prohibits state-sponsored genetic counseling programs from making referrals for abortions unless a physician certifies that the life of the mother would be endangered if the fetus were carried to term (Mo. Rev. Stat. § 191.320).

Thus, commentators have expressed concern that legislatively established conscience clauses for genetic counselors is just the newest wave of measures to restrict access to abortion for fetal anomalies (Stern 2014; Thomson-Deveaux 2014).

The Tension Between Laws Governing Prenatal Genetic Testing and Abortion

Importantly, commentators have observed that the restriction of abortion is occurring concurrently with the expanding access to prenatal genetic testing, effectively "disassociat[ing] … abortion [from] healthcare." (Rebouché and Rothenberg 2012). Rebouché and Rothenberg (2012) have noted that "for those who would choose abortion, the ability to screen and to test prenatally for genetic anomalies is expanding while abortion access, especially near or after viability, is contracting." Further, Jeffrey Botkin explains that based on the limited case law related to the constitutionality of state law prohibiting wrongful life and wrongful birth torts (discussed in more detail in the Section entitled "Tort Law/Liability Considerations for Preimplantation and Prenatal Genetic Diagnosis"), there is little legal support for a right to abort a fetus based on the results of prenatal genetic diagnosis (Botkin 2003). He clarifies that although "women have a right to decide whether they wish to remain pregnant at all[,] they might not have the right to decide whether they wish to remain pregnant with a specific fetus."

Nowhere is the tension between genetic diagnosis and abortion policies more obvious than with the question of funding. Although federal law requires states to extend eligibility for pregnancy-related care to pregnant women with incomes up to 133 % of the federal poverty level, how states interpret what is "necessary for the health of the pregnant woman and the fetus" (Hall and Berlin 2014) or what are considered "essential benefits" under the Affordable Care Act (ACA) is not necessarily consistent. For example, as of 2014, 36 states and the District of Columbia—out of 44 Medicaid programs—cover genetic screening services through their Medicaid programs (Ranji et al. 2009; Rebouché and Rothenberg 2012). In direct contrast, as previously mentioned, the Hyde Amendment explicitly prohibits the expenditure of federal funds—including Medicaid funds—for abortion except in circumscribed cases involving rape, incest, or danger to the life of the pregnant woman (*Harris v. McRae*, 448 U.S. 297 [1980]). This is no small point: Medicaid is the single largest payer of maternity-related services in the country (King 2011). Moreover, commentators have observed that the passage of the ACA in 2010 will intensify the tension concerning whether genetic testing and abortion qualify as routine reproductive medical care. Rebouché and Rothenberg argue that the former does, while the latter does not:

> [T]he ACA will practically reduce health care insurance coverage for abortions at the same time that it provides incentives to test and screen as part of routine maternal health care and preventative services. On the one hand, the ACA excludes abortion as an essential benefit and requires the strict segregation of federal funds for new exchange plans offering abortion coverage. On the other hand, the ACA includes prenatal care as an essential benefit and will cover a range of prenatal services, including genetic screening and testing (Rebouché and Rothenberg 2012).

Constitutional Law and Preimplantation Genetic Diagnosis

This Section will explore whether there is a constitutional right to access preimplantation genetic diagnosis and the extent to which the state may infringe this right by regulating the intervention. This analysis will build, in large part, on the previous section's analysis of the constitutional dimensions of pregnancy termination for fetal anomaly discovered via prenatal genetic diagnosis.

Access to Preimplantation Genetic Diagnosis

Concerns arising around questions of access to preimplantation genetic diagnosis (PGD) and the acceptable limits on patient autonomy are similar (if not the same) to those that arise, generally, in the context of assisted reproductive technologies (ART). Most commentators in favor of allowing access to ever-evolving technological advancements rely on the tenets of reproductive autonomy and bodily integrity to support the right of individuals to undergo procedures associated with ART, including PGD. In contrast, others argue that the state has an interest in intervening in an individual's access to PGD on behalf of the unborn child.

Thus, in considering the constitutional considerations that arise around PGD, two interrelated questions must be considered. First, is there a constitutional "right" to assisted reproduction (and PGD, in particular)? If so, may the state nevertheless regulate assisted reproduction, generally, and PGD, specifically?

What right do individuals have to assisted reproduction? Notably, at the federal level, there is no fundamental or constitutionally protected right to medical care (Gunnar 2006; Swendiman 2012), except where, like prisoners, individuals are dependent upon the government for their basic needs (*Farmer v. Brennan*, 511 U.S. 825 [1994]). Therefore, any attempt to extend a right to prenatal care to include a right to ART would likely be legally futile.

Thus, there can be no "right" to assisted reproduction technologies, or PGD in particular, without recognition of a basic "right" to procreation. Proponents of a constitutional right to procreation have premised its existence on the recognized right to seek the termination of a pregnancy. But, as discussed in the Section entitled "Pregnancy Termination for Fetal Anomalies," that latter right is categorically limited and ever-constricting. For example, the Supreme Court has found that parental consent requirements for minors (*Ohio v. Akron Center*, 497 U.S. 502 [1990]; *Planned Parenthood of S.E. Pennsylvania v. Casey*), waiting periods (*Webster v. Reproductive Health Services*, 492 U.S. 490 [1989]; *Hodgson v. Minnesota*, 497 U.S. 417 [1990]), and prohibition of specific types of pregnancy termination procedures altogether (*Gonzalez v. Carhart*) were not "substantial obstacles" to a woman's ability to obtain an abortion.

However, most scholars agree that the Supreme Court would, at the least, recognize a constitutional right to reproduce through sexual intercourse, at least for married couples, based on Supreme Court decisions addressing the right to avoid procreation using contraceptives and to terminate a pregnancy prior to a certain point (*Griswold v. Connecticut*, 381 U.S. 479 [1965]; *Eisenstadt v. Baird*, 405 U.S. 438 [1972]; *Roe v. Wade*; *Planned Parenthood of S.E. Pennsylvania v. Casey*). In particular, advocates of the right to procreate point to the Supreme Court's statement that "[i]f the right of privacy means anything, it is the right of the individual, married or single, to be free from unwarranted governmental intrusion into matters so fundamentally affecting a person as the decision whether to bear or beget a child." (*Eisenstadt v. Baird*). Similarly, although the Supreme Court in *Casey* decided that the government may make laws to protect the life of the mother and demonstrate respect for the embryo after viability, it also held that "personal decisions relating to marriage, procreation, contraception, family relationships, child rearing, and education" are "central to the liberty protected by the Fourteenth Amendment." Consequently, proponents of the principles of procreative liberty and parental autonomy argue that if a procedure is necessary to achieve biological reproduction, governmental efforts to regulate the procedure are subject to heightened judicial review.

Significantly, however, the 1942 Supreme Court decision *Skinner v. Oklahoma* represents the only time the US Supreme Court has directly addressed an affirmative right to reproduce, referring to it as a "basic liberty." (316 U.S. 535 [1942]) Under the Oklahoma statute in effect at the time which authorized sterilization for any criminal convicted of two or more felonies involving "moral turpitude," Oklahoma instituted sterilization proceedings against Jack Skinner. Skinner had previously been convicted, twice, of armed robbery and of stealing chickens. The Court, in deciding that the statute violated the Equal Protection clause, described the right to have offspring as "a right which is basic to the perpetuation of a race." However, as one commentator noted, "[i]mportantly… the statute received strict scrutiny because of the combination of the irreparable harm done [the permanence of sterilization] to an important liberty interest and the unequal way in which the state infringed upon that interest—not simply because the statute affected procreation" (Meyer 2009).

Despite finding that individuals' interest in procreation is at least a protected liberty interest, courts have upheld the state's role in restricting this interest. In some cases, in fact, the Supreme Court has permanently prevented individuals from procreating, in order to serve other "important" state interests of health, safety, and education. For example, in the 1927 decision *Buck v. Bell*, the Court held that the Virginia statute which authorized sterilization of Carrie Buck, an institutionalized "feeble minded" woman, did not deny her the right to due process and the equal protection of the laws as protected by the Fourteenth Amendment (274 U.S. 200 [1927]). Although shocking, this Supreme Court precedent remains: the case has never been overturned. Presumably, no state would sterilize an individual without his or her consent in a similar situation. However, this case may still be used to demonstrate the principle that the state may, pursuant to its police powers to protect public safety and health, require individuals to sacrifice some degree of procreative liberty, even before conception. And, in fact, the court in *Roe v. Wade* cited *Buck v. Bell* in its assertion that one does not have "an unlimited right to do with one's body as one pleases."

Thus, the right to procreate is not unassailable, and consequently, the right to make other decisions related to the act of procreation is legally unclear. The Supreme Court has not yet addressed whether there is a constitutional right to utilize assisted reproductive technologies, including IVF and PGD. In other words, uncertainty about the right to use assisted reproductive technologies persists because of the dearth of direct case law regarding whether there is a constitutional right to procreate, let alone a constitutional right to undergo PGD. Legal scholars are divided on the issue. Jeffrey Botkin has argued that despite the constitutionally protected right to seek an abortion until a certain point, "there is not a parallel constitutional right to obtain any and all information on which a termination decision might be based"—including information gleaned through preimplantation genetic testing (Botkin 2003). However, Jamie King has noted that, "in the absence of a compelling state interest, the state should not deny infertile couples the ability to obtain fertility treatment" (King 2008). Similarly, John Robertson has reasoned that "the state should not be able to deny [infertile persons] fertility treatment on the basis of harm that would not justify similar limitations on the rights of fertile persons to reproduce" (Robertson 2004). However, this does not mean that the government has the obligation to provide the services or resources.

Despite the lack of Supreme Court jurisprudence regarding the existence of a right to procreate—let alone to utilize ART and prenatal genetic diagnosis to do so—there are a select number of decisions at the state level that imply such a right. The most well-known, *Lifchez v. Hartigan*, was decided by an Illinois federal court in 1990 (735 F. Supp. 1361 [1990]). The court struck down a provision of the Illinois Abortion Law which required that no person "shall sell or experiment upon a fetus produced by the fertilization of a human ovum by a human sperm unless such experimentation is therapeutic to the fetus produced," on the ground that the statutory language was so vague that it might deter physicians from providing amniocentesis, genetic screening of in vitro embryos, and other interventions. Thus, the court held that the statute violated the Fourteenth Amendment principle of due process. Further, the court held that the statute infringed a woman's right of privacy and reproductive freedom by intruding on "a woman's zone of privacy," stating that "[i] t takes no great leap of logic to see that within the cluster of constitutionally protected choices that includes the right to have access to contraceptives, there must be included within that cluster the right to submit to a medical procedure that may bring about, rather than prevent, pregnancy." Notably, this has been the only federal court case addressing whether there is a right to choose not to implant an embryo, end a pregnancy, or avoid procreation altogether based on information regarding the fetus or embryo.

In determining the extent to which the state may intervene in the provision of assisted reproductive technologies, it is necessary to note the distinction between different forms of ART. For example, IVF "assists" reproduction, and therefore one may argue that it qualifies for the protections assured under cases such as *Skinner*. On the other hand, PGD allows individuals to control the kinds of children they have. Thus, although the right to the former may be protectable, the right to the latter may not.

The question of whether there is a right to use ART to further the (limited) right to procreate is further complicated by the fact that, at its core, use of PGD implicates the "right" to destroy (or at least, not implant) certain embryos while implanting others. Preimplantation genetic diagnosis, "therefore, presupposes an outcome of excess embryos and potential destruction in a way that is different from a woman who resorts to abortion only when she learns unwanted news about a fetus" (Mutcherson 2008). Whether the state may therefore compel implantation of these embryos is discussed in the following Section.

The Role of the State in Regulating Preimplantation Genetic Diagnosis

Thus, although there is a recognized right to procreate, states may regulate procreation under its police powers, in order to protect public health and safety (*Skinner v. Oklahoma*; *Buck v. Bell*). With high-profile stories like the 2009 "Octomom" saga and other accounts of high order multiple births, questions have arisen about the patient's right to demand (or a physician's right to provide) certain reproductive services, including unlimited implantation of embryos, and the state's role in regulating assisted reproduction (Daar 2012). Recent reports of children born through ART with cognitive delays, low birth weight, or birth defects indicate the importance of assessing the role and obligations of physicians to advise, monitor, and protect (Kaira et al. 2011; Hansen et al. 2005). For example, recently released studies have demonstrated a higher rate of stillbirth for children born from assisted reproductive technologies (Merritt et al. 2014).

Generally, courts will apply strict scrutiny to "any regulation of procreation that distinguishes socially disfavored groups for different treatment" under the Equal Protection clause of the Constitution (Meyer 2009). Where regulation applies equally to everyone, courts will still look at whether the law serves a legitimate governmental interest before permitting the state to infringe on a person's right to procreate.

To what extent the state may regulate embryo implantation and other aspects of ART hinges on when the state's "right" of governmental intervention on behalf of embryos begins. In the context of PGD, unlike in the abortion cases, the embryo is outside the woman's body. Thus, in a court's balancing of the privacy rights of the woman against the right of the state to intervene on behalf of the embryo, it follows that the woman's privacy interest may not be as strong before embryo implantation as it is after implantation. Accordingly, under current Supreme Court jurisprudence, legislation mandating limits on embryo transfer or other uses of ART does not absolutely frustrate an individual's liberty interest in procreation and serves the state's interest in protecting the health and welfare of the resulting fetus. For example, a law that forces a woman to undergo repeated egg retrieval procedures in order to avoid the creation of excess embryos (which may then be frozen or destroyed) may not unduly burden the health of a woman seeking IVF and PGD.

Moreover, to the extent that interventions requiring the "literal disembodiment of reproduction"—IVF, PGD, etc.—represent the medicalization of the procreative process, the state may choose to exercise its regulatory power in limiting access to and use of these interventions (recall that there is no constitutional right to medical care) (Suter 2008). Scholars assert that use of assisted reproductive technologies do not "directly implicate the values—bodily integrity, marital intimacy, or integrity of the family unit—that are central to the privacy cases" (Massie 1995). Thus, it may follow that any constitutionally protected interest in pregnancy termination—which is based on these very values—does not extend to the right to make decisions or pursue interventions that involve embryos prior to implantation. For example, at least one court, in addressing the disposition of frozen embryos created for IVF, has noted that the disposition of an embryo "does not implicate a woman's right of privacy or bodily integrity in the area of reproductive choice" (*Kass v. Kass*, 696 N.E.2d 174 [N.Y. 1998]). However, Carl Coleman has argued that:

> [The] fact that ARTs require medical interventions does not mean they fall outside the scope of constitutional protection. After all, the right to abortion is a right to a medical procedure; the fact that terminating a pregnancy requires medical intervention has never been thought to be inconsistent with recognizing abortion as a constitutional right (Coleman, Assisted reproductive technologies and the constitution, 2002b).

Importantly, a hypothetical law—based on the state's legitimate interest in protecting potential life—requiring that all embryos be immediately transferred (rather than be cryopreserved or destroyed) would not withstand constitutional scrutiny, because generally, prior to viability, the state's interest in fetal life is not strong enough to compel a woman to continue (or begin) a pregnancy she wishes to terminate. For example, in cases involving the disposition of excess IVF embryos, courts have determined that the individual's interest in avoiding parenthood is greater before embryo implantation than after implantation (*Kass v. Kass*, 696 N.E.2d 174 [N.Y. 1998]). Thus, generally, when there is contractual ambiguity, courts prioritize the right not to be a parent over the interests of the gamete donor that wishes to use an embryo for procreative purposes. In such cases, no court has compelled implantation of an embryo against the wishes of an unwilling spouse (or ex-spouse).

Some commentators have raised the possibility of parental responsibility to use preimplantation genetic diagnosis for the medical benefit of future children—with concomitant legal repercussions if the potential parents do not (Malek and Daar 2012). It is frequently debated whether there is a legal and moral duty to use PGD for the medical benefit of future children, in an effort to avoid harm. For example, Janet Malek and Judith Daar have explained that an ethical and legal case can be made in favor of using PGD when potential parents are aware that a possible future child is at substantial risk of inheriting a serious genetic condition. This debate implicates our understanding of the best interest standard, notions of disability and discrimination, and could even affect tort liability. Moreover, Kirsten Smolensky notes that, where the mother fails to abort or engage in prenatal genetic interventions, any right to sue the mother for wrongful life would comes up against the mother's bodily integrity right (for more on "wrongful life" claims, see the Section entitled "Tort Law/Liability Considerations for Preimplantation and Prenatal Genetic Diagnosis") (Smolensky 2008).

Two brief and final points: first, despite their similar uses, the state's role in overseeing Preimplantation genetic diagnosis is greater than for prenatal genetic diagnosis (although the state's interest in regulating abortion is even greater). This may be explained in a number of ways, including the latter's invocation of a woman's bodily integrity and the routine and ingrained nature of prenatal genetic diagnosis in prenatal care (Mutcherson 2008). Second, as is often the case with new technologies and treatments, PGD can be expensive, and distributive justice, equality, and access questions may arise.

Current Oversight of Preimplantation and Prenatal Genetic Diagnosis

In determining the extent to which preimplantation and prenatal genetic diagnosis is and may be regulated, commentators have noted its precarious position: it "sits at the intersection of two technologies with a confusing regulatory status: assisted reproduction and genetic testing" (Genetics and Public Policy Center 2004).

With regard to regulation of assisted reproduction, compared to most medical interventions, current oversight mechanisms do little to protect potential parents' health and safety. Most laws and regulations relevant to access to and use of assisted reproductive technologies do not set the minimum standards for obtaining informed consent, standardizations for medical and psychological screening procedures, or requirements that programs offer psychological counseling before and during treatment (New York State Task Force on Life and the Law 1998).

However, assisted reproduction is not entirely the "wild west" of medicine. Various statutes, regulations, and court decisions govern the use of ART, including the federal Fertility Clinic Success Rate and Certification Act of 1992 (FCSRCA), which requires standardized reporting of pregnancy success rates to the Centers for Disease Control and Prevention (CDC) and tasks the CDC to develop a model program for states for certification of embryo laboratories (Daar 2012). However, as of 2008, no state had enacted the model program (King 2008). The CDC does not oversee the certification of such laboratories itself, because the federal government does not have direct jurisdiction over the practice of medicine; instead, the individual states oversee the practice of medicine within their jurisdictions. However, states have been relatively reluctant to legislate the practice of assisted reproduction: "[i]n general, state law regulates the relationships that form around ART (between and among patients, physicians, and third party donors and surrogates) rather than the medical practices used within the field" (Daar 2012). Only a few states have passed legislation related to ART, and those often focus on determination of parentage (Genetics and Public Policy Center 2004). In the absence of state laws, non-binding state-issued reports and guidance documents recommend that new fertility treatments be thoroughly researched and approved by institutional review boards and that measures be taken to minimize high order multiple births (New York State Task Force on Life and the Law 1998).

In 2004, the Food and Drug Administration (FDA) promulgated federal standards for registration and regular inspections of all US assisted reproduction programs (Rebar and DeCherney 2004). These regulations also set requirements for donor eligibility and testing and screening for gamete and embryo donors (SART 2006). Furthermore, the FDA regulations establish "good tissue practice" to control the spread of communicable diseases (21 CFR § 1271).

There are also no federal or state laws that directly regulate the use of preimplantation or prenatal genetic testing, nor has any state passed such laws. Until recently, the FDA has exercised limited jurisdiction over regulation of preimplantation and prenatal genetic tests (designated as "home brew" tests when the laboratories develop their own tests), although sometimes the products used by clinical laboratories to perform genetic tests are regulated as medical devices (Genetics and Public Policy Center, 2010). However, the FDA has recently indicated an interest in more active regulation of laboratory developed tests (LDTs)—diagnostic tests developed and performed by a laboratory, including genetic tests, tests for rare conditions, and companion diagnostics—as devices (Hamburg 2013). Moreover, the Center for Medicare and Medicaid Services (CMS) currently implements the Clinical Laboratory Improvement Amendments of 1988 (CLIA). The CLIA program regulates laboratories that perform testing on patient specimens—including genetic tests—in order to ensure that test results are analytically valid. However, "CMS has not taken a position regarding whether laboratories that engage in the genetic analysis component of [preimplantation genetic diagnosis] are subject to regulation as clinical laboratories" under CLIA (Genetics and Public Policy Center 2004).

In 2008, Congress enacted the federal Prenatally and Postnatally Diagnosed Conditions Awareness Act, which enumerates requirements for post-diagnosis treatment and education. However, the law does not address how and when an individual may access prenatal genetic testing for Down syndrome and other conditions.

In the absence of federal or state regulation regarding access to and the use of preimplantation and prenatal genetic diagnosis (as well as other ART interventions), professional societies and other policy-making bodies have recognized the need for assisted reproduction providers to self-regulate. The American Society for Reproductive Medicine (ASRM) periodically releases guidelines to its members, identifying its analysis and recommendations related to assisted reproductive technologies. In 2013, it published its recommendations for use of PGD for serious adult onset conditions (ASRM 2013). The Ethics Committee concluded that PGD is ethically justifiable when the conditions are serious and when there is no known intervention for the conditions, or the available interventions are either inadequately effective or significantly burdensome. Further, for less serious conditions or conditions of lesser penetrance, the Committee determined that PGD is ethically acceptable as a matter of reproductive liberty. However, these guidelines are voluntary and non-binding, although member clinics are strongly encouraged to adhere to the organization's Practice and Ethics Committee guidelines. ASRM members are required, as a condition of their membership, to report their clinical outcomes to the CDC under the FCSRCA.

Similarly, in 2007, the American Congress of Obstetricians and Gynecologists (ACOG) released a set of "Clinical Management Guidelines" on screening for fetal chromosomal abnormalities (ACOG 2007). The guidelines recommend access to prenatal screening for particular genetic abnormalities for all pregnant women, regardless of age. These guidelines are also voluntary.

Tort Law/Liability Considerations for Preimplantation and Prenatal Genetic Diagnosis

Despite its rapidly growing impact in the marketplace—for example, the global market for noninvasive prenatal genetic testing is expected to grow approximately 37 % by 2019 (Transparency market research 2014)—there are currently no consistent liability rules specific to the provision of (or the failure to provide) preimplantation or prenatal genetic diagnosis. To the extent that states have addressed liability regarding the use of or access to these technologies, variation between the laws is often due to the fact that generally tort law has evolved on a state-by-state basis.

Despite the dearth of statutory law and regulations that govern the use of preimplantation or prenatal genetic diagnosis, IVF facilities and physicians that provide these interventions have been sued for genetic misdiagnosis on a number of types of claims under state common law—primarily informed consent and negligence. Informed consent claims are based on the failure of health care providers and entities to disclose information regarding medical options. In the case of preimplantation and prenatal genetic diagnosis, such claims may include the failure to disclose the risk of fetal abnormality, birth defects, or even undesirable—but not health endangering—traits in the resulting child. Informed consent claims have generally been based on: (1) failure to properly inform patients of the inherent errors associated with the PGD process, (2) failure to inform patients of a facility's minimal experience in performing PGD, and (3) failure to inform patients of PGD as an option (as of 2010, "no court has yet recognized a duty on the part of physicians to inform patients about" preimplantation genetic diagnosis) (Amagwula et al. 2012; Wevers 2010).

Negligence (or medical malpractice) claims are based on negligent testing, selection, and implantation of IVF embryos, often grounded in a provider's failure to detect a genetic anomaly or warn of the potential for genetic anomaly (Wevers 2010). Most often, facilities and providers have been sued under wrongful birth and wrongful life causes of action, after the birth of a child with a genetic anomaly. Wrongful birth claims arise when parents object to the birth of an unwanted or unplanned child. In such cases, the parents allege that the physician failed to warn them of the risk of conceiving or giving birth to a child with a serious genetic disorder, arguing that the birth of an ill or disabled child caused the parents harm (Botkin 2003). More than half of states permit wrongful birth actions (Rebouché and Rothenberg 2012). Wrongful life claims are those in which the child plaintiff (as represented by the child's parents) claims that the child would have been better off never having lived at all, and but for the physician's negligence, would not in fact have lived. Most jurisdictions refuse to recognize this cause of action (Crockin). In *Zepeda v. Zepeda*, the court worried that finding for the son in his wrongful life suit against his father would encourage others to "seek damages for being born of a certain color, another because of race; one for being born with a hereditary disease, another for inheriting unfortunate family characteristics; one for being born into a large and destitute family, another because a parent has an unsavory reputation" (190 N.E.2d 849 [Ill. App. 1963]).

Tort law claims—particularly those based in negligence—give rise to a number of ethical concerns, including questions about disability, parents' duties to use preimplantation and prenatal diagnosis, and genetic enhancement (Cohen 2008; Botkin 2003; Coleman, Conceiving harm, 2002a; Parens and Asch 2000). These issues are beyond the scope of this chapter, but are worth considering when determining the extent that our liability rules do and should influence social outcomes.

Recent court decisions have brought to light the liability concerns that can arise in the provision of preimplantation and prenatal genetic testing services. A select number of cases representing the various negligence and informed consent claims are discussed below (Amagwula et al. 2012).

Negligence: wrongful birth. In the largest individual award in Washington state history, in 2013 a jury awarded 50 million dollars to a couple whose son was born with "unbalanced chromosome translocation," leading to profound mental and physical disabilities (Ostrom 2013). The parents brought a wrongful birth case against the medical center and lab, alleging that the lab missed the translocation because the medical center mishandled the genetic test and failed to send vital information to the lab. The couple claimed that, had they known of the genetic defect, they would have ended the pregnancy.

Negligence: wrongful birth and wrongful life. In 2011, a couple undergoing IVF gave birth to a child with cystic fibrosis despite undergoing PGD (*Grossbaum v. Genesis Genetics Inst., LLC,* 2011 WL 2462279 [D.N.J. 2011]). The couple alleged that New York University IVF facilities and Genesis Genetics, a company that specializes in providing PGD laboratory services, were negligent in their embryo screening program. The parents were known carriers of cystic fibrosis and underwent IVF with PGD with the sole intention of avoiding having a child with the disease. After IVF of ten eggs by NYU personnel, biopsies of each embryo were sent to Genesis Genetics for PGD testing. The report faxed to the NYU IVF facility identified the embryos numbered 8 and 10 as "Carrier maternal—OK to transfer." Embryologists and an endocrinologist at NYU substituted embryo number 7, which had been identified as "Carrier at worst," for embryo 10. The NYU defendants subsequently implanted embryos 7 and 8. Two weeks after their child's birth, the daughter was diagnosed with cystic fibrosis. The Grossbaums sought damages for emotional distress, cost and expenses of medical care, and continuing care for the child after the age of majority.

Negligence and informed consent. In another case, a couple alleged that IVF providers at Columbia University and Columbia-Presbyterian Medical Center failed to conduct a PGD test to ascertain whether the donor egg had genetic diseases (*Paretta v. Medical Offices for Human Reproduction*, 195 Misc. 2d 568 [N.Y. Sup. Ct. 2003]). The couple's child was born with cystic fibrosis. The couple alleged that they were told that the donor did not have a history of mental illness or genetic diseases and that they were never given information about the potential for cystic fibrosis. The

New York Supreme Court stated that the parents would be permitted to "vigorously pursue recovery" for monetary damages resulting from caring for a child with cystic fibrosis. The parties later settled for 1.3 million dollars before trial.

Informed consent: failure to inform patients of preimplantation genetic diagnosis as an option. Although the case was never decided on the merits but was dismissed due to lack of jurisdiction, *Coggeshall v. Reproductive Endocrine Associates* represents a situation in which parents sued an IVF clinic for failure to inform them of the option for preimplantation genetic testing (376 S.C. 12 [2007]). After their child was born with Down syndrome, the couple sued the fertility clinic in Charlotte, North Carolina that provided the IVF services, alleging that the clinic's failure to offer IVF patients the option of PGD led to "substantial financial expenses." They claimed that they should have been informed of the option for PGD before their initial IVF cycle.

Negligence: wrongful life. In an unpublished 2009 case, parents who underwent IVF with PGD to screen for Fabry disease alleged misdiagnosis against the facility at the University of Southern California (*Bergero v. USC Keck School of Medicine*, 2009 WL 946874 [L.A. County Super. Ct. 2009]). The couple sought the IVF facility's services in order to decrease the chance of giving birth to a male child affected with the X-linked disease. An embryo—which was one of the presumed female carrier embryos—was successfully implanted. However, upon ultrasound and prenatal amniocentesis, a male fetus with Fabry disease was later identified. Regardless, the plaintiffs decided to carry the fetus to term. The parents alleged that the facility failed to inform the parents that they had only performed IVF with PGD on "one or two" previous occasions. The parties later settled out of court for an undisclosed sum.

Conclusion

As this chapter demonstrates, the legal questions that arise as one considers the regulation and oversight of, access to, and use of preimplantation and prenatal genetic diagnosis are increasingly complex and nuanced. They arise as tort law claims involving providers' malpractice and/or negligence and failure to provide informed consent. And they arise as constitutional questions of law, focusing on the various rights and interests at play, including those involving a woman's ability to terminate a pregnancy for fetal anomaly, prospective parents' desire to procreate by utilizing PGD, and the state's interest in protecting potential life.

Federal and state legislators, regulators, and judges have attempted to balance countervailing interests in diverse (and not always effective) ways. On the one hand, states are passing abortion restrictions at an increasing pace; on the other, they are doing very little to adequately and consistently regulate access to and use of prenatal and preimplantation genetic diagnosis. Moreover, as the development and utilization of assisted reproductive and genetic technologies proliferate, they may outpace law and policymakers' ability to appropriately respond. Consequently, law and policymakers must continue to endeavor to ensure that the law properly reflects (sometimes conflicting) ethical values in the wake of evolving technology.

References

Amagwula BS et al. Preimplantation genetic diagnosis: a systematic review of litigation in the face of new technology. Fertil Steril. 2012;98:1277–82.

American College of Obstetricians and Gynecologists (ACOG). Screening for fetal chromosomal anomalies. 2007. http://www.guideline.gov/content.aspx?id=10921. Accessed 23 May 2014.

An overview of abortion in the United States. Guttmacher Inst. 2014. http://www.guttmacher.org/presentations/abort_slides.pdf. Accessed 22 May 2014.

Botkin JR. Prenatal diagnosis and the selection of children. Fla State Univ Law Rev. 2003;30:265.

Boonstra HD, Nash E. A surge of state abortion restrictions put providers-and the women they serve-in the crosshairs. Guttmacher Institute Policy Review. Winter 2014;17(1):9–14, 18. Available online at http://www.guttmacher.org/pubs/gpr/17/1/gpr170109.pdf.

Cohen IG. Intentional diminishment, the non-identity problem, and legal liability. Hast L J. 2008;60:347.

Coleman CH. Assisted reproductive technologies and the constitution. Fordham Urb L J. 2002a;30:57–70.

Coleman CH. Conceiving harm: disability discrimination in assisted reproductive technologies. UCLA L Rev. 2002b;50:17.

Corrigan LM. Fetal anomalies, undue burdens, and 20-week abortion bans. Science Progress. May 23, 2013. http://scienceprogress.org/2013/05/fetal-anomalies-undue-burdens-and-20-week-abortion-bans/. Accessed 23 May 2014.

Crockin SL. Overview of court decisions involving reproductive genetics. Genetics & Public Policy Center. http://www.dnapolicy.org/resources/Overviewofcourtdecisions_Crockin.pdf. Accessed 17 June 2014.

Daar J. Federalizing embryo transfers: taming the wild west of reproductive medicine? Colum J Gender L. 2012;23:257–325.

Eckholm E. Abortion providers in Texas sue over a restrictive rule that could close clinics. NY Times. 20 Apr 2014.

Eckholm E. Court panel upholds Texas law on abortion. NY Times. 27 Mar 2014.

Ethics Committee of the American Society for Reproductive Medicine. Use of preimplantation genetic diagnosis for serious adult onset conditions: a committee opinion. Fertil Steril. 2013;100:54–7.

Genetics and Public Policy Center. Preimplantation genetic diagnosis: a discussion of challenges, concerns, and preliminary policy options related to the genetic testing of human embryos. 2004. http://www.dnapolicy.org/images/reportpdfs/PGDDiscussionChallengesConcerns.pdf. Accessed 22 June 2014.

Genetics & Public Policy Center. Reproductive genetic testing. 2010. http://www.dnapolicy.org/policy.international.php?action=detail&laws_id=63. Accessed 22 June 2014.

Gunnar WP. The fundamental law that shapes the United States health care system: is universal health care realistic within the established paradigm? Ann Health L. 2006;1:151.

Hall E, Berlin M. Using medicaid to support preterm birth prevention: five case studies. 2014. http://www.marchofdimes.com/materials/partner-using-medicaid-to-support-preterm-birth-prevention-five-case-studies.pdf.

Hamburg MA. Commissioner's address. June 2, 2013. http://www.fda.gov/NewsEvents/Speeches/ucm354888.htm. Accessed 22 June 2014.

Hansen M et al. Assisted reproductive technologies and the risk of birth defects – a systematic review. Hum Reprod. 2005;20:328–38.

Hill BJ. Legislative restrictions on abortion. Virtual Mentor. 2012;14:133.

Kaira SK et al. Ovarian stimulation and low birth weight in newborns conceived through in vitro fertilization. Obstet Gynecol. 2011;118:863–71.
King JS. Not this child: constitutional questions in regulating noninvasive prenatal genetic diagnosis and selective abortion. UCLA L Rev. 2012;60:2.
King JS. And genetic testing for all… the coming revolution in non-invasive prenatal genetic testing. Rutgers L J. 2011;42:599.
King JS. Predicting probability: regulating the future of preimplantation genetic screening. Yale J Health Pol'y L Ethics. 2008;8:283.
Kliff S. The landscape of abortion bans, in one must-see map. Washington Post. March 28, 2013. http://www.washingtonpost.com/blogs/wonkblog/wp/2013/03/28/the-landscape-of-abortion-bans-in-one-must-see-map/. Accessed 23 May 2014.
Lee SJ et al. Fetal pain: a systematic multidisciplinary review of the evidence. JAMA. 2005;294:947–54.
Malek J, Daar J. The case for a parental duty to use preimplantation genetic diagnosis for medical benefit. Am J Bioeth. 2012;12:3–11.
Massie AM. Regulating choice: a constitutional law response to professor John A. Robertson's children of choice. Wash Lee L Rev. 1995;52:135.
Merritt TA et al. Impact of ART on pregnancies in California: an analysis of maternity outcomes and insights into the added burden of neonatal intensive care. J Perinatol. 2014;34:345–50.
Meyer M. States' regulation of assisted reproductive technologies: what does the U.S. Constitution allow? The Nelson A. Rockefeller Inst of Gov't. 2009. http://www.rockinst.org/pdf/health_care/2009-07-States_Regulation_ART.pdf. Accessed 5 May 2014.
Monthly state updates: major developments in 2013 (as of 12/31/2013). Guttmacher Institute. http://www.guttmacher.org/statecenter/updates/2013/dec.html. Accessed 22 May 2014.
Monthly state updates: major developments in 2014 (as of 5/1/2014). Guttmacher Institute. May 1 2014. http://www.guttmacher.org/statecenter/updates/. Accessed 22 May 2014.
Mutcherson KM. Making mommies: law, pre-implantation genetic diagnosis, and the complications of pre-motherhood. Colum J Gender L. 2008;18:313.
Nash E, et al. Laws affecting reproductive health and rights: 2013 state policy review. 2013. http://www.guttmacher.org/statecenter/updates/2013/statetrends42013.html. Accessed 22 May 2014.
National Women's Law Center 2013. State level abortion restrictions: an extreme overreach into women's reproductive health care; 2014. http://www.nwlc.org/sites/default/files/pdfs/2013_state_legislation_factsheet_1-27-14.pdf. Accessed 22 May 2014.
New York State Task Force on Life and the Law. Assisted reproductive technologies: analysis and recommendations for public policy. 1998.
Non-invasive prenatal testing (NIPT) market (maternit21 plus, verifi, harmony, panorama, nifty, prenatest and bambnitest) – global industry analysis, size, share, growth, trends and forecast – 2013–2019. Transparency Market Research. 2013. http://www.transparencymarketresearch.com/noninvasive-prenatal-diagnostics-market.html. Accessed 21 June 2014.
Ostrom CM. $50m awarded over birth defect; test said baby would be ok. The Seattle Times. 11 Dec 2013.
Parens E, Asch A. The disability rights critique of prenatal genetic testing: reflections and recommendations. In: Parens E, Asch A, editors. Prenatal testing and disability rights. Washington, DC: Georgetown University Press; 2000. p. 13–4.
Pazol K, et al. Abortion surveillance – United States, 2009. Centers for Disease Control and Prevention. 2012. http://www.cdc.gov/mmwr/preview/mmwrhtml/ss6108a1.htm?s_cid=ss6108a1_w. Accessed 23 May 2014.
Ranji U, et al., Henry J Kaiser Fam Found. State medicaid coverage of perinatal services: summary of state findings. 2009:14. http://www.kff.org/womenshealth/upload/8014.pdf. Accessed 21 May 2014.
Rebar RW, DeCherney AH. Assisted reproductive technology in the United States. N Engl J Med. 2004;350:1603–04.

Rebouché R, Rothenberg K. Mixed messages: the intersection of prenatal genetic testing and abortion. How L Rev. 2012;55:983.
Robertson JA. Procreative liberty and harm to offspring in assisted reproduction. Am J L Med. 2004;30:7.
Smolensky KR. Creating children with disabilities: parental tort liability for preimplantation genetic interventions. Hast L J. 2008;60:299.
Society for Assisted Reproductive Technology (SART). Summary of "eligibility determination for donors of human cells, tissues, and cellular and tissue-based products". 2006. http://www.sart.org/news/article.aspx?id=337. Accessed 22 June 2014.
State policies in brief: state funding of abortion under medicaid. Guttmacher Institute. May 1, 2014. http://www.guttmacher.org/statecenter/spibs/spib_SFAM.pdf. Accessed 23 May 2014.
State policies in brief: state policies on later abortions. Guttmacher Institute. May 1, 2014. http://www.guttmacher.org/statecenter/spibs/spib_PLTA.pdf. Accessed 22 May 2014.
State policies in brief: targeted regulation of abortion providers. Guttmacher Institute. May 1, 2014. http://www.guttmacher.org/statecenter/spibs/spib_TRAP.pdf. Accessed 22 May 2014.
Stern A. A disturbing trend: conscience clauses threaten genetic counseling. Huffington Post. April 2, 2014. http://www.huffingtonpost.com/alex-stern/a-disturbing-trend-consci_b_5066570.html. Accessed 23 May 2014
Suter SM. The "repugnance" lens of *Gonzalez v. Carhart* and other theories of reproductive technologies. George Wash L Rev. 2008;65:1514–98.
Swendiman KS. Health care: constitutional rights and legislative powers. Congressional Research Service. 2012. http://fas.org/sgp/crs/misc/R40846.pdf. Accessed 22 June 2014.
Thomson-Deveaux A. Fetal abnormalities: the next minefield in the abortion wars? The Am Prospect. 2014. http://prospect.org/article/fetal-abnormalities-next-minefield-abortion-wars. Accessed 22 May 2014.
U.S. Department of Health and Human Services. Federal health care conscience protection statutes. http://www.hhs.gov/ocr/civilrights/understanding/ConscienceProtect/. Accessed 22 June 2014.
Wevers K. Prenatal torts and pre-implantation genetic diagnosis. Harv J L Technol. 2010;24:257.

Part III
Alternative Social Perspectives

Chapter 9
Ethical Issues

Mary B. Mahowald

Ethical Issues: The Burden of Choice

The subtitle of this book identifies a key problem in addressing ethical issues in prenatal and preimplantation testing: the meaning of "choice." It also raises questions about why and for whom such choices may be a burden. These issues are relevant to ethics because the ability to choose is indispensable to morally responsible decision-making. Respect for autonomy, a key principle of biomedical ethics, assumes the presence of the ability to choose in ethical decisions. However, this ability carries with it the burden of responsibility for what we decide, regardless of whether the results are good or bad for us or for others. The burden of moral responsibility is reduced, possibly even eliminated, to the extent that the capacity for choosing is not present or fully developed in specific individuals or in specific circumstances. Impediments or limitations to autonomy arise, for example, from social pressures, time constraints, and inability or lack of understanding of the full implications of decisions to be made. To the extent that the capacity for choosing is absent or deficient, other ethical principles have greater import.

In this chapter, we discuss the meaning of choice and describe how it relates to the principle of respect for autonomy as well as other basic principles of biomedical ethics. We also examine what these principles mean and how they apply in different circumstances to those who are affected by or make decisions about prenatal and preimplantation testing. While addressing these ethical issues, we cannot escape the fact that such decisions affect developing human embryos or fetuses, whose moral status, if any, is interminably controversial among philosophers and theologians

M.B. Mahowald, Ph.D. (✉)
Department of Obstetrics and Gynecology and MacLean Center for Clinical Medical Ethics, University of Chicago, 5841 Maryland Avenue, MC 2050, Chicago, IL 60615, USA
e-mail: mm46@uchicago.edu

J.P. Galst, M.S. Verp (eds.), *Prenatal and Preimplantation Diagnosis*,
DOI 10.1007/978-3-319-18911-6_9

as well as patients and practitioners. Although the primary goal of prenatal and preimplantation testing is to identify and select some embryos or fetuses for initiation or continuation of pregnancy, disagreement about the ethics of testing arises because of its inevitable connection with post-test decisions about the disposition of the undesired embryos or fetuses. While acknowledging that none of the diverse philosophical positions about the moral status of human embryos and fetuses is uncontroversially definitive, we begin by simply identifying the different positions that are ethically relevant to those who support them.

In contrast to the different philosophical positions, different religious views about the ethics of prenatal and preimplantation testing tend to be definitive because they follow from clear but rationally unprovable beliefs about the moral status of human embryos and fetuses. Legal rulings about testing can also be definitive because they stipulate such positions as their starting point; these, however, may differ from jurisdiction to jurisdiction, and are subject to change from time to time. Subsequent chapters in this book deal with religious and legal aspects of prenatal and preimplantation testing.

Basic Ethical Principles

In all seven editions of their classic work, *Principles of Biomedical Ethics*, Tom Beauchamp and James Childress identify the basic principles applicable to healthcare and medical research as respect for autonomy, beneficence, nonmaleficence, and justice (Beauchamp and Childress 2013). Unfortunately, the meanings of these principles are rather abstract, which allows for diverse but valid interpretations of them. Despite this potential diversity, the terms "beneficence" and "nonmaleficence" (derived from the Latin terms for "doing good" and "not doing harm") are familiar to clinicians who are trained in the importance of both principles as well as the relation between them. "First, do no harm" is thus commonly recognized as prioritizing nonmaleficence over beneficence wherever the potential benefit does not clearly outweigh the potential harm or burden (Beauchamp and Childress 2013). Both principles are also construed as primarily applicable to patients, and only secondarily, if at all, to those affected by decisions regarding patients, such as family members or clinicians. Rarely if ever are respect for autonomy, beneficence and nonmaleficence construed as applicable to those who are not directly affected, such as the public-at-large, who may be affected but far less significantly, as, for example, through the shared social costs of caring for individuals unrelated to them.

The principle of respect for autonomy is relatable but not equivalent to the role of "informed consent" in health care. The latter mainly refers to the institutional or legal process by which competent patients are required to voluntarily authorize their treatment after being told of its potential risks and benefits to them (Beauchamp and Childress 2013). Because the rules governing this process are socially defined, its requirements are subject to change in different institutional and legal settings, and fulfillment of these requirements is not necessarily consistent with the more demanding meaning of respect for autonomy.

The more demanding meaning of the principle of respect for autonomy carries with it the need for clarity regarding the meaning of both terms, and in the context of this book, their relationship to "choice." "Respect," for example, does not necessarily imply compliance with someone's choices; it may simply mean acknowledgment of the fact that someone has made a conscientious autonomous decision. People who disagree with each other about a particular issue may nonetheless respect each other's positions even while maintaining their disagreement. A clinician who chooses to offer preimplantation testing to her patients may thus respect the choice of a colleague not to do so, and vice versa. It is regrettable, therefore, that respect for autonomy has in some quarters been uncritically construed as necessarily implying compliance with the autonomous decision of another. Clinicians who define their role as one of simply carrying out the wishes of the patient exemplify this tendency, an "instrumentalist" conception of the practitioner's role (Mahowald 2006). Patients who regard their clinicians as morally obligated to comply with any of their wishes also exemplify it.

The term "autonomy" generally refers to the capacity to make a rational and informed decision; whether this capacity is exercised in particular situations is a different matter. As already suggested, if a decision is not rational, informed, or if it is determined by factors beyond one's control, the decision lacks autonomy even though the term "choice" may be used in describing it; in such situations, the principle of respect for autonomy is not applicable. Beneficence and nonmaleficence then become paramount, and either or both of these principles call for efforts to overcome the impediments to genuine choice and respect for autonomy as well as other ways of "doing good" and "avoiding harm."

The term "burden" relates to the principle of nonmaleficence because burdens are often harms to be avoided, or at least limited, if possible. In addition to the burden of responsibility that is associated with autonomy, autonomous choices can entail burdens in two other ways: the difficulty and/or anxiety of making decisions, and the consequences of their implementation. Obviously, these consequences may be beneficial as well as burdensome. How to weigh and prioritize the anticipated benefits and burdens while also respecting autonomy presents the ethical challenge of determining how to apply all three principles to specific cases. Attention to the particularities of each case is thus essential to its ethical assessment.

Another factor relevant to the ethical assessment of specific cases is the intention of the person or persons who make choices about what should or should not be done. There is thus a distinction between objective and subjective morality: the former refers to the act or omission in itself; the latter refers to the person who commits or omits the act, i.e., the moral agent. An act may be wrong in itself without the agent being morally responsible, or fully responsible, for its wrongness. This would occur, for example, if someone lacked the cognitive capacity to understand the implications of an intervention. It would also occur if someone were misinformed or uninformed about the consequences of a decision, or coerced or pressured to act in a way that is objectively immoral.

The basic bioethical principle of justice mainly refers to the way in which harms and benefits are distributed among all of those affected by particular decisions.

At times, for example, justice may require treating one patient before others because of the former's more urgent need. It also requires patients themselves to weigh the import of their decisions on others. Accordingly, in addition to patients, who are obviously most affected by decisions about their own health care, the other principles are applicable to those directly involved with patients, including family members as well as clinicians.

On grounds of justice, it may also be argued that social and economic burdens and benefits to those who are not directly affected are ethically relevant to decisions by and about patients. This principle obviously requires a prioritizing among those affected, ordering the applicability of the other principles by assessing the disparate impact of harms and benefits as well as the autonomous choices of individuals.

Inevitably, adequate consideration of the principles of beneficence, nonmaleficence and justice returns us to the thorny issue already mentioned, the moral status, if any, of human embryos or fetuses involved in prenatal or preimplantation testing. With prenatal testing the question arises with regard to abortion of in vivo embryos or fetuses that have been identified as undesired. With preimplantation testing, it relates to disposal of in vitro embryos that have been identified as undesired. At times, there may be disagreement among those who are personally involved, e.g., the progenitors of the embryos, and then the issue that must be addressed is whose autonomous decision is to be given priority.

Who Is the Patient?

Pregnant women are clearly patients because they are directly, physically affected by decisions made about continuing or discontinuing their pregnancies. This is true even when the pregnancy is undertaken for another through "surrogate gestation" (Mahowald 2000). Women who choose preimplantation testing to avoid an unwanted condition in their offspring are also patients in that they are directly, physically affected through the procedures required to produce in vitro embryos. Chervenak and McCullough argue that fetuses become patients who, as such, deserve treatment whenever a woman decides to continue her pregnancy, or, absent such a decision, when the developing fetus has achieved viability (Chervenak and McCullough 1994). In their view, embryos or fetuses involved in prenatal or preimplantation testing are not patients because they do not meet either criterion.

Although Chervenak and McCullough focus on "patienthood" rather than "personhood" in discussing embryos and fetuses, others equate the two, either attributing or denying a right to life at different stages of development (Mahowald 2006). "Personhood" is then seen as conferring a right to life that may only be justifiably disrupted on grounds of preserving another's life. There is a huge range of positions on the onset of personhood (Mahowald 1995). Some argue, for example, that even in vitro embryos are persons (George and Gomez Lobo 2005; Noonan 1970), while others maintain that the personhood that carries with it a right to life commences only at birth (Warren 2000). Still others hold that personhood is not achieved until or unless an individual has the capacity to reason and communicate, i.e., until sometime in early childhood; only then is the individual recognized as a moral agent who, as such, bears responsibility for his or her decisions (Engelhardt 1996; Tooley 1997).

Some positions about human embryos and fetuses ignore the issue of personhood while holding similar positions about their moral relevance to prenatal and preimplantation testing. These positions include (a) denial that human embryos or fetuses have any moral relevance to such decisions (Kuhse and Singer 1982; Tooley 1997), (b) affirmation that they have the same moral relevance as born humans (George and Gomez Lobo 2005; Noonan 1970), (c) claims that their moral status increases through the course of development but full moral status is only achieved at birth (Gillespie 1977; Robertson 1994), and (d) assertions that a specific point or stage of development (e.g., onset of brain activity, sentiency, viability) is associated with specific moral responsibility (Chervenak and McCullough 1994; Sass 1994; Steinbock 1992). Each of these positions leads to a different weighing of how the principles of biomedical ethics apply to specific cases.

Obviously, the principle of respect for autonomy is not applicable to embryos or fetuses, regardless of where they are (in vivo or in vitro), and regardless of their stage of development. For those who subscribe to position (a), neither are the principles of beneficence and nonmaleficence applicable to fetuses or embryos—at any stage of development. Those who subscribe to positions (c) and (d) believe that the principles of nonmaleficence and beneficence are applicable to developing fetuses, but the degree of applicability depends on the degree of moral status attributed to them at different stages of development. Although the possibility of fetal pain is a controversial issue, some authors argue that the possible development of sentiency carries a moral onus to avoid infliction of pain even in the context of abortions performed after late term prenatal testing (Steinbock 1992). Viability is a developmental threshold that others identify as morally relevant regardless of whether fetuses are regarded as having a right to life. Chervenak and McCullough, for example, maintain that viability makes the fetus a patient whose welfare clinicians are obliged to support independently of the pregnant woman's wishes (Chervenak and McCullough 1994). Nonetheless, short of having reached the milestones of development specified by those who hold positions (c) or (d), the principles of nonmaleficence and beneficence are inapplicable to fetuses.

Termination of unwanted in vitro embryos obtained through preimplantation testing is generally seen as ethically uncontroversial because it bypasses the thorny issue of abortion. It does so, however, only if abortion is defined as termination of pregnancy, as it is in clinical texts (Cunningham et al. 2009; Mosby's Medical Dictionary 2009), and not as termination of the embryo or fetus, as it is often viewed popularly, regardless of whether one is "prolife" or "prochoice." For those who subscribe to position (b), even in vitro embryos are viewed as persons or as having moral status equal to that of born human beings. For them, destruction of in vitro embryos is abortion. It is possible but highly unlikely that rejection of testing on grounds of opposition to abortion is avoidable through donation of unwanted in vitro embryos to women who agree to gestate them (sex selection might be the reason one party rejects the embryos while another wants them). Even freezing embryos would be rejected by those in group (b)—on grounds that the process reduces the probability of further development.

Regardless of whether preimplantation testing is construed as bypassing the necessity of abortion to avoid an unwanted birth, this mode of testing carries with it the emotional as well as physical advantage to a woman of avoiding termination of a pregnancy already established within her. This clear benefit must be weighed against the more invasive and expensive procedures of hormonal stimulation, ova retrieval and embryo transfer associated with in vitro fertilization (with partner's sperm), all of which are required in conjunction with preimplantation testing. The principles of nonmaleficence and beneficence are obviously relevant to determination of which mode of testing may be used to avoid a particular condition in offspring, but how the risks and benefits of one method versus the other are weighed by individuals or couples contemplating such testing may vary considerably.

Applicability of the Principles to Different Moral Agents

Those who are indisputably persons may be called moral agents because they are capable of, and therefore responsible for, their own informed and autonomous decisions (Tooley 1997). In terms of ethics, the central figure and the primary moral agent in the context of prenatal and preimplantation testing is the woman who undergoes testing or whose embryos are tested in vitro. She is central in both situations because she is most affected by the decision to test, the test itself, and decisions made after test results are obtained. She is directly, physically affected by prenatal tests, which vary in their timing during pregnancy, their invasiveness and discomfort, risks (to her and/or to the fetus), their expense, the definitiveness of their results, and the conditions being tested. Although she is not physically affected by the process of preimplantation testing, she is directly, physically affected by the invasive process through which the embryos examined in vitro are obtained. She is also directly affected by the decision to terminate or continue her pregnancy after learning the results of the tests. Moreover, in most situations, she becomes the main caregiver for offspring to whom she gives birth after testing. As a moral agent, all of her autonomous decisions about the issue carry with them concomitant responsibility.

The possibility that gestational and genetic motherhood are medically separable introduces a complicating feature to the argument that the woman's autonomy has priority in prenatal and preimplantation testing (Ravin et al. 1997). Nonetheless, the claim that the autonomy of the person who is physically most affected by testing be given priority applies to this situation also. Accordingly, a woman who gestates an embryo or fetus for another woman may not be coerced to undergo prenatal testing even if she agreed to do so prior to her pregnancy. If she does undergo prenatal testing, neither may she be coerced about termination or continuation of her pregnancy. However, depending on the degree of harm to be prevented, coercion may be morally objectionable even in situations in which its rationale is prevention of harm to another. Giving priority to the autonomy of someone because he or she is most physically affected by a potential intervention does not necessarily imply that the person's decision is morally justified or admirable.

For those who support position (a), the ethical principle of respect for the woman's autonomy is paramount, but beneficence and nonmaleficence towards her are also relevant to clinical decisions involving her autonomous choices. As described in previous chapters, however, the medical risks or potential harms to women of some testing procedures may be construed as minimal; financial burdens, as well as the medical burdens entailed by the requirements of obtaining embryos for preimplantation testing, are in most cases significant burdens to be avoided, but women themselves are unable to avoid these if they choose such testing.

If the potential father accepts and intends to fulfill his responsibility for a child to whom his partner gives birth, respect for his autonomy in testing decisions is ethically relevant, but not as compellingly as is respect for the autonomy of the woman. Arguably, she has a moral obligation to consider his wishes while making her own decisions about testing. The autonomy of clinicians should be respected as well, albeit not as bindingly as that of either potential parent. In general, no clinician should be compelled to perform a procedure he or she believes is medically more harmful than beneficial to a patient, or an elective procedure to which the clinician objects on moral grounds. As is commonly the case, clinicians who, on moral or religious grounds, do not wish to comply with a patient's request for a medically unnecessary treatment can and should refer the patient to a clinician for whom compliance is not objectionable.

Applicability to Specific Cases: Principles Interpreted in Light of Variables

Although the basic bioethical principles, as principles, do not change, the variables of particular cases are clearly relevant to the interpretation and application of the principles. As already suggested, for example, respect for autonomy does not have the same import when the person whose autonomy is to be respected does not fully grasp the consequences of a particular choice as it does for someone who fully grasps the consequences. Moreover, what counts as benefits or burdens often differs for different individuals. Some potential parents, depending on their circumstances and preferences, may attribute less priority to the genetic link between them and their intended child than to their desire to raise a healthy child regardless of whether the child is genetically related to both of them. Depending on the condition that potential parents wish to avoid in offspring, they may choose gamete donation as a means of bypassing the need for either prenatal or preimplantation testing. Arguably, this option, if available, as well as that of prenatal or preimplantation testing, should be offered to women or couples who are considering either test as a means of insuring that their potential child is free of an identifiable but undesired trait.

Regardless of whether the person most affected is male or female, intended parent or not, respect for the autonomy of the one most affected by a particular decision is still the paramount ethical obligation in bioethics. At times, however, nonmaleficence or beneficence may have priority. For example, a clinician's obligation to respect the autonomy of a particular patient would be outweighed by the obligation to practice nonmaleficence if the patient chose a high-risk procedure likely to cause significant harm to him or her. Respect for someone's autonomous choice of a procedure might also be overridden on grounds of justice; for example, if the costs of the procedure, whether in time or money, were so exorbitant that the welfare of others might thereby be significantly impeded.

The variables that are ethically relevant to testing decisions include nonclinical as well as clinical factors, and the nonclinical factors cover a huge range of possibilities. It is virtually impossible for individual clinicians to identify all of the potentially relevant nonclinical features of cases in which they are involved. Case reports of specific procedures rarely identify some of the knowable and potentially relevant nonclinical variables. Moreover, even if clinicians were able to identify all of these, they would still be at a loss to identify their particular relevance to particular patients.

Consider, for example, the recent report of preimplantation testing for a nonsymptomatic 27-year-old woman with a known family history of Gerstmann–Straussler–Scheinker (GSS) syndrome (Uflacker et al. 2014). After learning through predictive testing that she had the mutation for the disease, the woman was presented with the option of prenatal or preimplantation testing as a means of insuring that any child to whom she might give birth would be free of the mutation she carried. The woman requested preimplantation testing of embryos formed from her and her husband's gametes. Not noted in the report is whether the woman was apprised of the possibility of ovum donation as a means of avoiding the condition she wished to avoid. Nor did the authors acknowledge the possible moral relevance of the foreshortened life span of the woman who knew she had the GSS mutation.

According to the National Institute of Neurological Disorders and Stroke (NINDS 2007), GSS is a rare, autosomal dominant disorder due to a specific mutation (F198S) in the prion protein gene (PRNP), which has high penetrance. Severe neurological degenerative symptoms first appear during adulthood, generally between 35 and 50 years of age, and progress inexorably until death within an average span of 2–10 years (NINDS 2007).

After successful preimplantation testing, two unaffected embryos were transferred to the woman. The case report does not indicate whether pregnancy was established and continued until the birth of a healthy child or children. We may nonetheless examine the case as one in which basic bioethical principles supported the use of preimplantation testing. Respect for the autonomy of the patient seems to have been given appropriate priority, and the benefits of preimplantation testing to her (and her husband) appear to outweigh the burden and cost of the associated medical interventions (ova stimulation, IVF, embryo transfer). Presumably, her own ethical considerations have taken into account the impact of her own dismal prognosis on her husband and her potential child. The report makes it clear that this particular patient was not only competent but well informed not only by her clinicians but also by knowing her own family history of the disease and possibilities for avoiding it in her children. Although the principle of justice hardly seems applicable to this case, it would support an argument to extend the benefits of preimplantation genetic diagnosis to patients in similar medical circumstances who lack the resources to follow a similar course. It may also be argued, based on the principle of justice, that prenatal testing and abortion of embryos that test positive for GSS is a less invasive and less costly way to avoid the birth of children affected with the disorder.

The condition identified through prenatal and preimplantation testing obviously presents an important and ethically relevant clinical variable in specific cases. For example, although testing for detection of and avoidance of such a severe adult-onset disorder as GSS seems to be ethically compelling, it may be less so than it would be for a condition such as Tay–Sachs disease or Lesch–Nyhan syndrome, in which symptoms appear during infancy. The rationale for the difference is that the avoidance of a late-onset disorder suggests a disvaluing of the life lived prior to the onset of symptoms. However, the burdens anticipated after the adult onset of symptoms, not only to the affected person but also to those who care for him or her, may outweigh the value of the life lived before the onset—for the affected person as well as those associated with him or her.

Moreover, preimplantation or prenatal testing for women who know that they or their partners are carriers for such severe disorders as GSS is more compelling than it would be for the testing of adult onset disorders whose symptoms are less severe, unpredictable, treatable, or correctible, as well as those that identify risk as opposed to certainty of onset. An example of the last category is testing for the BRCA1 or BRCA2 mutation, which greatly increases the lifetime risk of developing breast cancer. The *possibility* that an individual could live a full lifetime without being affected by an identified condition reduces the strength of an ethical argument to eliminate the possibility through preimplantation or prenatal testing.

In their earlier work, authors of the case report on preimplantation testing for avoidance of GSS in offspring proposed preimplantation testing for all couples in which both partners were carriers for cystic fibrosis (Tur-Kaspa et al. 2010). Each of the potential offspring of such couples has a 1 in 4 risk of being affected by the disease, and a 1 in 2 risk of being a carrier for it (Lester et al. 1995) Prior to the availability of preimplantation testing, carrier couples could only avoid these risks through prenatal testing and abortion of the undesired fetuses. Regardless of which mode of testing is used, however, the ethical rationale for avoiding unaffected carrier status is clearly less compelling than the rationale for avoiding the disease itself.

Based on the principles of beneficence and nonmaleficence, testing for GSS is more ethically compelling than testing for cystic fibrosis because of differences between the two conditions: cystic fibrosis is treatable, but not curable, and does not entail such severe and progressive neurological devastation as GSS. Nonetheless, cystic fibrosis severely impairs function of the lungs and other organs over an entire lifetime, while considerably limiting the life expectancy of those affected (Lester et al. 1995). Testing to avoid cystic fibrosis in offspring may thus be based on the principle of nonmaleficence, i.e., avoidance of harm to potential children. Some authors have claimed that this rationale implies a disvaluing of life lived with a particular impairment. Advocates for people with disabilities, for example, have opposed prenatal tests to avoid the birth of children with disabilities on this basis (Parens and Asch 2000).

If the woman's autonomy is paramount, both preimplantation and prenatal testing are defensible for arguably less severe disorders than those that involve incurable and devastating adult onset conditions such as GSS, Huntington's disease, and Creutzfeldt–Jakob disease. This includes conditions such as cystic fibrosis and also any early onset or late onset disorder that is identifiable through preimplantation or prenatal testing. Less defensible are interventions to avoid conditions that involve correctible disorders such as cleft lip and palate, and less defensible still are those involving healthy non-medical conditions. Sex identification is an obvious and highly controversial example in the latter regard (Mahowald 2000).

Some authors have argued for a parallel between sex selection and disability avoidance (Asch 2000). While generally supporting a woman's right to terminate her pregnancy, they oppose her doing so in order to prevent the birth of someone with a particular disability. To do so, they claim, is as little justified, as is testing and termination to avoid the birth of a child of the undesired sex. The implication of such a choice is then the wrongful assumption that life lived with a specific disability or sex identification is not worth living. Their only limitation to the priority of respect for women's autonomy is that women's choices not be based on sex selection or avoidance of disability in offspring.

As a *basic* bioethical principle, respect for autonomy applies to everyone capable of an informed and voluntary choice about a specific issue. In the context of preimplantation and prenatal testing, therefore, this principle applies not only to the patient, who is always a woman, but also to her male partner and her practitioners. With regard to the latter, when a particular intervention is not medically necessary for the patient, the practitioner is not obligated to perform it, and his or her autonomy should be respected. Arguably, neither prenatal nor preimplantation tests are necessary for the health of the woman who seeks such testing. Consequently, if the practitioner is morally or religiously opposed to such testing, he or she may decline to provide it, while referring the patient to someone who is capable of and not opposed to its provision.

Respect for the woman's autonomy is usually paramount because she is the person most affected by the intervention not only physically but also in terms of the long-term consequences of interventions or lack thereof. In contrast with her male partner, and regardless of whether he acknowledges responsibility for a particular pregnancy, the woman is the one who directly undergoes the discomfort and risk of procedures associated with preimplantation and prenatal testing; in most situations, she is also mainly responsible for care of children to whom she gives birth, regardless of their health needs, and regardless of whether their biological fathers are also involved in meeting those needs. This does not mean that respect for the autonomy of potential fathers is irrelevant to decisions about prenatal or preimplantation testing. However, depending on the extent to which the potential father can be relied on to address the needs of future children, the woman should *respect* his autonomy, even while not obliged to comply with his decision. In other words, she should consider his wishes, and weigh them in forming her own informed, autonomous decision about testing or not testing. On this point, the difference between an ethics of obligation and an ethics of virtue is relevant; the latter refers to behavior that is morally commendable; the former to behavior that is morally mandatory. Thus, regardless of whether the woman makes her decision in a morally commendable manner, her choice trumps those of her partner if they do not agree.

Degrees of Moral Obligation, Virtue, and the Burden of Choice

The preceding section suggests how different circumstances affect the morality of specific decisions about prenatal and preimplantation testing on the part of a woman, her partner, and practitioners. These different factors point to conclusions that are not definitive statements about whether a specific decision is right or wrong; they do suggest, however, that some decisions are morally better or worse than others, even when some of the morally relevant features are the same. For any and every specific case, the basic principles of bioethics are relevant moral considerations whose interpretation and applicability must be determined in light of the variables involved.

To assist in applying the principles to the huge array of potential variables that are ethically relevant to cases, the following brief list of questions may be asked to help determine the meaning and applicability of the basic principles to particular cases:

Respect for Autonomy

Whose choice has priority? Is the patient fully capable of autonomous decision-making?

Is the patient fully informed of the risks, probable consequences, alternatives, and costs of the procedures being considered?

Is the patient free of social, emotional and economic pressures in making her decision?

Have the informed choices of others involved been considered (male partner, practitioners)?

Beneficence and Nonmaleficence

What are the risks, expected harms and benefits—physical, emotional, social, economic—of the potential procedures and their probable consequences, and to whom do these apply?

What factors regarding the condition to be tested strengthen or weaken the case for testing: e.g., early onset or late-onset, treatable or incurable, health-related or non-health related?

What factors regarding the test alternatives are ethically relevant—e.g., cost, invasiveness, before or during pregnancy, sensitivity and specificity of result?

Justice

Is it just or fair to deny either mode of testing to some potential patients because they cannot afford it?

Is it just or fair to deny either mode of testing for specific conditions? If so, which ones and why?

Conclusion

Although the term "choice" is often understood in contemporary society as an unmitigated good, this understanding is mistaken because choice inevitably entails, as the title of the book indicates, a burden. Many benefits to women, their partners and society-at-large may be attributed to prenatal and preimplantation testing, and these arguably outweigh the risks, harms, and benefits associated with the pertinent procedures for those who seek them. Even if the ratio of benefits to harms supports such testing, what remains is the inevitable burden of psychological and moral responsibility for the consequences of one's choices. Women who choose to undergo prenatal or preimplantation testing as well as those who decline to undergo it when they could have done otherwise bear the major burden of responsibility for the consequences of their decisions. Their male partners as well as practitioners who provide or decline to provide testing also bear responsibility, albeit to a lesser degree, for the consequences of their decisions.

The burden of choice about prenatal and preimplantation testing thus involves all of those directly affected and capable of choice regarding the issue. The weight of this burden is also inseparable, albeit to a lesser degree still, from the balance of harms and benefits that arise for those who are indirectly affected by the choices of others. The meaning and obligation of respect for autonomy is thus inseparable from the principles of beneficence, nonmaleficense and justice. In their selection of a subtitle for their book, the editors had the wisdom to recognize this important interrelatedness between the first and primary bioethical principle, respect for autonomy, and the other basic principles of bioethics.

References

Asch A. Why I haven't changed my mind about prenatal diagnosis: reflections and refinements. In: Parens E, Asch A, editors. Prenatal testing and disability rights. Washington, DC: Georgetown University Press; 2000. p. 234–58.

Beauchamp TL, Childress JF. Principles of biomedical ethics. New York: Oxford University Press; 2013.

Chervenak FA, McCullough LB. Ethics in obstetrics and gynecology. New York: Oxford University Press; 1994.

Cunningham F, Kenneth Leveno J, Steven Bloom L, John Hauth C, Dwight Rouse J, Catherine Spong. Williams obstetrics. New York: McGraw-Hill Companies Inc.; 2009.

Engelhardt HT. Foundations of bioethics. New York: Oxford University Press; 1996.
George RP, Gomez Lobo A. The moral status of the human embryo. Perspect Biol Med. 2005; 48:201–10.
Gillespie NC. Abortion and human rights. Ethics. 1977;87:237–43.
Kuhse H, Singer P. The moral status of the embryo. In: Walters W, Singer P, editors. Test-tube babies. Oxford: Oxford University Press; 1982. p. 57–63.
Lester LA, Lemke A, Levinson D, Mahowald MB. The human genome project and women, cystic fibrosis: a case study. J Wom Health. 1995;4(6):623–35.
Mahowald MB. Person. In: Reich WT, editor. Encyclopedia of bioethics. New York: Macmillan; 1995. p. 1934–40.
Mahowald MB. Genes, women, equality. New York: Oxford University Press; 2000.
Mahowald MB. Bioethics and women: across the life span. New York: Oxford University Press; 2006.
Mosby's medical dictionary. 8th ed. Maryland Heights, MO: Elsevier; 2009.
National Institute of Neurological Disorders and Stroke. NINDS Gerstmann-Straussler-Scheinker disease information. Bethesda, MD: National Institutes of Health; 2007.
Noonan JT. An almost absolute value in history. In: Noonan J, editor. The morality of abortion. Cambridge: Harvard University Press; 1970.
Parens E, Asch A, editors. Prenatal testing and disability rights. Washington, DC: Georgetown University Press; 2000.
Ravin AJ, Mahowald MB, Stocking CB. Genes or gestation? Attitudes of women and men about biologic ties to children. J Wom Health. 1997;6:639–47.
Robertson J. Children of choice: freedom and the new reproductive technologies. Princeton, NJ: Princeton University Press; 1994.
Sass H-M. The moral significance of brain-life criteria. In: Beller FK, Weir RF, editors. The beginning of human life. Dordrecht: Kluwer; 1994.
Steinbock B. Life before birth. New York: Oxford University Press; 1992.
Tooley M. Abortion and infanticide. In: Dwyer S, Feinberg J, editors. The problem of abortion. 3rd ed. Belmont, CA: Wadsworth; 1997.
Tur-Kaspa I, Aljadeff G, Rechitsky S, Grotjan HE, Verlinsky Y. PGD for all cystic fibrosis carrier couples: novel strategy for preventive medicine and cost analysis. Reprod Biomed Online. 2010;21(2):186–95.
Uflacker A, Doralswamy PM, Rechitsky S, See T, Geschwind M, Tur-Kaspa I. Preimplantation genetic diagnosis (PGD) for genetic prion disorder due to F1985 mutation in the PRNP gene. JAMA Neurol. 2014;2014:E1–3.
Warren MA. Moral status: obligations to persons and other living things. Oxford: Oxford University Press; 2000.

Chapter 10
Religious Traditions

Rebecca Rae Anderson

"Religion" denotes an organized belief system with a name, an articulated doctrine, conventions and rituals, and usually some source of temporal authority residing in a person or a group. In current parlance "spirituality" often is used to describe an individual's acknowledgment of and relationship with the transcendent, in whatever form that may take, within or outside of an organized religious tradition.

All people, regardless of religious or spiritual leanings, hold moral convictions that influence their behavior and sense of integrity. Sources of these principles include family beliefs and traditions, cultural mores, and peer values, as well as religious and philosophical considerations. People often conflate their religious beliefs with their cultural mores, and may be surprised to learn that certain conventions have no basis in religious doctrine (for instance, female circumcision [Gele et al. 2012; Hayford and Trinitapoli 2011; Rouzi 2013]). Loyalty to a religious tradition typically is characterized by nonrational adherence, not by logical consistency or intellectual rigor, with scattered exceptions (Dutney 2007).

The moral convictions of an individual do not necessarily coincide with the religious or cultural traditions in which he or she is embedded. *Clinicians should be careful not to make assumptions about a patient's goals, values, beliefs, or preferences on the basis of denominational affiliation, cultural heritage, or other external indicia.* Unless a patient explicitly requests a limitation of scope, it is the duty of the clinician to mention all medically reasonable, legally available treatment alternatives to each patient—even if the clinician does not personally perform some of these interventions. *To do otherwise is to usurp the moral agency of the patient* (Anderson 2002). As the clinician and patient begin to discuss the options, the clinician should ask, "Does this raise moral or spiritual issues for you?" Failure to do so may result in lost opportunities to align interventions with patient goals and

R.R. Anderson, J.D., M.S., C.G.C. (✉)
College of Public Health, University of Nebraska Medical Center,
984365 Nebraska Medical Center, Omaha, NE 68198-4365, USA
e-mail: randerso@unmc.edu

J.P. Galst, M.S. Verp (eds.), *Prenatal and Preimplantation Diagnosis*,
DOI 10.1007/978-3-319-18911-6_10

preferences. It may result in guilt or blame, particularly if the desired outcome is not achieved. It may deprive patients of much-needed emotional support and solace.

The goal of the clinician should not be to interpret doctrine, or to undertake spiritual guidance, but rather to identify these issues in a timely fashion and make appropriate resources available. Many US religious denominations maintain websites on which doctrinal statements and guidance can be found. For observant believers, a review of denominational doctrines may resolve some issues, and raise others. But in general it is better to know the parameters of one's community of faith before embarking on life-changing reproductive interventions.

Interestingly, in many denominations, clergy and lay members alike are unaware of their church's doctrinal statements concerning reproductive matters. These statements can be surprisingly nuanced, and many give considerable latitude to the individual faced with difficult medical choices. Even if a denomination's doctrine is inflexible, believers are better served by knowing in advance so that they can make considered choices, rather than learning after the fact that they have unwittingly violated a religious precept.

For a patient who is an active member of a community of faith, conferring with his or her own clergy member is the ideal—but in some cases a patient will be reluctant to do so, for fear of being judged or directed toward a particular course. If that is the case, or if a patient is not currently active in a community of faith but identifies with an established faith tradition, the pastoral care staff of a local hospital may be able to assist, or may direct the patient to a local or regional resource for pastoral counsel. For a patient who does not identify with a particular faith tradition or whose compass is not faith based, conferring with a knowledgeable counselor can help the patient identify and reconcile his or her convictions, values, goals, and priorities. Obviously, patients in committed relationships should be attentive to the concerns of both members of the dyad.

Religious Traditions and Spiritual Pathways

Most of the world's major religions predate by millennia our current reproductive technologies. Still, traditional sacred texts and theological works often grapple with the central issues these technologies raise: the relationship between corporal and spiritual being, the boundaries of life and death, the importance of family and the implications of infertility, pregnancy loss, birth defects, the nature of hubris, the conditions of full membership in the community of faith, and the requisites of salvation. Believers seeking guidance about reproductive technologies must extrapolate from these texts, with the help of theologians and religious authorities, to apply ancient wisdom to contemporary problems.

Denominations with hierarchical structures, such as many Christian denominations, provide formal interpretations and issue directives to guide the faithful in engaging with new technologies. In some traditions such as the Roman Catholic Church these interpretations carry authority equal to the scriptures.

Other Christian denominations, such as the Southern Baptist Convention, are organized as coalitions of autonomous congregations. Although resolutions may be adopted by these conventions, they are not binding on participants. A growing trend in Christianity is the nondenominational church, which looks to sacred texts alone, or to trusted commentaries, for guidance.

The Jewish and Islamic traditions are characterized by a rich history of scriptural interpretation and application by religious scholars, continuing into the present. These interpretations, while given considerable weight, are not considered equal to scripture. Doctrinal applications diverge more or less markedly, reflecting different interpretations and priorities among writers and sects.

Still other religious traditions have no overarching organization, but rely on ancient writings, history, and emergent teacher-sages to maintain continuity of thought (Buddhist, Hindu).

Summaries

The following summaries reflect doctrines or doctrinal interpretations of major faith traditions as expressed by recent authorities. It is common in some religious traditions that respected authorities are not in accord. Divergences may reflect different branches of the faith (for instance Orthodox, Conservative, Reform Judaism), or they may reflect different priorities on the parts of religious scholars. More importantly, believers themselves may assign different priorities to various religious precepts and may have reached independent conclusions about the doctrinal issues in question. The summaries below cannot be considered authoritative, but rather they provide a point of departure for further discussion or inquiry.

The represented traditions are presented in the order of historical emergence. Within each summary, the discussion is organized to reflect the typical sequence in which issues are encountered by a patient and provider of reproductive services.

Hinduism

The Hindu faith began some 5000 years ago in the Indus Valley of the Indian subcontinent. Unsurprisingly many distinctive variations exist. Some recognize a number of deities while most consider the traditional deities as different aspects or manifestations of a singular, all-powerful force (*Brahman*). Holy texts include the *Vedas*, four volumes containing key hymns, prayers, rituals, beliefs, and values. Also important in Hindu thought is the epic narrative known as the *Mahabharata*. Although not a sacred text, it is known colloquially as the “Fifth Veda” (Bhattacharyya 2006). These mythic narratives serve as ethical case studies for believers (Desai 1989).

Ahimsa (avoiding harm, doing good), *Karma* (essentially the law of cause and effect), *Dharma* (ethical living), and *Samsara* (reincarnation) are consistent tenets of Hinduism. One's temporal deeds are believed to influence events in future lives, with self-awareness and recognition of oneness with the divine eventually leading to a cessation of the cycle of reincarnation (*moksa*) (Melton 1999). Ayurvedic medicine is the practice of first resort among many Hindus, although Western medical interventions generally are accepted (Bharadwaj 2006).

In Vitro Techniques

There are no religious bars to the use of in vitro interventions, particularly when the gametes of the couple are used, although there may be social disapprobation due to the introduction of a third party into the process of reproduction (Bharadwaj 2006). The disposition of unused embryos may pose a problem for some couples, owing to the dominant belief that the soul is present from the time of conception. There are literary precedents for embryo manipulation and cloning.

> [Ghandari] delivers a dark, solid mass of flesh – a dense ball of clotted blood. She is totally distraught. After two years of being pregnant, how is it that all she has produced is a clotted mass?
>
> …
>
> With his divine sight, Vyasa sees what has just taken place and comes swiftly to her aid.
>
> …
>
> Vyasa dictates various orders and Gandhari follows his instructions. She collects one hundred clay pots and fills them with *ghee* (clarified butter). Then she sprinkles the ball with cold water. Upon doing this, the ball of flesh falls apart into one hundred pieces – each an embryo the size of a thumb joint …. As Vyasa finishes placing the embryos into their clay pots, he informs her that there is one extra piece – the piece that will become her daughter. After each embryo is placed in the *ghee* filled pots, they are incubated in a warm, well-guarded place. After some time, the first of Gandhari's sons, Duryodhana, is born. His birth is soon followed by the births of ninety-nine other sons and one daughter.
>
> Bhattacharyya (2006)
> U.S.

Preimplantation Genetic Diagnosis

Preimplantation genetic diagnosis may be problematic due to embryo wastage for those who subscribe to the belief that a soul is present very early. A minority view holds that ensoulment does not take place until the seventh month; arguably both the majority and the minority texts envision development (and ensoulment) as a gradual process. Preimplantation genetic diagnosis with selective implantation would likely be considered more palatable than prenatal diagnosis followed by therapeutic abortion.

> [N]othing is said [in the traditional texts] to indicate that in its development the embryo undergoes a quantum leap, passing from one kind of human moral status (human being) to another (human person). On the contrary, in characteristic Hindu fashion, the language here

is in terms of progressive MANIFESTATION of a personhood previously only latent rather than origination of personhood *ab initio*.

Lipner (1989)
U.S.

Hindu and Buddhist commentators generally hold that the transmigration of consciousness, or incarnation, takes place at conception. From that point, the destruction of the conceptus 'incurs the karmic burden of killing' .... [T]he deliberate destruction of an embryo is tantamount to murder or, if a version of the principle of double effect is applied, perhaps manslaughter. From this point of view, sex selection, preimplantation genetic diagnosis (PGD) and any other destructive embryo research cannot be contemplated. They all involve the killing of an innocent person.

...

However, [a 'generationist' view] makes it possible to see personhood as something that develops more gradually, allowing for the legitimate destruction of embryos for the sake of particular types of infertility treatment or even research. Buddhist bio-ethics has a similar range of views. Some appeal to ancient Hindu embryology that regarded incarnation as taking place as late as the seventh month of pregnancy.

Dutney (2007)
Australia

Unimplanted Pre-embryos

Freezing unimplanted pre-embryos for future use or relinquishment to other infertile couples would be acceptable in the Hindu tradition. Deliberate destruction of unused pre-embryos could be problematic for those who believe in early ensoulment. Some hold that experimentation on early pre-embryos is also acceptable since it could result in benefit to others (cf. Talwar, 2012).

Prenatal Diagnosis

Prenatal diagnosis for the purpose of therapeutic intervention or preparedness is acceptable. Prenatal diagnosis for the purpose of sex selection or abortion of compromised fetuses generally would be thought to contravene Hindu principles (see Pregnancy interruption, below).

Prenatal Therapeutic Interventions

Avoiding harm (*ahimsa*) in relation to self and others supports therapeutic intervention intended to improve the health of the fetus.

Pregnancy Loss

Miscarriage, stillbirth, and infant death are considered the workings of karma, relating to both parents and the fetus. Stoic endurance and responsiveness to one's duties in the face of the misfortune are thought to bring one closer to final release.

> Karma means both action and fate. Hindus (as well as Buddhists and Jains) believe that every action leads to a series of reactions …. A folk story based on the Mahabharata illustrates this point. At the end of a great war, queen Gandhari is informed that all her hundred children are dead. She weeps and seeks a reason for this unfair situation, to which a sage replies, "In your last life, you sat on a stone under which there were a hundred turtle eggs. The eggs were crushed. So the mother-turtle cursed you that you too would experience the loss of a hundred children."
>
> Pattanaik (2014)
> India

Pregnancy Interruption and Fetal Reduction

The dominant Hindu view is that ensoulment occurs at or near the time of conception. Thus, abortion for any reason other than to spare the life of the mother is condemned. A minority view suggests that ensoulment or full personhood evolves gradually or is not conferred until the seventh month post-conception. No ready parallels exist in the Hindu tradition to support multifetal reduction on the premise that eliminating one or more fetuses will enable the rest to survive, although reduction presumably would be defensible to preserve the well-being of the mother.

> The early texts consider abortion to be a sin equal to the killing of a learned person. *Bhrunahatya*, the killing of a fetus, is a word also used for the murder of a Brahmin. The practice was condemned in the *Atharva Veda*, one of the four revealed sources of knowledge, as well as in the later *smriti* literature.
>
> Desai (1989)
> U.S.

> "Brunahathya" or feticide (abortion) has not been described or advocated by the Hindu faith. However, in special situations it was permitted to protect women whose lives were endangered by pregnancy.
>
> Zaidi et al. (2009)
> Pakistan

> [A]bortion could be regarded as thwarting the unfolding of the karma of both the unborn and the perpetrator(s) of the act.
>
> Lipner (1989)
> U.S.

Classical Hindu texts reflect an understanding of the developmental nature of a zygote, embryo, and fetus. Preserving the *Atharvan* theory of fetal development, the *Garbha Upanisad* reads as follows:

> By the second night after the union of semen and blood the foetus is of the form of a round lump called *Kalala*, at the eighth night it is of the form of a vesicle called *Budbuda*, after a fortnight it assumes the form of a spheroid – *Pinda*, in two months the head appears, in three months the feet, in four months the abdomen, heels, the pelvic portion appear, in the fifth month the spine appears, in the sixth month nose, eyes and ears develop; in the seventh month the foetus becomes endowed with life […]; in the eighth month it becomes fully developed ….

> The major tradition is found in *Caraka-Samhita.* […]
>
> The fetus is produced out of the Soul[.]… By entering into the uterus, it gets combined with the sperm and the ovum thereby reproducing Himself in the form of a fetus[.] … The state of mere existence of sperm and ovum prior to the combination of the Soul cannot be called as fetus. They are entitled to be known as fetus only when the Soul gets combined with them.
>
> Bhattacharyya (2006)
> U.S.

> The Hindu attitude to severely handicapped newborns reflects the interface of several doctrines, such as that of nonviolence, or *ahimsa*, and those of *karma* and *dharma* …. The handicapped could be viewed as working out their bad karma through their present condition. This view could, however, easily lead one into blaming their bad *karma* for their condition. If, however, we ask, "What is our *dharma* (duty), given that the other person's karma brought the person to his or her current state?" the question shifts the focus and is widely acknowledged to reflect the proper ethical response.
>
> Sharma (1996)
> U.S.

Judaism

Judaism, arising around 1000 BCE in the Levant, is the oldest of the three great monotheistic religions with common roots in the region. The *Torah* or *Pentateuch* (Genesis, Exodus, Leviticus, Numbers and Deuteronomy) is the bedrock sacred text, which together with books recording History, Wisdom, and Prophets comprise the 24 books of the Hebrew Bible, or *Tanakh.* Supplemental interpretive texts (*Midrash, Talmud*) also are given considerable weight. In response to contemporary issues on which Jewish law (*Halakh*) is not settled, scholars compose and publish *Responsa*, analyses of Jewish law which often provide a comprehensive review of relevant texts and prior opinions. The three main US branches of Judaism are the Orthodox, Conservative, and Reform traditions, with Orthodox being the most traditional and Reform the most liberal of the major branches. In Israel observant Jews are broadly categorized as traditional, religious, or Haredi (ultra-Orthodox). Jewish state laws relating to matters of the family are heavily influenced by religious considerations (Jotkowitz 2011). Some rabbis have begun to specialize in harmonizing medical practice with halachic law; some physicians are uneasy about rabbinical conditions driving medical interventions (Ivry 2013).

In Vitro Techniques

In vitro fertilization using spousal gametes is accepted by most authorities but some Orthodox may require elaborate safeguards.

> The Jewish majority's religious point of view … as formulated by the chief rabbis of Israel (one from the Ashkenazi sector of European origin and one from the Sephardic sector of

Oriental origin) supports both IVF and embryo transfer [using the gametes of the husband and wife].

Schenker (2008a)
Israel

Where healing was once effected primarily by means of prayer, Jewish tradition has for many centuries accepted the practice of medicine (*refu'ah*) as the correct *therapy*, the right response to disease. Medicine, our sources tell us, is a *mitzvah*; it is the way in which we most often fulfill our obligation to save life (*pikuach nefesh*). While it is surely a good thing to ask God's blessings upon those who are ill – and we do so in our liturgy – prayer is no longer sufficient therapy. As the talmudic saying puts it, "one who is in pain should go to the doctor": when we are ill, we must avail ourselves of the remedies devised through human wisdom and scientific knowledge and not place our exclusive reliance upon the hope that God will intervene into the workings of nature.

From all of this, it follows that the various technologies which enable the infertile to conceive ought to be understood as medicine. Our Committee has indeed taken this position with respect to artificial reproductive techniques in general and IVF in particular. Human infertility is a disease, not because it threatens the life and health of the infertile but because it frustrates our attainment of the goal – the *mitzvah* – of bringing children into the world. The scientific tools developed to cure this disease are therefore advances in *medicine* and should be welcomed, as we welcome other medical advances, as a positive good.

CCAR In Vitro Fertilization and the Mitzvah of Childbearing (1996)
U.S. Reform

Preimplantation Genetic Diagnosis

Fertilized eggs are not given full human status, particularly when not implanted. But reverence for potential humanity forbids casual treatment of zygotes. PGD for serious conditions, followed by selective implantation, appears to be accepted by most authorities.

One fundamental principle that is agreed upon by all branches of the Jewish faith is that full human status is not acquired until birth. Thus until then, the destruction of a product of conception does not constitute homicide culpable as murder. Although the Jewish law refuses to grant a full human inviolability to the unborn child from conception, it is clearly agreed that the potentiality for life must not be compromised except for the most substantial medical reasons. Man's creation 'in the image of God' confers infinite value on every human life and renders its destruction a capital offence. Since the preimplantation pre-embryo carries an extremely low probability of reaching the neonate stage and thus achieving full human status, it does not enjoy the same sacred title to life as the fetus or embryo; its status is similar to that of human semen. Nevertheless, the destruction of human seed or embryo is considered a grave violation of the law.

Schenker (2008b)
Israel

Recent scientific advances have made highly reliable preconceptual *(sic)* sex selection possible by using preimplantation genetic diagnosis (PGD) or sperm separation by flow cytometry combined with AIH or IVF. The requirement for a Jewish man to procreate by having a minimum of two children, a boy and a girl, is obligatory according to Jewish law.

According to both schools, Beit Shamai and Beit Hillel, in order to fulfil the obligation of procreation, at least one son is required. Therefore the application of sex preselection for non-medical indications may be of practical importance using the method of sperm separation or sex selection of pre-embryo by PGD. It is allowed in the state of Israel for balancing of family with some limitations.

Schenker (2008a)
Israel

In cases where the additional medical risk of IVF treatment is halakhically permissible in order to avoid bearing a child with a serious disease, another halakhic consideration arises as in vitro fertilization necessitates the creation and eventual destruction—even if only passively—of embryos that would not have existed through natural conception. In Jewish tradition, few voices argue that an unimplanted embryo has the legal status of a fetus in utero. Even if this analogy held, Rabbi Elliot Dorff argues that the embryo would surely be no more than [*maya b'almah*]—mere water—the status of a fetus before the fortieth day of gestation. Because the embryo exists outside the womb and implantation is necessary for birth to be possible, the argument follows that the embryos may passively be allowed to disintegrate in certain situations where benefit is likely. Other rabbis argue for a more restrictive position, namely that the laws of [*hash'hatat zera*]—wasted seed—should apply, making the destruction of embryos permissible only when necessary for reproduction or life-saving purposes. Though I believe that applying the laws of [*hash'hatat zera*] to unimplanted embryos constitutes an unnecessary expansion of a stringency intended for an altogether different purpose, I do assert strongly we must still appreciate that embryos have the potential to become life and thus deserve some degree of special care and protection from unnecessary destruction. In the words of Rabbi Dorff, "In our own day, when we understand that the fertilized egg cell has all the DNA that will ultimately produce a human being, we must clearly have respect for human embryos and even for human gametes alone (sperm and eggs), for they are the building blocks of human procreation."

…

Adding nuance to these broad positions, Rabbi Aaron Mackler notes that many modern halakhic authorities permit aborting a fetus with a severe genetic disease or deformity. If the disease screened for using PGD is so severe that, were the fetus to carry that disease the parents would abort, then certainly "selective non-transfer of an early in vitro embryo would be preferable to abortion of a more fully developed fetus in utero." Rabbi Shlomo Daichovsky implies a similar argument when he writes … "I would prefer the genetic screening of embryos prior to implantation than after implantation."

…

However, the standard should be set so that the disease screened for and its effects must be so horrible that no matter what possible genetic disadvantages the alternate embryo selected may carry, their impact cannot reasonably be understood as worse than the disease avoided. This brings us, then, to … [the following criteria:] high likelihood of disease presentation, fatality or debilitating condition, and the absence of effective treatment.

Popovsky (2008)
U.S. Conservative

Unimplanted Pre-embryos

Freezing of gametes and pre-embryos for future use is permissible, with safeguards to assure correct identity. Pre-embryos outside of the womb are not accorded the same level of protection accorded to embryos in utero; thus, destruction of unused pre-embryos does not equate with abortion. Some authorities permit experimentation with unused pre-embryos.

> Freezing of sperm and pre-embryos is permitted in Judaism only when all measures are taken to ensure that the father's identity will not be lost. The recent technology of oocyte freezing in order to preserve fertility is recommended by Rabbinical authorities.
>
> Schenker (2013)
> Israel

> Are frozen embryos…property in the usual sense and therefore subject to the laws governing the ownership and transfer of property, or does their status as potential human beings put them into a different category, with presumably more restrictive rules?
>
> Jewish law, as I understand it, would affirm what American courts have said, namely, that if both members of the couple are alive, both have a right to restrict the use of their embryos; neither may do that alone. If their original attempts at having children with IVF succeed and they do not want any more children, they may discard the remaining embryos; Jewish strictures on abortion do not apply because these embryos exist outside the uterus, where they have no chance of developing or even of remaining viable on their own once thawed. Because of that, I would permit the couple to donate their embryos to an infertile couple, but only subject to the cautions and restrictions described [elsewhere].
>
> Dorff (1998)
> U.S. Conservative

> In the case of frozen embryos, Israeli law allows transfer of such embryos to the wife up to 1 year after the death of her husband even in the absence of consent, while in cases where the wife has died the frozen embryos cannot be used. Posthumous reproduction is supported by Jewish law.
>
> Schenker (2008a)
> Israel

> Our *sho'el* [inquirer] is correct that the sources regard a human embryo of less than forty days gestation as *maya be`alma*, "mere water", and therefore not a "fetus" (*ubar*) at all. On this basis, a number of authorities are willing to rule more leniently on the question of abortion; that is to say, if we presume a prima facie halakhic prohibition against abortion, that prohibition either does not apply or is much less stringent with regard to a fetus at less than forty days following conception. By extension, we would expect an even more permissive attitude concerning an embryo which, because it exists outside the womb, is not defined as a "fetus." This is indeed the case. One leading contemporary halakhist rules that it is forbidden to set aside the laws of Shabbat in order to save the life of an embryo in a petri dish, even though we are permitted to violate Shabbat on behalf of a fetus. In a ruling which touches directly upon our own *she'elah*, R. Chaim David Halevy permits a hospital or clinic to discard "excess" embryos created for purposes of IVF, explaining that the prohibition against abortion relates only to the *fetus* and not to an embryo maintained outside the womb. A similar decision is rendered by R. Mordekhai Eliyahu.
>
> CCAR In Vitro Fertilization and the Status of the Embryo (CCAR 1996b)
> U.S. Reform

Prenatal Diagnosis

Diagnostic procedures intended to assist in caring for the mother and fetus are accepted. Diagnostic procedures undertaken with the intention of aborting fetuses with birth defects generally are unacceptable to Orthodox theologians, unless continuing pregnancy poses a serious threat to the life or health of the mother.

> There is no justification in the traditional sources for aborting a fetus for reasons having to do with the health of the fetus; only the mother's health is a consideration. As a result, some people object to performing amniocentesis at all, even when the intent is to determine whether to abort a malformed fetus. Others reason in precisely the opposite direction; they justify abortion of a defective fetus on the basis of preserving the mother's mental health where it is clear that the mother is not able to cope with the prospect of bearing or raising such a child.
>
> Many Conservative and Reform rabbis, and even a few contemporary Orthodox rabbis, have handled the matter in a completely different way. They reason that traditional sources recognize only threats to the mother's health as grounds for abortion because until recently it was impossible to know anything about the genetic and medical makeup of the fetus before birth. Our new medical knowledge, they say, ought to establish the fetus's health as an independent consideration.
>
> Although I personally agree with this last approach, there are problems with it. Aside from the fact that it would represent an innovation in the law, it raises the extremely difficult issue of determining what constitutes a sufficient defect to warrant abortion.
>
> Dorff (1998)
> U.S. Conservative

> According to the vast majority of rabbis of all streams of Judaism, however, an abortion of a fetus afflicted with Tay-Sachs would be warranted.
>
> …
>
> [W]here the child will be afflicted with the disease, the parents, given that knowledge, may decide to abort the fetus if they so choose. If they allow the fetus to be born, however, no active measures may then be taken to hasten its death … [p]alliative care must be administered … but aggressively treating the child with medications, machines, or surgery to prolong life is neither necessary or wise. One may even remove feeding tubes, for the child is like an adult with a terminal illness (that is, a *terefah*) who … must be offered normal food and liquids but not artificial forms of nutrition and hydration.
>
> Dorff (1998)
> U.S. Conservative

> Jewish tradition countenances abortion under certain conditions, and Reform tradition has dealt with it on a number of occasions. Thus, we have permitted abortion when results of aminocentesis for Tay-Sachs Disease suggested its desirability.
>
> Generally, we would support decisions on an individual basis. Some families thrive on crisis situations, others break down; one woman reacts differently from another. The possibility that the test results may lead to some abortions is not, in our view, reason to abstain from research in this area altogether. As its methods are refined and the odds for accurate predictions increase, the necessity for more and more difficult moral decisions will also increase. Indeed, the application of new knowledge will frequently present us with new problems.
>
> CCAR Linkage Analysis (1990)
> U.S. Reform

Prenatal Therapeutic Interventions

The directive to care for one's body and seek appropriate medical interventions applies with less force to the fetus (and even to the newborn, prior to 30 days), who has not attained full status. Since the fetus is considered a part of the mother, a beneficial intervention on behalf of the fetus likely would be accepted unless it poses undue risk to the mother. Experimental interventions are not required.

> [T]here is general agreement among rabbis who have written on these matters that a Jew need not use heroic measures to maintain his or her life but only those medicines and procedures commonly available in the person's time and place.
>
> ...
>
> Thus a person who is currently incurable (*terefah*) may choose to undergo experimental therapies in an attempt to overcome the illness. Even if the therapy brings with it the risk of advancing the time of dying, use of it is permissible if the intent is not to bring about death but rather to prolong life.
>
> On the other hand, a person with an incurable illness may also choose to have machines and medications withheld or withdrawn and to engage in hospice care, where only palliative treatment will be administered.
>
> Dorff (1998)
> U.S. Conservative

> *[O]nce we have learned to cure the disease through techniques of genetic engineering or other methods*, there would be, in my view, a positive obligation for people in the group at risk to undergo the test and a second, positive obligation on the part of those found to have the mutation to undergo the procedures necessary to correct it .... Jews have the duty to try to prevent illness if at all possible and to cure it when they can, and that duty applies to diseases caused by genes just as much as it does to diseases engendered by bacteria, viruses, or some other environmental factor.
>
> Dorff (1998)
> U.S. Conservative

> There is already general agreement among rabbis that the legitimacy of human intervention to effect cure extends to procedures within the womb as well. When used in this therapeutic way, genetic engineering is an unmitigated blessing.
>
> Dorff (1998)
> U.S. Conservative

Pregnancy Loss

Birth defects and pregnancy loss are not taken by theologians as signs of divine judgment against the parents, the infant, or the family. Texts and traditional practice infer that an aborted, miscarried, or stillborn infant has no spiritual status (although the remains, being human, are entitled to reverence and respect) (Anderson 2002). However, the many biblical passages equating fertility to God's favor make it difficult to avoid the corollary presumption that failure of fertility is an indication of disfavor or punishment.

Pregnancy Interruption and Fetal Reduction

Traditionally, abortion was mandatory when continuing pregnancy posed an imminent threat to the woman's life. Abortion was allowed when continuing pregnancy posed a serious threat to the woman's health. The Orthodox community tends to limit abortion to life-threatening circumstances while the Conservative and Reform communities define threats to maternal life and mental health more broadly, allowing termination for fetal anomalies when giving birth would pose a risk to the mother's mental health (Dorff 1998).

> God formed the man from the dust of the earth and breathed into his nostrils the breath of life and the man became a living 'nephesh' (soul) (Gen. 2:7).
>
> ...
>
> And if men strive together, and hurt a woman with a child, so that her fruit depart and yet no harm follow, he shall be surely fined, according as the woman's husband shall lay upon him; and he shall pay as the judges determine. But if any harm follow, then shall thou give life for life (Ex.21:22-23).
>
> ...
>
> The Jewish Talmudic law assumes that the full title to life arises only at birth, if "the greater part" of the fetus has already been delivered.
>
> This formulation of the attitude toward abortion in the classic sources of Jewish law implies that:
>
> (1) The only indication considered for abortion is a hazard to the mother's life.
>
> (2) Otherwise, the destruction of an unborn child is a grave offence, although not murder.
>
> (3) It can be viewed that the fetus is granted some recognition of human life, but it does not equal that of the mother's and can be sacrificed if her life is in danger.
>
> The Babylonian Talmud Yevamot 69 b states, "The embryo is considered to be 'mere water' until the fortieth day." Afterward, it is considered sub-human until it is born.
>
> Schenker (2013)
> Israel

Abortion on demand is repulsive to the ethics of the Halakha; however, as we have seen, in some situations a pregnancy may be terminated. If, for example, the mother's life is in danger, as is sometimes in case of multiple pregnancy [in which] a fetus is a Rodef; an aggressor who may even or must be killed in order to save the individual in danger. Most rabbis permit and even mandate abortion when the health or life of the mother is threatened. Some authorities are stringent and require the mother's life to be in actual danger, however remote that danger, whereas others permit abortion for a serious threat to the mother's health.

The question of multifetal pregnancy reduction was debated in the Responsa literature by rabbinical authorities. If the mother's life is in danger, each fetus is a Rodef and can be killed to save the mother. But if the danger is to the fetuses and not to the mother, each fetus is an aggressor and victim with equal status. In this case, it might not be permissible to put aside one soul for the sake of another. Searching for a legal analogy for this situation, some rabbis focused on the case of a group of people who are in mortal danger and who can be saved by sacrificing one innocent member of the group. Most Halakhic authorities agree that in such a case all must allow themselves to die rather than sacrifice an innocent person. If, however, it is absolutely certain that all would be lost unless one is forfeited, these same authorities would allow some innocent people to be selected randomly and sacrificed to save the others. This conclusion is applicable to cases of a viable person. In the case of fetuses who are already condemned to death, multifetal reductions might well be allowed. The number of fetuses to be destroyed is a medical question that should be decided by the doctors involved, who must determine the minimum number that need to be reduced to ensure a good prognosis for the mother and remaining fetus[es].

Schenker (2008b)
Israel

[S]enior religious authorities such as Rabbi Mordecai Eliyahu, late Chief Rabbi of Israel, and Rabbi Haim David Halevi, late Chief Rabbi of Tel Aviv, allow reducing the pregnancy to the extent necessary to ensure a good prognosis for the remaining fetuses. Similarly, there is a spectrum of views in halakhic Judaism concerning abortion. All agree that abortion is moral and required to save the life of the mother, and all agree that abortion on demand for the simple convenience of the mother is anathema. However, there is a strong position allowing abortion for serious considerations, especially when the resulting pregnancy will effect *(sic)* the mental health of the mother who must cope with a seriously compromised child. Thus, some halakhists will allow the abortion of a Tay-Sachs fetus.

Grazi and Wolowelsky (2010)
U.S.

[S]ome Orthodox rabbis have permitted selective abortions on the grounds of the mother's mental and/or physical health when more than three embryos implant in the uterus, and Conservative rabbis would undoubtedly do so as well. However, to avoid the need for selective abortions as much as possible, Jews in the first place should have only two, or at most three, zygotes implanted for IVF or ZIFT, and should use only two, or at most three, eggs for GIFT.

Dorff (1998)
U.S. Conservative

We agree with the traditional authorities that abortions should be approached cautiously throughout the life of the fetus. Most authorities would be least hesitant during the first forty days of the fetus' life …

From forty days until twenty-seven weeks, the fetus possesses some status, but its future remains doubtful (*goses biydei adam*; San. 78a; Nid. 44b and commentaries) as we are not sure of its viability. We must, therefore, be more certain of our grounds for abortion, but would still permit it.

It is clear from all of this that traditional authorities would be most lenient with abortions within the first forty days. After that time, there is a difference of opinion. Those who are within the broadest range of permissibility permit abortion at any time before birth, if there is a serious danger to the health of the mother or the child. We would be in agreement with that liberal stance. We do not encourage abortion, nor favor it for trivial reasons, or sanction it "on demand."

CCAR When is Abortion Permitted? (1985)
U.S. Reform

Severed limbs and fetuses are generally buried for two reasons; first in order to assure their dignified disposal as a part of a human body, and second, in order to prevent the ritual uncleanliness of priests who might come in contact with them (*Yad* Hil. Tumat Okhlin 16.8; *Shevut Yaaqov*, II, #10; Ket. 20b).

As there is no mandate to bury a fetus, and as it has not been viewed as a human being with its own soul, there is no objection to its use for medical experimentation. This has been the general view expressed by some traditional authorities (*Noda Biyehudah* II Yoreh Deah #209; Eliezer Waldenberg, *Tzitz Eliezer*, X, #25, Chapt. 8).

We should mention one additional negative argument which might be raised, i.e., not benefiting from the dead *(asur behana-ah)*. This, however, is not involved in our case, as this referred only to a deceased "person," a status which the fetus has not attained (*Shulhan Arukh* Yoreh Deah 364.1). The experimentation, which this scientist intends to conduct is, therefore, in keeping with Jewish tradition as well as with our interpretation of it.

CCAR Fetus Used for Experimentation (1984)
U.S. Reform

Pre-reformation Christianity

Roman Catholicism

Other Orthodox Christian traditions

Grounded in Judaism, Christianity arose with the birth, death, and resurrection in Israel of Jesus Christ (~3 BCE to ~32 CE). Believers hold him to have been at once fully human and fully divine, the Son of God and the Messiah predicted in Jewish theology. Christians have adopted the Jewish sacred texts along with a varying number of additional scriptures (*Old Testament*), and added to them narratives of Jesus's life and teachings (*New Testament*, consisting of the Gospels, Acts of the Apostles, Epistles, and Revelations) to form the *Holy Bible*. The Christian churches established in the early Common Era were centered in Rome and Constantinople. In the "Great Schism" of 1053–1054 theological and political disputes severed the Western (Roman) from the Eastern Orthodox churches (Greek, Russian, Antiochean, and others), although in many respects their theologies remain closely aligned. The material below denotes the stance of the Roman Catholic Church. Believers are expected to adhere to the declarations of Rome and may be excommunicated (forbidden to take communion) if they fail to do so. Reinstatement into the community of faith typically requires repentance of the sin in question (averring that, given the chance, one would behave otherwise in the same situation), and performing penance prescribed by the priest.

Other Orthodox traditions, while expressing serious reservations about certain aspects of reproductive technology, nevertheless may allow more latitude to believers in interpreting and applying principles of faith to contemporary issues.

The [Greek Orthodox] Church avoids specific rules or excommunications when dealing with bioethical matters, including those concerning assisted reproduction. Basically, She leaves them open, while, at the same time, She indicates the direction and ethos of approaching each specific case.

Nikolaos (2008)
U.S. Greek Orthodox

In Vitro Techniques

No form of in vitro fertilization is permitted by the Roman Catholic Church, even when using the gametes of the couple. The only licit method of conception is an act of sexual intercourse by a married heterosexual couple. The conjugal act must always be open to the transmission of life, and conception apart from the conjugal act is illicit. Artificial insemination in general is thus excluded, unless the technical intervention somehow serves not to replace the conjugal act but to assist it to achieve its natural purpose.

> [A]ll techniques of heterologous artificial fertilization, as well as those techniques of homologous artificial fertilization which substitute for the conjugal act, are to be excluded. On the other hand, techniques which act as an aid to the conjugal act and its fertility are permitted. The Instruction Donum vitae states: "The doctor is at the service of persons and of human procreation. He does not have the authority to dispose of them or to decide their fate. A medical intervention respects the dignity of persons when it seeks to assist the conjugal act either in order to facilitate its performance or in order to enable it to achieve its objective once it has been normally performed". And, with regard to homologous artificial insemination, it states: "*Homologous artificial insemination within marriage cannot be admitted except for those cases in which the technical means is not a substitute for the conjugal act, but serves to facilitate and to help so that the act attains its natural purpose*" *(emphasis added).*
>
> CFaith (2008)

> 41. Homologous artificial fertilization (that is, any technique used to achieve conception using the gametes of the two spouses joined in marriage) is prohibited when it separates procreation from the marital act in its unitive significance (e.g., any technique used to achieve *extracorporeal* conception) *(emphasis added).*
>
> USCCB (2009)

> It is often objected that the loss of embryos is, in the majority of cases, unintentional or that it happens truly against the will of the parents and physicians. They say that it is a question of risks which are not all that different from those in natural procreation; to seek to generate new life without running any risks would in practice mean doing nothing to transmit it. It is true that not all the losses of embryos in the process of in vitro fertilization have the same relationship to the will of those involved in the procedure. But it is also true that in many cases the abandonment, destruction and loss of embryos are foreseen and willed.
>
> …
>
> In many countries, it is now common to stimulate ovulation so as to obtain a large number of oocytes which are then fertilized. Of these, some are transferred into the woman's uterus, while the others are frozen for future use. The reason for multiple transfer is to increase the probability that at least one embryo will implant in the uterus. In this technique, therefore, the number of embryos transferred is greater than the single child desired, in the expectation that some embryos will be lost and multiple pregnancy may not occur. In this way, the practice of multiple embryo transfer implies a purely utilitarian treatment of embryos. One is struck by the fact that, in any other area of medicine, ordinary professional ethics and the healthcare authorities themselves would never allow a medical procedure which involved such a high number of failures and fatalities.
>
> CFaith (2008)

> Just as in general with in vitro fertilization, of which it is a variety, ICSI [Intra-Cytoplasmic Sperm Injection] is intrinsically illicit: it causes a complete separation between procreation and the conjugal act. Indeed ICSI takes place "outside the bodies of the couple through actions of third parties whose competence and technical activity determine the success of the procedure. Such fertilization entrusts the life and identity of the embryo into the power of doctors and biologists and establishes the domination of technology over the origin and destiny of the human person. Such a relationship of domination is in itself contrary to the dignity and equality that must be common to parents and children. Conception in vitro is the result of the technical action which presides over fertilization. Such fertilization is neither in fact achieved nor positively willed as the expression and fruit of a specific act of the conjugal union".
>
> CFaith (2008)

Preimplantation Genetic Diagnosis

Since all in vitro procedures are disallowed, preimplantation genetic diagnosis is illicit. The Church expressly rejects embryo selection for any indication.

> Certain attempts to influence chromosomic or genetic inheritance are not therapeutic but are aimed at producing human beings selected according to sex or other predetermined qualities. These manipulations are contrary to the personal dignity of the human being and his or her integrity and identity. Therefore, in no way can they be justified on the grounds of possible beneficial consequences for future humanity. Every person must be respected for himself: in this consists the dignity and right of every human being from his or her beginning.
>
> CFaith (1987)

> Embryos produced in vitro which have defects are directly discarded. Cases are becoming ever more prevalent in which couples who have no fertility problems are using artificial means of procreation in order to engage in genetic selection of their offspring …. In fact, techniques of in vitro fertilization are accepted based on the presupposition that the individual embryo is not deserving of full respect in the presence of the competing desire for offspring which must be satisfied.
>
> CFaith (2008)

> Preimplantation genetic diagnosis – connected as it is with artificial fertilization, which is itself always intrinsically illicit – is directed toward the qualitative selection and consequent destruction of embryos, which constitutes an act of abortion. Preimplantation genetic diagnosis is therefore the expression of a eugenic mentality that "accepts selective abortion in order to prevent the birth of children affected by various types of anomalies. Such an attitude is shameful and utterly reprehensible, since it presumes to measure the value of a human life only within the parameters of 'normality' and physical well-being, thus opening the way to legitimizing infanticide and euthanasia as well."
>
> CFaith (2008)

Unimplanted Embryos

Since all in vitro procedures are disallowed, creating and freezing embryos is illicit. At the same time, embryos that have already been brought into existence possess human dignity and may not be deliberately destroyed for any reason.

The question of whether it is ever permitted to implant an embryo that has already been produced through in vitro procedures is not entirely resolved. Some Catholics promote the idea of "rescuing" embryos destined for destruction by implanting them and raising the children. The 2008 statement "*Dignitas Personae*" (below) discourages this idea, but it has not been definitively ruled out (USCCB 2015, James LeGrys, personal communication).

> Cryopreservation is incompatible with the respect owed to human embryos; it presupposes their production in vitro; it exposes them to the serious risk of death or physical harm, since a high percentage does not survive the process of freezing and thawing; it deprives them at least temporarily of maternal reception and gestation; it places them in a situation in which they are susceptible to further offense and manipulation.
>
> …
>
> With regard to the large number of frozen embryos already in existence the question becomes: what to do with them? Some of those who pose this question do not grasp its ethical nature, motivated as they are by laws in some countries that require cryopreservation centers to empty their storage tanks periodically. Others, however, are aware that a grave injustice has been perpetrated and wonder how best to respond to the duty of resolving it.
>
> Proposals to use these embryos for research or for the treatment of disease are obviously unacceptable because they treat the embryos as mere "biological material" and result in their destruction. The proposal to thaw such embryos without reactivating them and use them for research, as if they were normal cadavers, is also unacceptable.
>
> The proposal that these embryos could be put at the disposal of infertile couples as a treatment for infertility is not ethically acceptable for the same reasons which make artificial heterologous procreation illicit as well as any form of surrogate motherhood; this practice would also lead to other problems of a medical, psychological and legal nature.
>
> It has also been proposed, solely in order to allow human beings to be born who are otherwise condemned to destruction, that there could be a form of "prenatal adoption". This proposal, praiseworthy with regard to the intention of respecting and defending human life, presents however various problems not dissimilar to those mentioned above.
>
> All things considered, it needs to be recognized that the thousands of abandoned embryos represent a situation of injustice which in fact cannot be resolved. Therefore John Paul II made an "appeal to the conscience of the world's scientific authorities and in particular to doctors, that the production of human embryos be halted, taking into account that there seems to be no morally licit solution regarding the human destiny of the thousands and thousands of 'frozen' embryos which are and remain the subjects of essential rights and should therefore be protected by law as human persons".
>
> CFaith (2008)

> In order to avoid the serious ethical problems posed by the freezing of embryos, the freezing of oocytes has also been advanced in the area of techniques of in vitro fertilization. Once a sufficient number of oocytes has been obtained for a series of attempts at artificial procreation, only those which are to be transferred into the mother's body are fertilized while the others are frozen for future fertilization and transfer should the initial attempts not succeed.
>
> In this regard it needs to be stated that cryopreservation of oocytes for the purpose of being used in artificial procreation is to be considered morally unacceptable.
>
> CFaith (2008)

Prenatal Diagnosis

Prenatal diagnosis is permitted in order to provide more appropriate supportive care for the fetus, mother, or family. For the purposes of pregnancy interruption it is illicit.

> When they do not involve disproportionate risks for the child and the mother, and are meant to make possible early therapy or even to favour a serene and informed acceptance of the child not yet born, these techniques are morally licit. But since the possibilities of prenatal therapy are today still limited, it not infrequently happens that these techniques are used with a eugenic intention which accepts selective abortion in order to prevent the birth of children affected by various types of anomalies. Such an attitude is shameful and utterly reprehensible, since it presumes to measure the value of a human life only within the parameters of "normality" and physical well-being, thus opening the way to legitimizing infanticide and euthanasia as well.
>
> John Paul II (1995)

> 50. Prenatal diagnosis is permitted when the procedure does not threaten the life or physical integrity of the unborn child or the mother and does not subject them to disproportionate risks; when the diagnosis can provide information to guide preventative care for the mother or pre- or post-natal care for the child; and when the parents, or at least the mother, give free and informed consent. Prenatal diagnosis is not permitted when undertaken with the intention of aborting an unborn child with a serious defect.
>
> 51. Nontherapeutic experiments on a living embryo or fetus are not permitted, even with the consent of the parents. Therapeutic experiments are permitted for a proportionate reason with the free and informed consent of the parents or, if the father cannot be contacted, at least of the mother. Medical research that will not harm the life or physical integrity of an unborn child is permitted with parental consent.
>
> USCCB (2009)

Prenatal Therapeutic Interventions

Prenatal interventions intended to promote the life or health of the fetus are permitted, even if investigative.

> As with all medical interventions on patients, one must uphold as licit procedures carried out on the human embryo which respect the life and integrity of the embryo and do not involve disproportionate risks for it but are directed towards its healing, the improvement of its condition of health, or its individual survival.
>
> CFaith (1987)

Pregnancy Loss

Pregnancy loss, stillbirth, and newborn death are not viewed by the Church as divine punishment or judgment. Although the spiritual status after death of the unbaptized fetus or neonate is uncertain, the Church recently stated that there is "reason to hope" that the soul of the innocent is united with God (International Theological Commission 2007). Baptism of a critically ill neonate is of central importance and can be performed by anyone, lay or clergy, "with the proper intention." Baptism is not performed in utero or *postmortem*, although blessings can be offered.

> 17. Except in cases of emergency (i.e., danger of death), any request for Baptism made by adults or for infants should be referred to the chaplain of the institution. Newly born infants in danger of death, including those miscarried, should be baptized if this is possible. In case of emergency, if a priest or a deacon is not available, anyone can validly baptize.
>
> USCCB (2009)

Pregnancy Interruption and Fetal Reduction

The human soul is considered to be present at the completion of fertilization, and abortion is considered a grave sin. Pregnancy interruption is not allowed for fetal indications. For "a proportionate reason" induction of delivery may be undertaken for a fetus past the age of viability; this is most often invoked for maternal indications but early delivery followed by expectant management of the newborn with a lethal anomaly may be accepted. Early delivery of a pre-viable fetus for maternal benefit is disapproved. A pregnant woman is permitted to end a pregnancy that directly endangers her life; however, the intervention must not have the "sole immediate effect" of ending the pregnancy. Moreover, if a woman has a life-threatening illness she is permitted to accept therapeutic interventions to preserve her own life, even if the secondary and unintended effects are fetal death or maternal infertility.

> From the moment of conception, the life of every human being is to be respected in an absolute way because man is the only creature on earth that God has wished for himself and the spiritual soul of each man is "immediately created" by God; his whole being bears the image of the Creator.
>
> CFaith (1987)

> [T]he human being is to be respected and treated as a person from the moment of conception; and therefore from that same moment his rights as a person must be recognized, among which is the inviolable right of every innocent human being to life.
>
> John Paul II (1995)

> [A] person who actually procures an abortion incurs automatic (latae sententiae) excommunication. The excommunication affects all those who commit this crime with knowledge of the penalty attached, and thus includes those accomplices without whose help the crime would not have been committed.
>
> John Paul II (1995)

> The moral gravity of procured abortion is apparent in all its truth if we recognize that we are dealing with murder and, in particular, when we consider the specific elements involved. The one eliminated is a human being at the very beginning of life. No one more absolutely innocent could be imagined. In no way could this human being ever be considered an aggressor, much less an unjust aggressor!
>
> John Paul II (1995)

The killing of innocent human creatures, even if carried out to help others, constitutes an absolutely unacceptable act.

John Paul II (1995)

From the ethical point of view, embryo reduction is an intentional selective abortion. It is in fact the deliberate and direct elimination of one or more innocent human beings in the initial phase of their existence and as such it always constitutes a grave moral disorder.

The ethical justifications proposed for embryo reduction are often based on analogies with natural disasters or emergency situations in which, despite the best intentions of all involved, it is not possible to save everyone. Such analogies can not in any way be the basis for an action which is directly abortive. At other times, moral principles are invoked, such as those of the lesser evil or double effect, which are likewise inapplicable in this case. It is never permitted to do something which is intrinsically illicit, not even in view of a good result: the end does not justify the means.

CFaith (2008)

While it is always morally illicit to kill an innocent human being, it can be licit, praiseworthy or even imperative to give up one's own life (cf. Jn 15:13) out of love of neighbour or as a witness to the truth.

John Paul II (1993)

45. Abortion (that is, the directly intended termination of pregnancy before viability or the directly intended destruction of a viable fetus) is never permitted. Every procedure whose sole immediate effect is the termination of pregnancy before viability is an abortion, which, in its moral context, includes the interval between conception and implantation of the embryo.

47. Operations, treatments, and medications that have as their direct purpose the cure of a proportionately serious pathological condition of a pregnant woman are permitted when they cannot be safely postponed until the unborn child is viable, even if they will result in the death of the unborn child.

48. In case of extrauterine pregnancy, no intervention is morally licit which constitutes a direct abortion.[1]

49. For a proportionate reason, labor may be induced after the fetus is viable.

USCCB (2009)

Islam

The Prophet Muhammad (~570 CE to 632 CE), Arabian Peninsula, is considered by Muslims to be the last and greatest of a series of prophets beginning with Adam and including Abraham, Moses, and the non-divine Jesus Christ. Muhammad is believed

[1] Note that Directive 45 defines an abortion as any procedure "whose sole immediate effect is the termination of pregnancy before viability." Thus, a procedure undertaken to end a tubal pregnancy would not meet the strict definition of an abortion, since its immediate effect is to avert maternal hemorrhage and possible death. As in Directive 47, the procedure has the direct purpose of curing a serious pathological condition in the mother and thus is permitted, even though the unwanted secondary effect is the death of the fetus. The termination is not "the means to an end" but rather the inevitable result of a procedure which cannot be postponed (Anderson 2002).

to have restored the proper understanding of the monotheistic tradition upon which the Jewish and Christian faiths are built. The divine revelations of Muhammad are recorded in the holy text, the *Qur'an* or *Koran* (Melton 1999). The *Sunna/Haddith*, compendia of Muhammad's teachings and practices, provide additional sources of Islamic law (*Shari'aa*), along with the unanimous opinion of prior scholars (*Igmaa*), and *Aaimaa*, reasoning by analogy (Aramesh 2009; Serour 2008). Scholarly interpretations and applications of Islamic law are known as *Fatwa*.

Sunni Islam is the more conservative of the major sects, comprising about 90 % of believers worldwide. Shi'a theology is somewhat more liberal; its believers comprise about 90 % of Iranian Muslims (Aramesh 2009).

> According to the Shiite theology, moral goodness and badness can be revealed by reason (*aghl*) on its own. Therefore, newly emerging jurisprudential and ethical issues (including bioethical ones) should be categorised and discussed in the light of both reason and scripture. According to the majority of Sunni schools, however, every jurisprudential topic, including bioethical issues, should be examined only on the basis of scripture and the prophetic tradition. Therefore, in dealing with newly emerging issues, one can use analogical deduction (*qiyas*) to find the most compatible response with the holy scripture.
>
> Aramesh (2009)
> Iran

In Vitro Techniques

No limitations are placed on in vitro interventions using the gametes of the married couple. The success of ICSI has enhanced the acceptability of and demand for assisted reproduction (Serour 2008). The use of donor gametes is controversial.

> The Sunni Islamic position on assisted reproduction clearly permits in vitro fertilization, using eggs from the wife with the sperm of her husband and the transfer of the fertilized embryos back to the uterus of the same wife. However, since marriage is a contract between the wife and the husband during the span of their marriage, no third party should intrude into the marital functions of sex and procreation. This means that a third party donor is not acceptable, whether he or she is providing sperm, eggs, embryos, or a uterus (as in surrogacy). As noted by Islamic legal scholar Ebrahim Moosa,
>
> > In terms of ethics, Muslim authorities consider the transmission of reproductive material between persons who are not legally married to be a major violation of Islamic law. This sensitivity stems from the fact that Islamic law has a strict taboo on sexual relations outside of wedlock (*zina*). The taboo is designed to protect paternity (i.e., family) which is designated as one of the five goals of Islamic law, the others being the protection of religion, life, property, and reason.
>
> Inhorn (2011b)
> U.S.

> [I]nfertile couples often dream of making a test-tube baby 'back home' for a variety of cultural, moral and psychological reasons. These reasons – including medical expatriotism, the language of medicine, co-religion and moral trustworthiness, donor phenotype, the comforts of home and discrimination – are rarely highlighted in the scholarly literature[.]
>
> Inhorn (2011a)
> U.S.

Preimplantation Genetic Diagnosis

Preimplantation genetic diagnosis is preferred over prenatal diagnosis. Its use for sex selection is disapproved by some authorities.

> The use of sperm sorting techniques or preimplantation genetic diagnosis (PGD) for non-medical reasons such as sex selection or balancing sex ratio in the family is guarded. These techniques are a better alternative to prenatal diagnosis, which necessitates abortion for sex selection. Most Muslims adhere to the view that human life requiring protection commences 2 weeks from conception and uterine implantation.
>
> ...
>
> Accordingly, decisions not to attempt replacement of embryos produced in vitro on the grounds that they show serious chromosomal or genetic anomalies, such as aneuploidy, cystic fibrosis, muscular dystrophy or haemophilia, are accepted. PGD is encouraged, where feasible as an option to avoid clinical pregnancy termination for couples at exceptionally high risk.
>
> Serour (2008)
> Egypt

> Sex selection technologies have been condemned on the ground that their application will discriminate against female embryos and fetuses, so perpetuating prejudice against the girl child and social devaluation of women .... However, universal prohibition would itself risk prejudice to women in many present societies, especially when births of sons or girls remain central to women's wellbeing.
>
> Serour (2008)
> Egypt

Unimplanted Pre-embryos

There are no objections to cryopreserving embryos for future use by married couples using their own gametes. Generally the relinquishment of unused embryos for use by other couples would be disapproved because maintenance of genetic lineage is of great importance. However, Iran (Shi'a) in 2003 enacted legislation permitting healthy married couples with excess embryos to donate them to other healthy married infertile couples. The donors remain anonymous and relinquish all ties to the embryos; the recipients assume full parental obligations.[2]

> Several embryos are usually produced during the procedure of in vitro fertilization (IVF) for the treatment of infertility of a couple who are legally married at the time. Many of them are not implanted in the wife's uterus. These are usually cryopreserved for possible future use if this cycle was not successful or if this couple wants to try another pregnancy. In Islam

[2] Donation is managed by licensed fertility clinics with attestations and judicial review. Identities of donors and recipients are confidential. The donor couple must be married; healthy in body, mind, and intellect; and free of addictions and incurable diseases. The recipient couple must be Iranian; married; infertile; healthy in body, mind, and intellect; free of addictions and incurable diseases; and capable of raising the child. The recipient parents are responsible for the child "such as responsibility of real parents." The law is silent concerning inheritance, lineage, and other issues (Tehran University of Medical Sciences, undated).

> these extra embryos cannot be implanted into another woman's uterus nor can they be used by either spouse if they get divorced or if one of the spouses dies as preservation of lineage is of prime importance in Islamic law. If this couple later on decides not to use their cryopreserved embryos, the frozen embryos are thawed and either left to die or destroyed. So the great majority of Muslim scholars agree that their use for research, which may bring potential therapeutic benefit, is better than letting them go to waste.
>
> Fadel (2012)
> U.S.

> The excess number of fertilized eggs can be preserved by cryopreservation. The frozen embryos are the property of the couple alone and may be transferred to the same wife in a successive cycle but only during the validity of the marriage contract.
>
> Serour (2008)
> Egypt

> The old threshold of 40 days and upwards from conception has been brought back to 14 days, because recent progress in embryology has established that individuality of the new being cannot begin before this date …. Embryo research, for advancement of scientific knowledge and benefit of humanity, is therefore allowed before 14 days after fertilization on surplus embryos donated for research with the free informed consent of the couple.
>
> Serour (2008)
> Egypt

Prenatal Diagnosis

Prenatal diagnosis is acceptable when the aim is preservation of maternal or fetal life or health. Pregnancy interruption for serious fetal indications is permitted by some authorities provided that it occurs prior to ensoulment (see Sect 3.4.6, below). Preimplantation diagnosis is considered preferable to prenatal diagnosis (see Sect. 3.4.2, above).

Prenatal Therapeutic Interventions

Prenatal therapeutic interventions are acceptable if directed toward the preservation of maternal or fetal life or health, or the correction of anomalies.

> The background concept is that gene therapy might be legitimate, not to promote advantage or privilege, but to redeem genetically or otherwise physiologically inherited disadvantage.
>
> Serour (2008)
> Egypt

Pregnancy Loss

Miscarriage, stillbirth, and infant death are thought to be in the hands of God. Islamic texts say that if a fetus is miscarried after 120 days (quickening, ensoulment) it should be prayed over and buried in a Muslim cemetery. However, cultures differ in their approach to pregnancy loss, with some traditions not recognizing personhood and not allowing Muslim burial unless the infant is liveborn and the *azan* (Muslim confession of faith) is whispered in its ear prior to death (Shaw 2014).

Pregnancy Interruption and Fetal Reduction

Abortion is disapproved at any gestational age; however, it may be tolerated in the event of maternal or fetal indications, particularly if it occurs prior to ensoulment. There are several interpretations concerning the timing of ensoulment.

> [T]here is a verse in the Quran that is generally understood to relate to this:
>
> Man We did create from a quintessence (of clay). Then We placed him as a drop (*nutfa*) in a place of rest firmly fixed. Then We made the drop into a clot that clings (*alaqa*). Then out of that We made a chewed lump (*mudgha*). Then We made out of that lump bones and clothed the bones with flesh. Then out of that We developed another creature. So blessed be God the best to create.
>
> This verse strongly indicates that the new creation (the person) exists only after some stage of embryonic development and not at the time of fertilization.
>
> Muslim scholars, on the basis of this verse, described early life as occurring in two phases: biological and human. They generally agree that ensoulment, the breathing of God's spirit into the fetus, differentiates biological life that starts at fertilization from human life.
>
> …
>
> Scholars have identified the timing of ensoulment based on a prophetic *hadith*:
>
> Each of you is collected in the womb of his mother for forty days then turns into a clot (*alaqa*) just like that (*mithla dhālika*) and turns into a lump (*mudgha*) just like that, and then Allah (God) sends an angel and orders him to write four things i.e. his career, his provision, his life duration, and whether he will be wretched or blessed (in the Hereafter), then the angel breathes the soul into him.
>
> This *hadith* mentions three 40-day stages of embryonic development before ensoulment occurs. Many scholars understand this to mean that ensoulment occurs at 120 days after conception. However some scholars understand the 'just like that' (*mithla dhālika*) to indicate that these three stages occur within the same time period, i.e., 40 days, at the end of which time ensoulment occurs.
>
> All Muslim scholars agree that embryonic life is entitled to respect even before ensoulment, becomes progressively more deserving of rights as the development proceeds and definitely acquires full rights after ensoulment.
>
> Fadel (2012)
> U.S.

> The parliament of the Islamic Republic of Iran also ratified the Act of Therapeutic Abortion in 2005 …. Under the new act, therapeutic abortion would be permissible within the first four months of pregnancy after confirmation of it *(sic)* by three experts and verification by the Legal Medicine Organization. The law would allow abortion to be performed when there are familial or genetic disorders of the fetus that would lead to psychological affliction or undesirable burden on the parents, or in the case of serious maternal disease…. [T]he new act resulted in numerous requests for abortion due to disabling fetal disorders. It should be mentioned that incidence of some congenital disorders such as haemoglobinopathies

(particularly ß-thalassaemia) is considerable due to the customary preference for consanguineous marriage. The proponents of the law emphasized the high cost and psychological trauma of children with birth defects.

Zahedi and Larijani (2008)
Iran

Should [high-order multiple pregnancy] occur in spite of all preventive measures, then multi-fetal pregnancy reduction may be performed applying the jurisprudence principles that necessity permits the prohibited and the choice of the lesser harm.

Serour (2008)
Egypt

Post-reformation Christianity

Protestant
Pentecostal
Evangelical
Church of Jesus Christ of Latter-Day Saints (Mormon)
Jehovah's Witness
Church of Christ, Scientist
Many others

Growing dissatisfaction with the theology and politics of the Roman Catholic Church led to the Protestant Reformation (generally 1517–1648, with fourteenth- and fifteenth-century antecedents) in which Martin Luther, John Calvin, and others advocated translating the scriptures into lay languages and recognizing the "priesthood of all believers," rejecting the putative spiritual authority of the Saints, the Pope, and the ordained priesthood, recognizing salvation through grace and faith (rather than through good works or purchase of *Indulgences* from the Church), and other reforms unacceptable to the Church of Rome. Eventually these groups established independent churches which came to be known as "protestant" denominations. To these were added, over the centuries, other faith communities with their roots in the Christian Bible but not in the original Protestant sects. Post-reformation Christians vary widely in their beliefs. All acknowledge the centrality of the Bible but some believe it to be the literal, infallible word of God while others believe it to be "the word of God in the words of men," a product of its culture of origin and subject to interpretation. Some denominations recognize additional sacred or authoritative texts (e.g., Church of Jesus Christ of Latter-Day Saints, Church of Christ, Scientist) (Melton 1999).

The doctrines of the *United Methodist Church* are given here as examples of mainstream Christian beliefs. The UMC is the second most populous protestant denomination in the USA, with some 7.4 million members. Although Baptists as a group are more numerous, Baptist congregations are autonomous and there is no central doctrinal authority. Wide variation of belief and practice is common between and within Christian denominations, particularly in the USA.

In Vitro Techniques

In vitro techniques involving the gametes of the parents are unlikely to pose a problem. The use of donor gametes is not officially prohibited or sanctioned. There is considerable concern about preimplantation genetic diagnosis as a possible invitation to eugenics.

> The quadrilateral, as its name implies, uses four sources for discernment: scripture, tradition, experience and reason. Scripture, considered primary, is reflected on, based on the question asked. If we are seeking the answer to the question, "Should I seek assisted reproductive technologies to become pregnant?" we would reflect on passages that relate to that question. Not an easy task for some of the questions we struggle with in the 21st century. Scripture may provide us with some core guiding principles about what it means to be human and created in God's image but doesn't speak to the specifics of assisted reproductive technologies.
>
> Next, we consider what the tradition of the church teaches us about the question we ask. What has guided Christians over the past millennia regarding this particular question we ask. This again may not be a substantial amount for issues of new and emerging technologies…
>
> Next, we consider our experience both as individuals and corporately as the people called Christians …. [W]e are challenged to understand and embrace the unique perspectives of our sisters and brothers who we are linked with under the common name of Christian.
>
> Finally, we use our God-given reason to test, confirm, challenge and ultimately articulate our answer to the question we are discerning.
>
> United Methodist Church (2005)

Preimplantation Genetic Diagnosis

Preimplantation genetic diagnosis is recognized as imperfect and seen as a possible invitation to eugenics or frivolous uses. Since the church has acknowledged the legitimacy of prenatal diagnosis and subsequent pregnancy interruption for serious, early-onset genetic conditions, it would not be opposed to preimplantation genetic diagnosis for similar conditions. It has grave reservations about the use of PGD for adult-onset conditions and disapproves it for sex selection.

> The new eugenics is not so much the negative eugenics of state coercion or the oldest positive eugenics of better baby contests, but rather the eugenics made possible by the emerging biotechnology sciences, such as Preimplantation Genetic Diagnosis. Parents, not the state are the new eugenicists. They, as never before, are confronted with choices about which children they should have based on an incomplete science pointing to the genetic links of many conditions.
>
> Preimplantation Genetic Diagnosis (PGD) is only one of many emerging genetic and reproductive technologies in need of broad public discussion and regulation, but we view PGD as a gateway technology. PGD, if permitted to continue unregulated, could pave the way to new eugenics, where children are literally selected and eventually designed according to a parent's desires and fears.
>
> Recent rapid developments in PGD indicate that we are stumbling down a slippery slope toward this future, rendering a policy response an urgent matter.
>
> …

> Today, two thirds of the fertility clinics in the world offering PGD are in the US. Some clinics are blatantly performing PGD for selection. Many other clinics have used PGD to avoid late-onset diseases like Alzheimer's and recently breast cancer. A growing number of couples are using PGD to select an embryo that would grow into a child intended to be a tissue match for its sibling. None of these applications was subject to formal regulatory review or public deliberation prior to their use. In the case of sex selection, the practice specifically violates the voluntary guidelines of the American Society of Reproductive Medicine .... [Robert] Edwards has predicted that "Soon it will be a sin for parents to have a child which carries the heavy burden of genetic disease. We are entering a world where we have to consider the quality of our children."
>
> ...
>
> The church needs to remind its members that as Christians we are called to stand apart from culture and rejoice that our identity comes from being 'adopted' by Christ and where we are all welcomed as children of God regardless of our genetic makeup.
>
> UMC Book of Resolutions 2012a, b #3184

Unimplanted Pre-embryos

The church contemplates and expressly permits freezing of embryos for future use by the couple. It cautions against creating more embryos than intended for implantation. It would likely approve of donating unused embryos to other infertile couples.

> We call for a ban on medical and research procedures that intentionally generate "waste embryos" that will knowingly be destroyed when the medical procedure or the research is completed. The exception to this is when ova (eggs) are being collected for use in in vitro fertilization. A woman is at risk for complications each time drugs are given to stimulate ovulation and ova are removed. Obtaining and fertilizing multiple ova may be justified to avoid the necessity of multiple attempts to obtain ova. The first attempt at IVF results in a living child less than 30 % of the time thus making multiple attempts necessary.
>
> UMC Book of Resolutions 2012a, b #3181

Prenatal Diagnosis

Prenatal diagnosis undertaken to improve the care of the mother and fetus would be approved without reservation. The church recognizes a clear duty to the unborn but gives equal or greater weight to the needs of the mother and family. Thus, prenatal diagnosis for serious genetic disorders, followed by selective termination, is within the discretion of the mother after consultation with her partner, physician, and pastor.

> For it was you who formed my inward parts;
> you knit me together in my mother's womb.
> I praise you, for I am fearfully and wonderfully made.
> Wonderful are your works; that I know very well.
> My frame was not hidden from you,
> when I was being made in secret,

intricately woven in the depths of the earth.
Your eyes beheld my unformed substance.
In your book were written all the days that were formed for me,
when none of them as yet existed.

Psalm 139:13–16 NRSV
Quoted in UMC (2005)

When an unacceptable pregnancy occurs, we believe that a profound regard for unborn human life must be weighed alongside an equally profound regard for fully developed personhood, particularly when the physical, mental, and emotional health of the pregnant woman and her family show reason to be seriously threatened by the new life just forming. We reject the simplistic answers to the problem of abortion that, on the one hand, regard all abortions as murders, or, on the other hand, regard abortions as medical procedures without moral significance.

… We believe that continuance of a pregnancy that endangers the life or health of the mother, *or poses other serious problems concerning the life, health, or mental capability of the child to be*, is not a moral necessity. In such cases, we believe the path of mature Christian judgment may indicate the advisability of abortion. We support the legal right to abortion as established by the 1973 Supreme Court decision. We encourage women in counsel with husbands, doctors, and pastors to make their own responsible decisions concerning the personal and moral questions surrounding the issue of abortion. (*emphasis added*)

UMC Book of Resolutions 2012 #2025

We recognize and affirm the full humanity and personhood of all individuals with mental, physical, developmental, neurological, and psychological conditions or disabilities as full members of the family of God. We also affirm their rightful place in both the church and society.

UMC Book of Discipline 2012 ¶162(I)

Prenatal Therapeutic Interventions

Any medically sound intervention intended to cure or ameliorate the effects of a disease or disability would be approved, provided that it does not involve germ-line manipulation, which is deemed excessively risky. Enhancements are expressly disapproved.

We welcome the use of genetic technology for meeting fundamental human needs for health and a safe environment.

…

Human gene therapies that produce changes that cannot be passed to offspring (somatic therapy) should be limited to the alleviation of suffering caused by disease. Genetic therapies for eugenic choices or that produce waste embryos are deplored.

UMC Book of Discipline 2012 ¶162(O)

We support human somatic gene therapies (recombinant DNA therapies that produce genetic changes in an individual which cannot be passed to offspring) that prevent or minimize disease and its effects. But we believe these therapies should be limited to the alleviation of suffering caused by disease …. We oppose human germ-line therapies (those that result in changes that can be passed to offspring) because of the possibility of unintended consequences and of abuse. With current technology it is not possible to know if artificially introduced genes will have unexpected or delayed long-term effects not identifiable until the genes have been dispersed in the population.

We oppose both somatic and germ-line therapies when they are used for eugenic purposes or enhancements, that is, to provide only cosmetic change or to provide athletic or social advantage ….

UMC Book of Resolutions 2012 #3181

Pregnancy Loss

Miscarriage, stillbirth, and infant death are not considered signs of divine punishment. Baptism, while desirable for an imperiled infant, is not essential for salvation. All such fetuses and infants are considered to be with God.

Death is never a sign that God has abandoned us, no matter what the circumstances of the death might be …. We encourage the use of medical technologies to provide palliative care at the end of life when life-sustaining treatments no longer support the goals of life, and when they have reached their limits. There is no moral or religious obligation to use these when they impose undue burdens or only extend the process of dying.

UMC Book of Discipline 2012 ¶161(M)

Pregnancy Interruption and Fetal Reduction

As noted above (see 3.5.4), the church acknowledges the right of a woman to end a pregnancy when her life or the prospects of the fetus are seriously compromised. This is not to be undertaken lightly. There are no doctrinal statements concerning selective reduction. However, if the choice of abortion can be made in the face of fetal compromise or "when the physical, mental, and emotional health of the pregnant woman and her family show reason to be seriously threatened by the new life just forming" (UMC Resolution #2025), then by implication selective fetal reduction could be acceptable as a means of preserving the prospects of the remaining fetuses.

Our belief in the sanctity of unborn human life makes us reluctant to approve abortion.

But we are equally bound to respect the sacredness of the life and well being of the mother and the unborn child.

We recognize tragic conflicts of life with life that may justify abortion, and in such cases we support the legal option of abortion under proper medical procedures[.] … We cannot affirm abortion as an acceptable means of birth control, and we unconditionally reject it as a means of gender selection or eugenics (see Resolution 3184).

We oppose the use of late-term abortion known as dilation and extraction (partial-birth abortion) and call for the end of this practice except when the physical life of the mother is in danger and no other medical procedure is available, or in the case of severe fetal anomalies incompatible with life.

…

We commit our Church to continue to provide nurturing ministries to those who terminate a pregnancy, to those in the midst of a crisis pregnancy, and to those who give birth.

> …
>
> [A] decision concerning abortion should be made only after thoughtful and prayerful consideration by the parties involved, with medical, pastoral, and other appropriate counsel.
>
> UMC Book of Discipline 2012 ¶161(J)

Conclusion

Andrew Dutney concluded his 2007 examination of best practices concerning religion and ART with the following advice:

- Be prepared for patients' concerns to take an unexpectedly religious turn from time to time, and for the likelihood that their religious orientation will be expressed in clumsy, unsophisticated ways.
- Be aware of the major religious traditions represented in the community and how those traditions have responded to developments in ART.
- Do not assume that a particular couple will have an attitude that mirrors the official view of the religion with which they identify.
- Do not try to 'correct' apparent wrong-headedness ('This is God's judgment on us because of the termination I had when I was nineteen') but be supportive of the patient's gradual 'reframing' of faith in the light of the experience of infertility ('God has also given us access to ART and the wonderful people in this [Reproductive Medicine Unit] and is with us as we work through this IVF cycle together').
- Identify people in the community to whom patients could be referred for spiritual support or counsel; for example, ministers or priests who have personal knowledge of the experience of infertility.

Dutney (2007)
Australia

Dutney's guidelines provide a sound and hopeful template with which to engage patients during a profoundly trying time in their lives. Providers who follow his advice are likely to have a smoother journey with their religious patients.

References

Anderson RR. Religious traditions and prenatal genetic counseling. Omaha, NE: University of Nebraska Medical Center, Munroe Meyer Institute; 2002. p. 198.

Aramesh K. Iran's experience with surrogate motherhood: an Islamic view and ethical concerns. J Med Ethics. 2009;35:320–2.

Bharadwaj A. Sacred conceptions: clinical theodicies, uncertain science, and technologies of procreation in India. Culture, Medicine and Psychiatry. 2006;30:451–65.

Bhattacharyya S. Magical progeny, modern technology: a Hindu bioethics of assisted reproductive technology. Albany NY: State University of New York Press; 2006. p. 161.

Central Conference of American Rabbis (CCAR). ccarnet.org. "Fetus used for experimentation". 1984. CCAR Responsa www.ccarnet.org/responsa/carr-34-35. Accessed 20 Oct 2014

Central Conference of American Rabbis (CCAR). ccarnet.org. "When is abortion permitted?" Central Conference of American Rabbis. 1985 www.ccarnet.org/responsa/carr-23-27/. Accessed 20 Oct 2014

Central Conference of American Rabbis (CCAR). ccarnet.org. "In Vitro Fertilization and the Mitzvah of Childbearing." Central Conference of American Rabbis. 1996. www.ccarnet.org/responsa/rr21-no-5758-3/. Accessed 20 Oct 2014

Central Conference of American Rabbis (CCAR). ccarnet.org. "In Vitro Fertilization and the Status of the Embryo." Central Conference of American Rabbis. 1996. www.ccarnet.org/responsa/rr21-no-5757-2/. Accessed 20 Oct 2014

Central Conference of American Rabbis (CCAR). ccarnet.org. "Linkage analysis." Plaut WG, Washofsky M. 1990. Teshuvvot for the 1990's. www.ccarnet.org/responsa/trf-no-5752-6-305-308. Accessed 20 Oct 2014

Congregation for the Doctrine of the Faith (CFaith). Respect for Human Life (*Donum Vitae*). The Vatican; 1987.

Congregation for the Doctrine of the Faith (CFaith). Instruction *Dignitas Personae* on certain bioethical questions. The Vatican; 2008.

Desai PN. Health and Medicine in the Hindu Tradition. Chicago, Il: The Park Ridge Center; 1989. p. 153.

Dorff EN. Matters of life and death: a Jewish approach to modern medical ethics. Philadelphia, PA: The Jewish Publication Society; 1998. p. 456.

Dutney A. Religion, infertility and assisted reproductive technology. Best Practice & Research Clinical Obstetrics and Gynaecology. 2007;21(1):169–80.

Fadel HE. Developments in stem cell research and therapeutic cloning: Islamic ethical positions, a review. Bioethics. 2012;26(3):128–35.

Gele AA, Kumar B, Harsløf Hjelde K, Sundby J. (2012). Attitudes toward female circumcision among Somali immigrants in Oslo: a qualitative study. Int J Womens Health. 2012;4:7–17.

Grazi RV, Wolowelsky JB. Orthodox Judaism does not necessarily prohibit all multifetal reductions. Fert Steril. 2010;94(4), e67.

Hayford SR, Trinitapoli J. Religious differences in female genital cutting: a case study from Burkina Faso. J Sci Study Relig. 2011;50(2):252–71.

Inhorn MC. Diasporic dreaming: return reproductive tourism to the Middle East. Reproductive Biomedicine Online. 2011a;23:582–91.

Inhorn MC. Globalization and gametes: reproductive 'tourism', Islamic bioethics, and Middle Eastern modernity. Anthropology & Medicine. 2011b;18(1):87–103.

International Theological Commission of the Roman Catholic Church. The hope of salvation for infants who die without being baptised. The Vatican; 2007.

Ivry T. Halachic infertility: rabbis, doctors, and the struggle over professional boundaries. Med Anthropol. 2013;32(3):208–26.

John Paul II. The splendor of truth (*Veritatis Splendor*). The Vatican; 1993.

John Paul II. The gospel of life (*Evangelium Vitae*). The Vatican; 1995

Jotkowitz A. Surrogate motherhood revisited: maternal identity from a Jewish perspective. J Relig Health. 2011;50:835–40.

Lipner J. In Coward H, Lipner J, Young K, Hindu ethics: purity, abortion, and euthanasia. New York, NY: State University of New York Press; 1989. p. 139.

Melton JG. Encyclopedia of American Religions, Sixth Ed. Gale Research. Farmington Hills MI, 1999. 1243 p.

Moosa E. Human cloning in Muslim ethics. Fall: Voices Across Boundaries; 2003. p. 23–6.

Nikolaos M. The Greek orthodox position on the ethics of reproductive medicine. Reproductive Bioethics Online. 2008;17(3):25–33.

Pattanaik D. Infertility in Hindu mythology; 2014. http://blog.drmalpani.com/2014/03/infertility-in-hindu-mythology-dr.html. Accessed 15 Oct 2014.

Popovsky M. Choosing our children's genes: the use of preimplantation genetic diagnosis. Responsum approved by the Committee on Jewish Law and Standards, 28 May 2008. https://www.rabbinicalassembly.org/sites/default/files/public/halakhah/teshuvot/20052010/Popovsky_FINAL_preimplantation.pdf. Accessed 10 Oct 2014

Rouzi AA. Facts and controversies on female genital mutilation and Islam. Eur J Contracep Reprod Health Care. 2013;18(1):10–4.

Schenker JG. Assisted reproductive technology: perspectives in Halakha (Jewish religious law). Reproductive BioMedicine Online. 2008a;17(3):17–24.
Schenker JG. Human reproduction: Jewish perspectives. Gynecol Endocrinol. 2013;29(11): 945–8.
Schenker JG. The beginning of human life. Status of embryo. Perspectives in halakha. J Assisted Repro Genet. 2008b;25:271–6.
Serour GI. Islamic perspectives in human reproduction. Reproductive BioMedicine Online. 2008;17(3):34–8.
Sharma A. The Hindu tradition: religious beliefs and healthcare decisions. Religious traditions and healthcare decisions handbook series. Chicago, IL: Park Ridge Center for the Study of Health, Faith and Ethics; 1996.
Shaw A. Rituals of infant death: defining life and Islamic personhood. Bioethics. 2014;28(2): 84–95.
Talwar P. Manual of assisted reproductive technologies and clinical embryology. New Delhi: Jaypee Bros Medical Publisher Ltd; 2012. p. 900.
United Methodist Church. Spiritual discernment: a guide for genetic and reproductive technologies. West Palm Beach, FL: United Methodist Church; 2005. p. 112.
United Methodist Church. The Book of Discipline of The United Methodist Church. Nashville, TN: United Methodist Publishing House; 2012a.
United Methodist Church. The Book of Resolutions of the United Methodist Church. Nashville, TN: United Methodist Publishing House; 2012b.
United States Conference of Catholic Bishops, Inc. (USCCB). Ethical and religious directives for Catholic health care services. Washington, DC: United States Conference of Catholic Bishops, Inc.; 2009.
Zahedi F, Larijani B. National bioethical legislation and guidelines for biomedical research in the Islamic republic of Iran. Bull World Health Org. 2008;86:630–4.
Zaidi S, Ramarajan A, Qiu R, Raucher M, Chadwick R, Nossier A. Sexual rights and gender roles in a religious context. International Journal of Gynecology and Obstetrics. 2009;106:151–5.

Chapter 11
Disability Perspectives

David Wasserman

There is no single "disability" perspective on prenatal diagnosis. Rather, there are a variety of concerns, about the process by which such diagnosis is offered, accepted, reported, and acted upon; about the assumptions about disability that inform decisions on whether to offer, accept, and act upon the diagnosis; about the actual consequences or expressive significance of decisions to test and terminate; and about the understanding of parenting and family reflected in those decisions. Some of these concerns apply, or are directed, to the institutions that develop and offer tests; others to the prospective parents responsible for their "uptake." These concerns are all heightened by the advent of noninvasive and comprehensive prenatal diagnosis.

This chapter reviews these distinct but related concerns. I summarize them at the outset, then discuss each in detail. The capital letters preceding each indicate whether they are directed toward institutional practices (IP), parental decisions (PD), or both.

1. (IP) The process by which prenatal diagnosis is offered to prospective parents (a) leaves inadequate opportunity for reflection about whether to test and how to respond to the results; (b) is biased in its presentation of the diagnosed conditions; and (c) treats termination as the default option for "positive" results. Although earlier testing will allow more time for reflection, its lack of risk and intrusion may also discourage reflection. More comprehensive testing will make meaningful reflection far more difficult.
2. (IP, PD) Both the health professionals who offer prenatal diagnosis and the prospective parents to whom it is offered generally lack adequate information about life with any of the conditions for which testing has been done. This is likely to be even more of a problem as diagnosis becomes less invasive, more

D. Wasserman, J.D., M.A. (✉)
Clinical Center, Department of Bioethics, National Institutes of Health,
10 Center Drive, Bethesda, MD 20814, USA
e-mail: david.wasserman@nih.gov; dtwasserm@gmail.com

J.P. Galst, M.S. Verp (eds.), *Prenatal and Preimplantation Diagnosis*,
DOI 10.1007/978-3-319-18911-6_11

comprehensive, and cheaper, since it will then be performed for a wide range of rare conditions, in the absence of such indications as family history.

3. (IP) (a) Tests for genetic and chromosomal anomalies are developed and introduced not, or not only, to increase "reproductive choice"; but in the expectation that the high uptake of those tests will result in a significant reduction in the number of children born with the conditions tested for. (b) This expectation reflects and expresses the view that it is desirable to greatly reduce the number of people with those conditions. (c) Existing people with those conditions may reasonably regard this view as objectionable. (d) A policy encouraging prospective parents to select against those conditions is in tension, if not incompatible, with policies seeking to achieve social equality and greater inclusion for people with disabilities.
4. (PD) Even if they are well informed about life with the diagnosed conditions prospective parents fall short of the most attractive ideal of parenthood in choosing to employ prenatal diagnosis for selection purposes. This ideal reflects the belief that prospective parents should not set standards for "admitting" children into their families any more than actual parents should set standards for retaining them. This can be an extremely demanding ideal, and is better taken as aspirational rather than as a basis for criticizing parental decisions.

None of these concerns rest on beliefs about the moral status of the embryo or fetus. Many, though by no means all, of the critics of prenatal disability testing have been pro-choice, and few have sought legal restrictions on disability-based termination. The concerns about informed consent and misinformation are widely shared by others who find it unproblematic to terminate a pregnancy for disability. But critics also believe that such important decisions should be made without pressure, with accurate information, and with adequate opportunity for counseling and reflection.

Since the introduction of prenatal testing, there has been widespread concern about its use for sex selection (Wertz and Fletcher 1998). Several countries, not including the USA, actually ban its use for that purpose (Dickens 2002). Until recently, however, most critics of sex selection have not seen their opposition as having implications for disability selection. Indeed, most have recognized an exception for sex-linked diseases and disabilities (Council of Europe 1996). Critics of disability selection have argued that it is objectionable for many of the same reasons as sex-selection, i.e., in reinforcing prejudice against a disfavored group and in judging a potential person on the basis of a single characteristic (Asch 2003). Some feminist critics of sex selection now take this comparison seriously (Hall 2013).

As the range of diagnosable conditions expanded, many critics worried that testing would be used to select against trivial abnormalities, e.g., club feet, or for desired traits, e.g., high intelligence and musicality. These critics generally favored drawing a line between "serious" diseases and disabilities, which should be tested for, and all the rest, which should not be subject to testing (Botkin 1995). Disability critics, in contrast, are wary of line-drawing, fearing the stigmatizing effects on those having "serious" conditions and suspecting that the lines drawn reflect misinformed or exaggerated views about the severity of many disabilities (Asch 2003). Some argue that "the cure for testing is more testing"; that allowing tests for any condition or trait, significant or trivial, undesired or desired, would result in recognition that prenatal selection was not a strictly medical procedure and would make testing for disabilities less stigmatizing, even if it remained popular (Wasserman 2003; Gavaghan 2007).

The issue of line-drawing has been greatly complicated by the advent of microarray testing and whole genome testing, which do not target a single condition for which the fetus is "at risk." Rather, these tests reveal a variety of genetic changes which vary widely in known clinical significance. It is difficult to draw lines for the analysis and disclosure of findings from these tests, and yet clearly tempting, to avoid information overload, confusion, and anxiety (Bernhardt et al. 2014; Donley et al. 2012; Klugman et al. 2013).

The Concept of Disability and the Social Model

Before discussing the objections to prenatal selection against disability in more detail, it will be useful to say something about the concept of disability. Only a minority of those conditions classified as disabilities can be diagnosed prenatally by genetic testing, since most arise from environmental causes or interactions—a point I emphasize later. But the way in which disability is conceptualized is relevant to policies, practices, and individual decisions about prenatal testing and termination.

Two common features stand out in official definitions of disability created by the World Health Organization, the UK Disability Discrimination Act, and the Americans with Disabilities Act. There must be (1) an impairment [or a perceived impairment] and (2) some personal or social limitation associated with that impairment. The notion of a limitation encompasses restrictions on such "basic" actions as moving one's arms or legs (Nordenfelt 1997); on daily activities such as dressing and toileting; and on social activities, such as working. The classification of a physical or mental variation as an impairment may be statistical, based on the average in some reference group; it may be biological, based on an account of human functioning; or it may be normative, based on a conception of what is good for human beings (Tremain 2006). Most often, it involves some combination of these.

The most controversial aspect of the definition of disability is the relationship between the two elements—the impairment and the limitation. At one extreme are definitions that imply, or are read to imply, that impairments are the sole causes of limitation. At the other extreme are definitions that seem to treat the physical and social environment as the sole cause of disability. Between these extremes are definitions that regard the impairment and environment as interacting to cause limitation. For example, an individual with a mobility impairment who uses a wheelchair is limited in getting from place to place by the interaction of his inability to move his legs and the lack of ramps and wide doors in the buildings he frequents.

For simplicity's sake, disability scholars and philosophers of disability refer to two models of disability. As summarized in the *Stanford Encyclopedia of Disability* entry "Disability: Definitions, Models, Experience":

> The *medical model* understands a disability as a physical or mental impairment of the individual and its…consequences. It regards the limitations faced by people with disabilities as resulting primarily, or solely, from their impairments. In contrast, the *social model* understands disability as a relation between an individual and her social environment: the exclusion of people with certain physical and mental characteristics from major domains of social life. Their exclusion is manifested not only in deliberate segregation, but in a built environment and organized social activity that preclude or restrict the participation of people seen or labeled as having disabilities. In their extreme forms, the medical and social models serve to chart the space of possible relationships between impairment and limitation more than to reflect the actual views of individuals or institutions…. The medical model is rarely defended but often adopted unreflectively by health care professionals, bioethicists, and philosophers who ignore or underestimate the contribution of social and other environmental factors to the limitations faced by people with disabilities.

I simplify further for this chapter, treating the social model of disability as holding that the physical and social environment is a primary source of the limitations and disadvantages faced by many, if not all, people with impairments.

The attribution of disadvantage to social (environmental) barriers may matter less to prospective parents than to policy makers. If a future child with an impairment is likely to be excluded or stigmatized, there may be little its parents can do to prevent or even mitigate those disadvantages; for their purposes, they may be as much a given as if they were hard-wired genetically. For policy makers, however, it would be highly objectionable to promote prenatal selection against disability as the least expensive or difficult means of preventing discrimination against people with disabilities and the costs of fully including them in society. Indeed, defenders of prenatal testing who argue that it is compatible with the social equality of people with disabilities often stress that it must be accompanied by policies that support equality and inclusion for existing people with disabilities (see below).

With this background, I turn to an assessment of the specific objections to prenatal selection against disability outlined in the introduction.

The Critiques in Detail

1. *The process by which prenatal diagnosis is offered to prospective parents (a) leaves inadequate opportunity for reflection about whether to test and how to respond to the results; (b) is biased in its presentation of the diagnosed conditions; and (c) treats termination as the default option for "positive" results.*

Reproductive testing gives women options that were never available to them previously. Before ultrasound and karyotyping were introduced almost a half-century ago, women faced, at most, an unconditional choice about whether or not to continue a pregnancy. Since the advent of testing, that decision can be conditioned on ever more fetal attributes.

It is debatable, however, whether these options have really increased women's autonomy, i.e., their capacity to make independent decisions based on their own values.

Research over the past 15 years raises serious questions about whether consent to prenatal testing and selective abortion can be regarded as truly informed and voluntary.

It should not be surprising that many reproductive health professionals share the general views of nondisabled people about the overwhelming burdens of raising children with disabilities. Whether or not the mere offer of a prenatal test is itself directive (Clarke 1992), conveying the expectation that a prospective parent will terminate if the result is positive may make it difficult for pregnant women to continue a pregnancy, especially if the result is accompanied by one-sided information about disability. Several studies suggest that when reproductive health professionals do talk to their patients about the reasons for prenatal testing and termination, they tend to focus narrowly on the medical issues associated with disability (Klein 2011; Lippman and Wilfond 1992; Skotko 2005; Wertz 2000). They emphasize "the array of potential medical complications and physical limitations that may occur in children with the condition" (Lippman and Wilfond 1992, p. 936). A 2011 literature review concluded that a high proportion of reproductive clinicians held extremely negative attitudes towards life with a disability, which they communicated to their patients (Klein 2011). Other research suggests that such negative information has a significant impact on decisions about whether to terminate in the face of positive test results.

As reproductive testing becomes routine and comprehensive, issues of informed consent become more acute. In 1997, Press and Browner reported that women were being presented with prenatal testing as part of routine prenatal care, as "just another blood test." Many were not told that the test concerned fetal health, not maternal health; nor were they told that the results would not help them or their doctor to manage their pregnancy or to improve the health of their fetus. The option of abortion after positive results was rarely mentioned. A 2009 study suggests the continuing failure to explain the implications of prenatal testing to pregnant women: "Approximately one half of the women surveyed who underwent both ultrasound and biochemical screening did not foresee that they might ultimately be confronted with the need to make the decision about whether or not to terminate the pregnancy" (Seror and Ville 2009). In a 2009 study (Gottfreðsdóttir et al. 2009a), a woman explained her decision in these terms: "I just thought, well this is something you do when you are pregnant" (p. 716). The frequent absence of clear discussion should trouble conscientious health professionals, because it means that pregnant women are often led to obtain information they may not want to have, and to make decision they may not want to make.

The introduction of noninvasive tests may further increase pressure to utilize prenatal testing, because it lacks the risk or discomfort of invasive procedures (Hill et al. 2014a). Noninvasive testing may also discourage reflection and discussion on the implications of testing. An invasive procedure with a risk of miscarriage may "concentrate" the mind of prospective parents in a way that a simple blood draw does not. Moreover, as recent research suggests, pregnant women may be more likely to abort in the face of positive results from a noninvasive than an invasive test because of the fetal age at the time that they learn of the results: they are far less likely to have developed an attachment to an 8- than a 22-week old fetus, making the decision to abort that much easier (Hill et al. 2014b; Lewis et al. 2014).

Although some may view such attachment as an impediment to clear decision-making, disability critics would argue that it highlights the stakes involved in abandoning an intended pregnancy because of an unwelcome discovery about the fetus. At the same time, early testing offers a greater opportunity for reflection than later, invasive testing. One reason for the pressure to schedule an abortion after positive chorionic villus sampling (CVS) or amniocentesis results is the advanced stage of pregnancy at which those results are available, approaching the (expanding) stage of fetal viability. In contrast, results from noninvasive tests frequently will be available before the second trimester, offering considerably more opportunity for counseling and reflection. It remains to be seen how often this opportunity will be taken by prospective parents, and how it will weigh against the ease of testing and comparative lack of attachment.

2. *(IP, PD) Both the health professionals who offer prenatal diagnosis and the prospective parents to whom it is offered generally lack adequate information about life with any of the conditions for which testing has been done . This is likely to be even more of a problem as diagnosis becomes less invasive, more comprehensive, and cheaper, since it will it will then be performed for a wide range of rare conditions, in the absence of such indications as family history.*

Clearly, many health professionals, bioethicists, and laypeople believe that being born with a disability is almost always damaging and often disastrous for the child, her parents, and her siblings. Their assumption is that parents must give up other important life goals; that nondisabled children are neglected as parents focus on the needs of the child with the disability; that mothers especially must forsake or curtail other interests to "cope with" their child; and that resources of time and money are often strained to the breaking point (Botkin 1995; Wertz and Fletcher 1993a, b). Despite parental commitment and increased social acceptance, life with a disability is regarded as almost always of lesser quality than life without one (Brock 2005; Buchanan et al. 2000; Green 2008). Research suggests that some of these views are shared by prospective parents who accept prenatal testing (Gottfredsdottir and Arnason, 2011).

But are these assumptions warranted? A stable disability is not equivalent to acute illness or sudden injury, in which an active disease process or unexpected change in physical function disrupts life's routines. Most people with conditions such as spina bifida, achondroplasia, Down syndrome, and many other mobility and sensory impairments perceive themselves as healthy, not sick, and describe their conditions as "givens" of their lives—the equipment with which they meet the world. The same is true for many people with chronic conditions such as cystic fibrosis, diabetes, hemophilia, and muscular dystrophy. These conditions include intermittent flare-ups requiring medical care and adjustments in daily living, but they do not render the person as unhealthy as most of the public—and members of the health profession—often imagine.

Some proponents of prenatal testing and termination insist that critics ignore the fact that some conditions for which tests are available can be lethal in early childhood (e.g., Tay-Sachs), and can impair cognitive, physical, and sensory capacities to an extreme degree (e.g., Trisomy 13 or 18)—making it unclear how the child could have rewarding interactions in any environment. Nonetheless, the vast majority of diagnosable impairments are neither lethal in early childhood nor so capacity-limiting. The availability of tests for such rare conditions hardly supports selection against all significant disabilities; it merely reinforces the case that prospective parents should make testing decisions based on a careful assessment of information about specific impairments and on how a child's particular condition will influence their parental goals.

Most research on the well-being of people with disabilities relies on self-reports, and those reports do not confirm the grim views of third parties. Most people with disabilities report a quality of life similar to people without disabilities (Albrecht and Devlieger 1999; Gill 2000; Goering 2008; Saigal et al. 1996). However, the interpretation of self-reported well-being is complex and disputed (Barnes 2009; Menzel et al. 2002; Schwartz et al. 2007), and it raises questions about the extent to which appraisals of well-being should rely solely on subjective self-appraisal. This is not, or not entirely, an empirical question; it depends on our conception of well-being in the context of procreation, at which time the individual in question is not (yet) capable of self-appraisal, desire-formation, or the experiences of pleasure and pain.

Existing studies of families paint a more complex picture than that found in most medical and bioethical literature. Many studies do find that parents of children with significant disabilities face considerable stress and hardship at various stages in their children's lives. Thus, Gerstein et al. (2009) note that "a wealth of research continues to suggest that families of children with ID [intellectual disabilities] face increased stressors … Levels of stress have been found to be higher in parents of children with ID than in their typically developing counterparts." Eisenhower et al. (2009) find that mothers of children with developmental delays have poorer physical health outcomes, as well as the poorer mental health outcomes already shown in extensive research. The challenges may be greatest for parents of adult children with psychiatric disabilities, where "a body of research suggests that older parents of adults with serious mental illness experience on average, higher levels of burden and elevated health and mental health symptoms" (Aschbrenner et al. 2010).

Yet there is also considerable research, including some of the studies just cited, suggesting that these negative findings need to be qualified in several ways. First, the findings are not uniform. Some studies find that families of children with significant disabilities fare on average about as well as other families (Ferguson 2001; Walker et al. 1987). Some find that the additional challenges facing parents of children with disabilities are largely attributable to external factors like a lack of support services, or to preexisting family, social, or economic circumstances (Hatton et al. 2010). And some find that although families with disabled children face additional challenges, they experience equal or distinct rewards. This is true even for parents of adult children with serious psychiatric disabilities, "while later stages of the life course may involve unprecedented difficulties, they may also present unique opportunities for positive parenting experiences, including personal growth and a greater awareness of family strengths" (Aschbrenner et al. 2010).

A 2002 review of the existing research on families of disabled children noted that evidence of positive outcomes may have been overlooked because of the prevailing emphasis on negative ones. "If we ask negatively phrased questions, we are not very likely to get positive answers…" (Hastings and Taunt 2002, p. 117). Taking up this challenge 5 years later, Blacher and Baker (2007) found that "the expression of common benefits across families with and without disability, despite differences in negative impact…tempers the exclusively negative perspective that has characterized earlier literature on family and disability" (p. 343).

Prospective parents with disabilities themselves have the personal experience enabling them to reject the exaggerated assumptions about disability held by many people without disabilities. They are often harshly confronted with those assumptions in deciding to have children. And yet, having experienced a variety of challenges related to their disabilities, from frequent hospitalization to pervasive stigma, they have a wide range of responses to testing and termination (Gottfreðsdóttir et al. 2009b; Skotko 2005). Some refuse testing, some use it only for preparation, some test and terminate, much like their nondisabled counterparts, and some choose not to reproduce (Boardman 2014; Kelly 2009; Walsh-Gallagher et al. 2012).

Decision making of prospective parents is unlikely to be enhanced by providing clinical detail about each of the conditions for which testing has been done. The sheer number of conditions that can now or soon be tested for, and the diagnostic and predictive limitations of many of those tests, make a comprehensive consent process virtually impossible. What is needed is not more detail, but a broader focus, from the severity of the diagnosed condition to the expectations of the prospective parents in having a child, and how they think a child's motor, cognitive, emotional, or sensory impairment might affect that experience. Genetic counselors and other reproductive health professionals should try to assess the knowledge, attitudes, and values of pregnant women and their partners concerning reproductive testing, termination, and raising a child with a disability. And prospective parents must be able to obtain information about a subject they may know very little about, i.e., what it is like to raise a child with a particular impairment. If prospective parents have a chance to reflect on and respond to such questions, professionals may be in a much better position to discuss their concerns about the effect of impairments on parental goals and experiences (The Boston Women's Health Book Collective 2008).

In 2008, the US Congress took a major step in making that information available to pregnant women by enacting, with wide bipartisan support, the Prenatally and Postnatally Diagnosed Conditions Awareness Act (known as the "Kennedy-Brownback Act"). The act requires the federal government to arrange for the collection and dissemination of evidence-based, up-to-date information about the conditions subject to diagnosis. This information encompasses "the range of outcomes for individuals living with the diagnosed condition, including physical, developmental, educational, and psychosocial outcomes." Such information may provide a powerful corrective to the "bad news" typically delivered to pregnant women whose fetuses are diagnosed with the tested conditions.

The Act may have an even greater impact on prenatal decision making if it helps reframe how women and their partners view their choices after positive test results (Asch and Wasserman 2009). Information on the range of outcomes for individuals living with the diagnosed condition may help pregnant women and their partners see their decision as one about parenting a child who will have a disabling trait, not about "preventing disability." Indeed, studies of prospective parents with disabled family members (cited above) suggest that those who see disability in the context of full human lives are less likely than other prospective parents to terminate a fetus with a diagnosed ability. They may be better able to envision the whole of a future life that is too easily obscured by its diagnosed "part" (Asch and Wasserman 2005).

The Act, however, has a built-in limitation: it mandates better information only for women who have already been tested and received positive results, not for women deciding whether to be tested. The information collected will likely come too late in the process to reframe prenatal decision making. A woman who has already been led to regard such testing as a routine part of reproductive health care may have difficulty in seeing the testing as a prelude to a decision about what kind of child she is willing to parent. She might not want to make that decision, and, if she had understood the test's purpose before consenting to it, she might have refused to put herself in a position where she had to make such a choice.

Education about disability should begin much earlier, for a much broader population of individuals contemplating having children, reproductive health professionals, and the general public. In order for this information to be meaningfully integrated into the decision making of prospective parents, the processes by which prenatal testing is now offered may have to be restructured. It will be a formidable challenge to offer and provide this information in an increasingly complex and congested informed-consent process, especially one that frequently begins at the very first encounter with reproductive health professionals.

3. *(IP) (a) Tests for genetic and chromosomal anomalies are developed and introduced not, or not only, to increase "reproductive choice"; but in the expectation that the high uptake of those tests will result in a significant reduction in the number of children born with the conditions tested for. (b) This expectation reflects and expresses the view that it desirable to greatly reduce the number of people with those conditions. (c) Existing people with those conditions may reasonably regard this view as objectionable. (d) A policy encouraging prospective parents to select against those conditions is in tension, if not incompatible, with policies seeking to achieve social equality and greater inclusion for people with disabilities.*

Unlike the difficult, complex, often confused decisions of individuals and couples, which need not "send a message" to anyone regarding the lives of disabled persons, official policies and practices can indeed send a message of inferiority. This would be obvious for race or sex. Imagine a state-funded research program to identify genetic variants associated with dark complexion or African ancestry, designed to enable prospective parents to terminate fetuses with those variants. Such research would rightly be denounced as eugenic and racist. The fact that there is no popular concern over similar research programs to promote selection against disability suggests that—even if there are important differences between disability and race as minority characteristics—the expressive significance of such practices and policies has been overlooked. Whether or not they identify with or celebrate their disabilities, people with disabilities may reasonably be troubled by state or professional sponsorship of programs that treat the birth of people with conditions like theirs as a highly undesirable outcome.

Two approaches have been proposed for weakening the expressive force of the connection between prenatal testing and selection against disability. First, prenatal testing can be used more frequently to arrange appropriate medical and social services for children expected to have disabilities. Although the dominant use of prenatal or preimplantation genomic testing is, and will remain, to decide about pregnancy termination or embryo selection, its clinical utility is not limited to those decisions. An early diagnosis of intellectual or developmental disabilities can significantly benefit prospective parents who intend to continue the pregnancy regardless of the diagnosis. There is a growing recognition that prenatal diagnosis of these conditions can spare parents a painful and expensive diagnostic odyssey after birth. It can also facilitate early intervention, which can be helpful, even critical, in achieving better outcomes for some conditions (Lopez-Rangel et al. 2008; Makela et al. 2009). Further, even when testing only yields probabilities, it may help identify environmental factors that increase risk or exacerbate symptoms. Thus, prenatal testing can be used to promote early intervention, heightened vigilance, improved treatment, and greater continuity of care. The professional and societal expectation that some parents will chose to bear children with diagnosed impairments, as well as the specific arrangements reflecting that expectation, may well reduce the proportion of women and couples choosing to terminate after such a diagnosis (Le Dref et al. 2012).

A second, more controversial measure would be to allow prenatal testing for any genetically detectable condition or trait, whether or not it was associated with disease or disability. Such an unrestricted policy could support reproductive choice without singling out disability as a basis for selective embryo transfer or pregnancy termination (Asch 2003; Gavaghan 2007; Wasserman 2003). That policy would avoid the heightened stigmatization likely to result from the line-drawing, now widely advocated (Botkin 1995; Wertz 2000) to limit testing to more "serious" or "severe" disabilities. The more restricted the list of conditions subject to testing, the more stigmatizing testing will be for people living with those conditions.

The comparative virtue of this approach—of permitting any and all available testing—is that it would give no official or privileged role to disabilities in the determination of whether to offer testing or termination. Perhaps it would make little practical difference. Most prospective parents might well test only for disabilities (which would limit the costs of unrestricted testing), because they share prevailing attitudes toward disability, and because there may be fewer reliable tests for characteristics besides sex and disability. But this is not all that matters in gauging the expressive significance of a prenatal testing regime. A policy that did not treat disabilities as providing a presumptively stronger basis for selection than any other trait or variation would emphatically disavow the exceptionalism about disability that has dominated prenatal testing since its inception. It would "send the message" that disability did not give prospective parents a privileged reason to screen out embryos or terminate a pregnancy, that disabilities were just some among the myriad variations that might be relevant to some prospective parents in deciding whether to bring a child into the world.

At the same time, an unrestricted testing policy might appear to endorse a consumerist approach toward parenting; to express the view that embryos and fetuses, if not children, were valuable objects to be carefully selected To choose a policy of unrestricted testing is to treat this as a lesser evil than the heightened stigmatization of those disabilities subject to testing under a more restrictive policy.

An unrestricted policy would also permit selection *for* disability, a controversial issue in the recent bioethics literature. Most criticism of such selection concerns the welfare of the children chosen or its impact on aggregate well-being. Despite their skepticism about standard objections to creating children with disabilities, many disability advocates are reluctant to endorse their deliberate creation. Sometimes, the skepticism reflects doubts about "disability neutrality"—the view that there is nothing worse in having a disability than in lacking it (Bickenbach 2013, p. 168–98; Wasserman and Asch 2013, p. 139–67). But it may also reflect misgivings about the selection of a child based on any detectable trait—disability, sex, skin- or eye-color (Asch and Wasserman 2005; see next section).

4. *(PD) Even if they are well informed about life with the diagnosed conditions prospective parents fall short of the most attractive ideal of parenthood in choosing to employ prenatal diagnosis for selection purposes. This ideal reflects the belief that prospective parents should not set standards for "admitting" children into their families any more than actual parents should set standards for retaining them. This can be an extremely demanding ideal, and is better taken as aspirational rather than as a basis for criticizing parental decisions.*

Choosing a future child on the basis of any trait—whether positive or negative—arguably falls short of what Asch and Wasserman (2005) call an ideal of "unconditional welcome." This ideal is the counterpart for prospective parents of the ideal of unconditional love or commitment for actual parents. Prospective parents can hardly be expected to make an unconditional commitment toward an early-term fetus, let alone towards any or all of the embryos in an IVF array. The ideal of unconditional welcome enjoins them to *anticipate* the commitment they would make on becoming parents by not conditioning their willingness to bear and raise a child on the expected presence or absence of virtually any trait. Asch and Wasserman argue that this posture distinguishes prospective parents from prospective friends and lovers, who may and should exercise selectivity in choosing to form their intimate relationships. It also suggests a role for prospective parents continuous with that of actual parents, whose attachment to their children is expected to be even less dependent on the loss or acquisition of important traits than the attachment to a friend or lover.[1]

[1] A somewhat different argument against selectivity is offered by Herissone-Kelly (2009). He argues that in assessing the prospects for a future child, the prospective parent must "imaginatively inhabit" the lives of those children. Like an actual parent, she must identify with each of their lives, an identification that precludes selecting against any life the child herself would find acceptable (pgs. 256–257). Although he rejects comparisons among lives in choosing future children, Herissone-Kelly adopts a non-comparative standard for selection. His "Principle of Acceptable Outlook" holds that the future life must be expected to be acceptable to the individual living it (259–261). The proviso merely appears to express in subjective terms a life-worth-living requirement. The internal perspective otherwise provides no moral basis for selection.

The use of admissions criteria affect the moral and psychological character of any association. Even within exclusive associations, with high standards and competitive admission, there is a tension between those admission standards and the equality expected among members, expressed in an ideal of collegiality. Many a member of an academic admission committee has remarked, only half in jest, that he or she would never have been admitted under prevailing standards. More poignantly, institutions that raise their standards often relegate their older members to a kind of second-class citizenship. This kind of tension may be worth bearing to maintain and enhance the excellence of academic institutions. But it would be toxic in a family.

Imagine a family formed during an era of rapidly improving genetic testing, in which the capacity to detect predispositions to disease and disability grew ever more comprehensive, discriminating, and accurate. The prospective parents avail themselves of the latest selection technology in having children spaced 2 or 3 years apart. Each child, if he knew about the selection process, would have the disturbing awareness that he might well have been selected against on the latest round; that he would no longer pass muster. This would not, of course, preclude the parents from displaying unconditional and equal love for all their actual children, to the extent that any parents can. But it would result in a profound moral and psychological tension.

Mary Ann Baily (2000) and others have criticized the ideal of unconditional welcome for one of the same reasons Asch and Wasserman endorse it: the fact that any child can pose unexpected challenge. These critics argue that this fact provides a reason *for* selection, not *against* it: it gives prospective parents a way to "improve their odds." Asch and Wasserman (2005) counter that the attempt to do so by prenatal testing exaggerates the singular challenges of disability, mistakenly assuming that it is additive, and creates a false sense of security.

Unconditional welcome is no more compatible with parental selection *for* disability than against it. Parents should recognize that disability is only one of a child's attributes, and that possessing or not possessing a disability does not in itself guarantee a child's potential for having a satisfying relationship with her parents or a rewarding and productive life outside the family. An impairment is just one source of possible affinity with parents who share it, just as it is only one source of possible lack of affinity with parents who lack it. In neither case should it be a basis for prenatal selection.

The ideal of unconditional welcome is not in tension with the social model, which understands disability as a relational characteristic (Kukla and Wayne, 2011). It is doubtful that most health professionals and prospective parents involved in routine prenatal testing *see* diagnosed disabilities in relational terms, as conditions that are disadvantageous because of an unaccommodating environment. For those who do—for example, those who are successfully raising a disabled child but decline to have another child with the same disability because of realistically estimated costs—the critique would apply with lesser force, and the departure from the ideal of unconditional welcome would be less significant. In the extreme case of prospective parents living under a regime that killed those with significant disabilities, the critique would not apply at all.

Others argue that the ideal of unconditional welcome is too narrow (Ruddick 2000) or too demanding—particularly on women (Gedge 2011). Ruddick argues that it is only one, i.e., the "maternal" model, of three reasonable models of parenthood. It is not clearly superior to two others: the "familial"—where decisions about a child are based on its role in, and likely impact on, the family as a whole; and the "projectivist" model, where decisions are based on whether the traits of a child are compatible with the goals or projects of its prospective parents. Asch and Wasserman (2005) argue that the familial model is rarely incompatible with unconditional welcome, which is an ideal both for parents and families. The perceived incompatibility, they argue, arises largely from exaggerated or unsupported beliefs about the adverse impact of children with significant disabilities on other family members. The projectivist model is indeed incompatible with the ideal of unconditional welcome, but it is arguably too inflexible and self-oriented in treating the creation and rearing of a child as an individual "project." Moreover, a projectivist parent may be thwarted by a non-disabled child who turns out to be able but not willing to participate in valued family activities, who simply rejects the parents' values and projects.

There are two responses to the demandingness objection. The first, more general one, is that unconditional welcome is offered as an ideal, one to which prospective parents should aspire even if they will inevitably fall short (Wasserman and Asch 2005). For example, a couple may decide with deep misgivings not to have a child very likely to predecease them, or at risk of unemployment and institutionalization in surviving them. Such a decision may be unduly pessimistic, but if made with serious reflection and careful research, it is hardly one for which the couple should be criticized. The more specific worry, that the burden of welcoming will fall disproportionately on the mother, seems realistic as a practical concern but not as an objection to the ideal. A moral ideal should not be rejected because of the risk that it will be abused or distorted by social prejudice.

Challenges for the Future

Some observers fear a slippery slope in prenatal genetic testing, from diagnosing disease and disability to selecting desired (nonmedical) traits (Henn 2000). But for the near future, at least, the fear of "genetic consumerism" seems greatly exaggerated. Not only is the detection of genetic variations predisposing to such traits likely to remain elusive, but parental expectations for their children's biological endowment are generally modest (Wasserman 2003)—"as long as it has ten fingers and ten toes." This expectation, however, is double-edged. It reveals a lack of perfectionist aspirations, but also an anxiety about babies with more or less than the standard complement of fingers—or any significant disability. That anxiety will only be exacerbated by the multiplex genetic testing that will soon become the standard of care. It may be comforting for bioethicists and disability advocates to be reminded that we all carry potentially lethal, disabling, and disease-causing genes, but it is likely to be anything but comforting to prospective parents. One benefit to the prospect of universally available noninvasive prenatal testing, which both proponents and critics of testing can acknowledge, is that it will afford prospective parents the opportunity to decide whether they want to be tested at all, and if so, what kind of information they want. It may also prompt them to examine their goals, expectations, and hopes in becoming parents.

Providing guidance for prospective parents in making decisions about reproductive issues presents three kinds of challenges for reproductive health professionals. First, they must respect their patients' values about procreation and parenting—values that initially may be inchoate and confused. Second, they will need to make increasingly complex medical information available to those patients, information whose relevance may be uncertain to all parties. Third, they need to be prepared to help prospective parents deal with several kinds of uncertainty, from the clinical significance of ambiguous genetic findings to the practical challenges of raising a child with a disability. Meeting these challenges will require three very different kinds of knowledge: about the patients seeking to begin or enlarge their families, about the complex genetics of a growing number of medical conditions, and about the experience of parents and children living with these conditions. No one health professional, or small team of professionals, can expect to have sufficient knowledge about all possible scenarios. But care providers will need to know how to obtain and make information available to anxious patients who may know as little about the difficulties and rewards of raising children with various medical conditions as they know about the genetics of those conditions.

Disclaimer & Acknowledgment wherever you deem it appropriate: The views expressed in this chapter are the authors' own. They do not reflect any position or policy of any U.S. governmental entity, including the National Institutes of Health or the Department of Health and Human Services. Many, though not all, of the views expressed in the chapter reflect collaborative work with the author's late friend and colleague Adrienne Asch, who developed the most powerful and cogent critiques of reproductive testing for disability.

References

Albrecht GL, Devlieger G. The disability paradox: high quality of life against the odds. Soc Sci Med. 1999;48(8):977–88.

Asch A. Disability, equality and prenatal testing: contradictory or compatible? Fla State Univ Law Rev. 2003;30(2):315–42.

Asch A, Wasserman D. Where is the sin in synecdoche: prenatal testing and the parent-child relationship. In: Wasserman D, Wachbroit R, Bickenbach J, editors. Quality of life and human difference: genetic testing, health care, and disability. New York: NY, Cambridge; 2005. p. 172–216.

Asch A, Wasserman D. Informed consent and prenatal testing: the Kennedy-Brownback Act. Virtual Mentor. 2009;11(9):721–4.

Aschbrenner KA, Greenberg JS, Allen SA, Seltzer MM. Subjective burden and personal gains among older parents of adults with serious mental illness. Psychiatr Serv. 2010;61(6):605–11.

Baily MA. Why I had amniocentesis. In: Parens E, Asch A, editors. Prenatal testing and disability rights. Washington, DC: Georgetown; 2000. p. 64–71.

Barnes E. Disability, minority, and difference. J Appl Philos. 2009;26(4):337–55.

Bernhardt BA, Kellom K, Barbarese A, Faucett WA, Wapner RJ. An exploration of genetic counselors' needs and experiences with prenatal chromosomal microarray testing. J Genet Couns. 2014;23(6):938–47.
Bickenbach J. Disability and the well-being agenda. In: Bickenbach J, Felder F, Schmitz B, editors. Disability and the good human life. New York: Cambridge; 2013. p. 168–98.
Blacher J, Baker BJ. Positive impact of intellectual disabilities on families. Am J Ment Retard. 2007;112:330–480.
Boardman FK. Knowledge is power? The role of experiential knowledge in genetically 'risky' reproductive decisions. Sociol Health Illn. 2014;36(1):137–50. doi:10.1111/1467-9566.12048.
Botkin JR. Fetal privacy and confidentiality. Hastings Cent Rep. 1995;25(5):32–9.
Brock DW. Preventing genetically transmitted disabilities while respecting persons with disabilities. In: Wasserman D, Wachbroit R, Bickenbach J, editors. Quality of life and human difference: genetic testing, health care, and disability. New York: NY, Cambridge; 2005. p. 67–100.
Buchanan A, Brock DW, Daniels N, Wikler D. From chance to choice: genetics & justice. Cambridge: New York, NY; 2000.
Clarke A. Is non-directive genetic counseling possible? Obstet Gynecol Surv. 1992;47(5): 304–5.
Collective TBW'sHB. Prenatal testing. In: Our bodies, ourselves: pregnancy and birth. New York: Touchstone/Simon & Schuster; 2008. p. 109–27.
Council of Europe. Convention for the protection of human rights and dignity of the human being with regard to the application of biology and medicine: convention on human rights and biomedicine. Strasbourg: Council of Europe, Directorate of Legal Affairs; 1996.
Dickens BM. Can sex selection be ethically tolerated? J Med Ethics. 2002;28(6):333–6.
Donley G, Hull SC, Berkman BE. Prenatal whole genome sequencing. Hastings Cent Rep. 2012;42(4):28–40.
Eisenhower AS, Baker BL, Blacher J. Children's delayed development and behavior problems: impact on mothers' perceived physical health across early childhood. Soc Sci Med. 2009; 68(1):89–99.
Ferguson P. Mapping the family: disability studies and the exploration of parental response to disability. In: Albrecht GL, Seelman KDD, Bury M, editors. Handbook of disability studies. New York, NY: Sage; 2001. p. 373–96. doi:10.4135/9781412976251.n15.
Gavaghan C. Right problem, wrong solution: a pro-choice response to 'expressivist' concerns about preimplantation genetic diagnosis. Camb Q Healthc Ethics. 2007;16(1):20–34. doi:10.1017/S096318010707003X.
Gedge E. Reproductive choice and the ideals of parenting. Int J Fem Approaches Bioeth. 2011;4(2):32–47.
Gerstein ED, Crnic KA, Blacher J, Baker BL. Resilience and the course of daily parenting stress in families of young children with intellectual disabilities. J Intellect Disabil Res. 2009; 53(12):981–97.
Gill CJ. Health professionals, disability, and assisted suicide: an examination of empirical evidence. Psychol Public Policy Law. 2000;6(2):526–45.
Goering S. 'You say you're happy, but…': contested quality of life judgments in bioethics and disability studies. J Bioeth Inq. 2008;5(2-3):125–35.
Gottfreðsdóttir, Helga, and Vilhjálmur Árnason. "Bioethical concepts in theory and practice: an exploratory study of prenatal screening in Iceland." *Medicine, Health Care and Philosophy* 14.1 (2011): 53-61.
Gottfreðsdóttir H, Björnsdóttir K, Sandall J. This is just what you do when you are pregnant: a qualitative study of prospective parents in Iceland who accept nuchal translucency screening. Midwifery. 2009a;25(6):711–20.
Gottfreðsdóttir H, Björnsdóttir K, Sandall J. How do prospective parents who decline prenatal screening account for their decision? A qualitative study. Soc Sci Med. 2009b;69(2):274–7.
Green R. Babies by design: the ethics of genetic choice. New Haven: Yale; 2008.
Hall MC. Reconciling the disability critique and reproductive liberty: the case of negative genetic selection. Int J Fem Approaches Bioeth. 2013;6(1):121–43.

Hastings RP, Taunt HM. Positive perceptions in families of children with disabilities. Am J Ment Retard. 2002;107:116–27.
Hatton C, Emerson E, Graham H, Blacher J, Llweellyn G. Changes in family composition and marital status in families with a young child with cognitive delay. J Appl Res Intellect Disabil. 2010;23:14–26.
Henn W. Consumerism in prenatal diagnosis: a challenge for ethical guidelines. J Med Ethics. 2000;26(6):444–6.
Herissone-Kelly P. Two varieties of "better-for" judgments. In: Roberts MA, Wasserman DT, editors. Harming future persons: ethics, genetics and the nonidentity problem. Dordrecht: Springer; 2009. p. 249–63.
Hill M, Compton C, Karunaratna M, Lewis C, Chitty L. Client views and attitudes to non-invasive prenatal diagnosis for sickle cell disease, thalassaemia and cystic fibrosis. J Genet Couns. 2014a;1–10.
Hill M, Suri R, Nash EF, Morris S, Chitty LS. Preferences for prenatal tests for cystic fibrosis: a discrete choice experiment to compare the views of adult patients, carriers of cystic fibrosis and health professionals. J Clin Med. 2014b;3(1):176–90.
Kelly SE. Choosing not to choose: reproductive responses of parents of children with genetic conditions or impairments. Sociol Health Illn. 2009;31(1):81–97.
Klein DA. Medical disparagement of the disability experience: empirical evidence for the "expressivist objection". AJOB Prim Res. 2011;2:8–20.
Klugman S, Suskin B, Spencer BL, Dar P, Bajaj K, Powers J, Reichling J, Wasserman D, Dolan SM, Merkatz IR. Clinical utility of chromosomal microarray analysis in prenatal diagnosis: report of first 6 months in clinical practice. J Matern Fetal Neonatal Med. 2013;6(1):1333–8.
Kukla R, Wayne K. Pregnancy, birth, and medicine, The Stanford Encyclopedia of Philosophy, Edward N. Zalta, editor. http://plato.stanford.edu/archives/spr2011/entries/ethics-pregnancy/.
Le Dref G, Grollemund B, Danion-Grilliat A, Weber JC. Towards a new procreation ethic: the exemplary instance of cleft lip and palate. Med Health Care Philos. 2012;1–11.
Lewis C, Hill M, Chitty LS. Non-invasive prenatal diagnosis for single gene disorders: experience of patients. Clin Genet. 2014;85(4):336–42.
Lippman A, Wilfond BS. Twice-told tales: stories about genetic disorders. Am J Hum Genet. 1992;51:936–7.
Lopez-Rangel E, Mickelson ECR, Lewis MES. The value of a genetic diagnosis for individuals with intellectual disabilities: optimising healthcare and function across the lifespan. Br J Dev Disabil. 2008;54:69–82.
Makela NL, Birch PH, Friedman JM, Marra CA. Parental perceived value of a diagnosis for intellectual disability (ID): a qualitative comparison of families with and without a diagnosis for their child's ID. Am J Med Genet A. 2009;149A:2393–402.
Menzel P, Dolan P, Richardson J, Olsen JA. The role of adaptation to disability and disease in health state valuation: a preliminary normative analysis. Soc Sci Med. 2002;55(12):2149–58.
Nordenfelt L. The importance of a disability/handicap distinction. J Med Philos. 1997; 22:607–22.
Prenatally and Postnatally Diagnosed Conditions Awareness Act, 2008, S.1810: 110–374.
Press N, Browner CH. Why women say yes to prenatal diagnosis. Soc Sci Med. 1997;45:979–89.
Ruddick W. Ways to limit prenatal testing. In: Parens E, Asch A, editors. Prenatal testing and disability rights. DC, Georgetown: Washington; 2000. p. 95–107.
Saigal S, Feeny D, Rosenbaum P, Furlong W, Burrows E, Stoskopf B. Self-perceived health status and health-related quality of life of extremely low-birth-weight infants at adolescence. JAMA. 1996;276:453–9.
Schwartz CE, Andresen EM, Nosek MA, Krahn GL. Response shift theory: important implications for measuring quality of life in people with disability. Arch Phys Med Rehabil. 2007;88(4): 529–36.
Seror V, Ville Y. Prenatal screening for Down syndrome: women's involvement in decision-making and their attitudes to screening. Prenat Diagn. 2009;29(2):120–8.

Skotko BG. Prenatally diagnosed Down syndrome: mothers who continued their pregnancies evaluate their health care providers. Am J Obstet Gynecol. 2005;192:670–7.
Tremain S. Reproductive freedom, self-regulation, and the government of impairment in utero. Hypatia. 2006;21(1):35–53.
Walker LS, Ford MB, Donald WD. Cystic fibrosis and family stress: effects of age and severity of illness. Pediatrics. 1987;79:239–46.
Walsh-Gallagher D, Sinclair M, Mc Conkey R. The ambiguity of disabled women's experiences of pregnancy, childbirth and motherhood: a phenomenological understanding. Midwifery. 2012;28(2):156–62.
Wasserman D. A choice of evils in prenatal testing. Fla State Univ Law Rev. 2003;30(2): 295–313.
Wasserman D, Asch A. Understanding the relationship between disability and well-being. In: Bickenbach J, Felder F, Schmitz B, editors. Disability and the good human life. New York: Cambridge; 2013. p. 139–67.
Wertz DC. Drawing lines: notes for policymakers. In: Asch A, Parens E, editors. Prenatal testing and disability rights. Washington, DC: Georgetown; 2000. p. 261–87.
Wertz DC, Fletcher JC. A critique of some feminist challenges to prenatal diagnosis. J Womens Health. 1993a;2(2):173–88.
Wertz DC, Fletcher JC. Fatal knowledge? Prenatal diagnosis and sex selection. Hastings Cent Rep. 1993b;19(3):21–7.
Wertz DC, Fletcher JC. Ethical and social issues in prenatal sex selection: a survey of geneticists in 37 nations. Soc Sci Med. 1998;46(2):255–73.

Chapter 12
Feminist Perspectives on Prenatal and Preimplantation Diagnosis

Deborah Blizzard

Introduction

> Antonio: We were just wondering if, if it is good to just leave a few things to, to chance?
> Geneticist: We want to give your child the best possible start. Believe me, we have enough imperfection built in already. Your child doesn't need any more additional burdens. Keep in mind, this child is still you. Simply, the best, of you. You could conceive naturally a thousand times and never get such a result.
> GATTACA, 1997
> Columbia Pictures

In 1997, film producer, writer, and director, Andrew Niccol, presented the film GATTACA to audiences. This futuristic film shows a life where genetic determinism has run amuck and preimplantation genetic diagnosis (PGD) and *therapy* are common. The protagonist God-birth (i.e., human without the benefit of preimplantation genetic therapy), Vincent, narrates, "[I] belonged to a new underclass, no longer determined by social status or the color of your skin. No, we now have discrimination down to a science" (IMDb Gattaca Quotes). The science fiction of GATTACA, and its victorious ending for Vincent, was one borne of courage, will, and the drive to succeed regardless of genetic predetermination. Niccol presented his story as a futuristic, and potentially fatalistic tale which, could, perhaps, be evaded. Today, in 2015, Niccol's story still resonates, and in some ways has come to fruition.

Concern over body politics, reproduction, and (re)creation of identity have been cornerstones of feminist scholarly debate. How ought we to reproduce our world and the people within it? What constitutes a person, a human, or a being with agency? If the personal is political, how far might the political define or invade the personal? Is the role of the state to govern in ways that produce *healthy* or *normal*

D. Blizzard, Ph.D. (✉)
Department of Science, Technology and Society, Rochester Institute of Technology, 92 Lomb Memorial Drive, Rochester, NY 14623-5604, USA
e-mail: dlbgsh@rit.edu

J.P. Galst, M.S. Verp (eds.), *Prenatal and Preimplantation Diagnosis*,
DOI 10.1007/978-3-319-18911-6_12

individuals, and, for that matter, who defines these traits? As science fiction has become more aligned with reality, we must continue to ask provocative, political, personal, and morally infused questions that are difficult to answer. As prenatal and preimplantation diagnostic technologies continue to evolve, these questions must be addressed and polices implemented.

This chapter highlights some of the major contributions of feminist literature to the debate over the use of the reproductive technologies of prenatal and preimplantation diagnosis. Beginning in earnest in the 1960s and gaining momentum in subsequent years, feminist scholarship examining prenatal diagnostic technologies has grown substantially. Utilizing bioethical concepts of patient autonomy and informed consent within flexible definitions of risk, this chapter reflects on some of the historical feminist concerns regarding prenatal diagnosis, and offers insights to the ways in which disease is defined, identified, and treated. As reproductive technologies move into the earliest stages of gestation[1] it is not surprising that reproductive diagnosis has literally moved outside the womb, before implantation occurs, a technique termed preimplantation genetic diagnosis, or PGD. Against a backdrop of bioethical understanding and feminist perspectives on prenatal diagnosis, this chapter explores how PGD may force its designers, users, and communities to (re)think how one should reproduce and *make babies*. By offering insights into the role of PGD in passing genetic deafness (a medicalized condition) from one generation to the next, and in family balancing (a nonmedical condition), the chapter concludes with a vision of a future in which regulation of reproductive technology will be needed despite shifting definitions of normalcy and acceptability.

Although many assume the decision not to carry an ill fetus or implant an abnormal embryo[2] to be relatively non-problematic, the decision becomes more difficult when the condition under scrutiny is seen differently by the individuals creating the child and the community which will receive the child. Different conditions have a variety of meanings in their local cultures. However, common to many cases is that parents who *choose* for or against specific traits for their would-be-child may face accusations of not exhibiting "unconditional love" by virtue of their involvement in altering (including ending) the pregnancy. Of particular concern for feminists is under what conditions are these decisions made? Are these decisions made of free will or do women feel pressured or coerced into undergoing diagnosis for given traits?

Although many cultures and subcultures in the USA may not value prenatal and preimplantation diagnosis, those that do accept it (even if they do not use it) tend to accept concepts of Western medicine, including the concept that there is a level of wellness that is identifiable and which individuals strive to attain. Within this context, desire to aid the ill, whether a living human or preimplanted embryo, is often shared by health care professionals in clinical and research settings. Unfortunately,

[1] For example over the counter pregnancy tests promise a correct response very soon after a missed menstrual period.

[2] For example, if the medical care provider follows the rule of beneficence it would be difficult to knowingly propagate genetic traits known to cause pain, suffering, and early death.

research and experimental clinical trials have not always led to desired outcomes. To avoid unwanted outcomes, federal policies and laws (and other internal and external policing bodies) are designed to reduce the potential for negative consequences of medical interventions.

In addition to laws and policies, medical professionals self-police their actions and attempt to uphold high ethical standards by consensus. Beyond the Hippocratic Oath, other more general philosophies also guide contemporary medical practice. Of these, the four guiding principles of bioethics are perhaps the best known: autonomy, beneficence, justice, and nonmaleficence (Munson 2011). Using these guiding principles, it is hoped that those creating technologies allowing reproductive choice, and those offering the procedures to patients, do so in a fair, honest, and respectful manner. However, this is a tall order in a USA that is multifaceted with competing politics, religions, and personal ideals.

Of the guiding principles of bioethics, those most controlled by the patient, autonomy and informed consent, must be examined in a discussion of prenatal diagnosis and PGD, particularly when the discussion is framed within feminist critiques. Although all four bioethical principles are negotiated between patients and medical providers, the issues of justice and beneficence highlight the ways in which the system treats the individual (justice) and the caregiver treats the individual (nonmaleficence). The remaining principles, autonomy and informed consent, are two parts of one unit in which the patient decides if she is acting of her own accord and if she feels fully informed to make a decision. Due to the philosophical and pragmatic importance of autonomy and informed consent within feminist perspectives of prenatal and preimplantation diagnosis, both require further discussion to understand how feminist critiques clarify and problematize these entrenched and valued concepts in Western medicine.

Autonomy

Individuals and the social organizations and cultural beliefs in which they exist base the philosophical concept of autonomy upon a number of assumptions. Autonomy, in simplest terms, implies that the individual can exist and make decisions without the intruding force of others. The autonomous individual, though he/she is socially linked to others, has the assumed ability to act on free will.

Such idealism has come under considerable critique, specifically within feminist debates that question the existence of one singular reality and the ability of one not to act in a manner that reflects implicit and explicit pressure to behave *appropriately*. Opponents to such idealism argue that we cannot remove an abstract individual from a value laden context and then assume that any further information is neither impacted by the history and assumptions of the individual, nor is free of the values of those who imparted the information. To illustrate, constructivists including philosopher Sandra Harding (1995), and sociologist Sal Restivo (1994), argue that there is no pure individual; individuals are the manifestation of multiple social interactions and thus make decisions based upon multiple standpoints that are constantly being shaped by those around them, the structures in which they exist, and the cultural nuances they implicitly accept. Yet Harding and other proponents of this approach do not favor an *anything goes* approach to reality and decision-making (c.f., Feyerabend 2010). Instead, she counters that other approaches, including strong objectivity, are more realistic in that the so-called objective reality that is created and consumed by a wide variety of individuals is in actuality an amalgamation of competing interests, assumptions, and knowledge (Harding 1991, 1995, 2003; Crasnow and Waugh).[3] Strong objectivity looks to the average understanding of a variety of people with different standpoints or worldviews but acknowledges that objective reasoning changes over time.

Even though most constructivists argue that the ideal of autonomous decision-making cannot be fully carried out in any truly objective manner; they do accept that in medical decision-making there are best practices that one can hope to attain when giving care to a patient. As medical anthropologist Rayna Rapp reminds readers, there is no such thing as *free choice*, there are only decisions. These decisions are embedded in social, cultural, and historically informed contexts (Rapp 2000). How these decisions are made, and under what duress, are foundational points for understanding feminist critiques to prenatal diagnosis, including PGD. Once the individual is accepted as an autonomous decision maker (though it is always a debated and evolving state), the idea of creating an environment in which he or she can consent to a procedure following clear information must be addressed and upheld: this process is termed *informed consent*.

Informed Consent and Risk

Following the human atrocities of World War II as well as learned concerns about science for science's sake (e.g., Nazi experimentation on prisoners and the Tuskegee Study on marginalized individuals) (Annas and Grodin 1995; Jones 1992), many Western individuals developed a healthy, if not reactionary, approach to science and the researchers that create and promote its use. Particularly in medicine, concern over the ability of a person to express willingness to undergo experimental or other bodily investigation, in part led to the Belmont Report (1978). This report makes clear that research on humans must only be undertaken after review of a study's purpose, benefits and risks by a properly constituted board. Vulnerable populations e.g., (pregnant women, children and prisoners) receive special protection in such reviews.

Although the ideals of autonomy and informed consent may be applauded, feminist perspectives and critiques elucidate the explicit and implicit ways in which women can intentionally and unintentionally be coerced into accepting technologi-

[3] Objectivity has been critiqued through a number of methods. Although here, I highlight Strong Objectivity, other forms include weak objectivity or standpoint theory, and interest-based objectivity.

cal interventions and diagnosis. Do women feel a subtle coercion to accept prenatal testing or to terminate a pregnancy with indications of disability? Are women affected by the intentions and desires of their family and social networks? Does the larger medicalization of *pregnancy as a condition* and the *baby as a reproductive product or outcome* suggest an abstract but known measure of acceptability?

Although the thought that patients, particularly pregnant patients, may face coercion in their decision-making may be repulsive, a closer investigation of informed consent that envisions a woman's desires within the larger social and cultural milieu in which she exists suggests that coercion is rarely black and white. While some forms of coercion may be clear, such as threatening harm to an individual who refuses to consent to a procedure, other more subtle forms of coercion are nebulous and difficult to identify. Many of these may be found within the rhetoric and cultural assumptions used in presenting reproductive technologies and the information they can deliver to the patient. One question then is: what *really happens* when women make reproductive decisions?

Other questions are raised by bioethicists, feminists, and others who examine possible outcomes of prenatal diagnosis and PGD and wonder where they may lead. A changing cultural and social calculus that measures the individual, the community, the unborn and the future child must balance the desires of the individual with that of the community in which she is located. For example, in the US individuals have rights; however, governing systems also limit those rights. Law, policy, and social normativity make boundaries that frame our reproductive decision-making. Although laws and policies that are informed and based in social and cultural assumptions of acceptability and civil society are *intended* to be clear, often their *multiple interpretations* and nuances make them difficult to apply in a given case.

This inherently flexible rhetoric about personal choice and social limitations includes a variety of approaches to using reproductive technologies. Whether one uses technologies for medical or nonmedical reasons, a key concern of many social scientists, and feminist scholars in particular, is what is it that we are creating or supporting, who or what constitutes the "we" that creates or supports its use, and under what circumstances? Informed consent relies on the individual to understand "risk" and make decisions based upon the level of risk associated with a potentially positive outcome. However, just as autonomy is contextually defined, so too is risk. What is risk and who determines how much risk is too much?

If human reproduction is among the most personal events an individual may undertake, it may be surprising to many that it leads to some of the most politicized outcomes. As such, a close examination of its use, justifications, and intended and unintended effects must be continually undertaken.

To illustrate the various ways in which risk is understood it is helpful to consider the case of fetal surgery (Blizzard 2007). As medical sociologist, Monica Casper notes, if we consider fetal surgery a women's health issue it is difficult to imagine how fetal surgery cannot be seen as threatening to women's body politics (Casper 1998). However, as I argue elsewhere, fetal surgery is not only about women's health politics, it is also about individual women trying to be the mothers they wish to be. Based upon our different framings of the issue, what counts as risk changes. In my earlier work I describe these complexities,

> In all cases, patient-mothers, their referring physicians, and often their larger social networks (including families and religious institutions) must negotiate and define multiple kinds of risk before deciding whether or not a particular procedure is acceptable. To appreciate the complexities behind medical decisions it is important to know how others *influence or create a context* in which consent is given and procedures delivered. Among other issues, the fetoscopy [in utero fetal surgery via endoscopic techniques] context includes individual beliefs, social norms, professional habits and legal restrictions. With each patient-mother and procedure these issues and countless others mix and match to form the context in which decisions are made (Blizzard 2007).

Like fetoscopy, the risk in deciding whether or not to undergo prenatal or preimplantation diagnosis is a burden that is carried by many who do not define risk in the same way (Blizzard 2005, 2007).

A Good Parent Creates a Good Baby?

Beyond medical risk, the issue of social risk, including the risk of not being seen as a good parent is an issue many individuals face. Bioethicists Arthur Caplan and Gregory Pence caution that we must be clear about what it means to alter or affect the development of a fetus prenatally, and suggest that good parenting involves active caretaking of the fetus, often through means that are readily identifiable in already born children (Caplan 1992; Pence 2000). To illustrate, Caplan argues that today mothers and fathers do many things to improve the likelihood that their unborn child will have the best chance of being born mentally, physically, and emotionally healthy. Whether it is singing to the unborn, playing classical music, or undergoing therapeutic massage, a woman who does such things is often seen as being a good mother-to-be—she uses her time, effort, and finances to create a loving and nurturing environment (Caplan 1992). She is actively being a good parent to her unborn and future child. The family unit is coming together to make the eventual arrival as successful as possible. The question that begs critical investigation is how different is actively altering a genotype from actively altering the environment in which the phenotype is expressed? Both theorists make a strong argument that biologically altering a would-be baby is not too far from what we are already doing and what is largely accepted as *good parenting*.

Pence, even more aggressively than Caplan, has argued that in fact we *owe* it to our future children to use all of the scientific advances available, even if this means that some embryos are not implanted, or by extension, born (Pence 2000). In his text, *Recreating Bioethics*, Pence challenges readers to imagine finding a letter to future generations in a time capsule (Pence 2000). The letter argues that predecessors were obligated not to pass on painful or lethal genetic conditions if they could be avoided. Pence's style, while not common in academic prose, effectively instigates critical thought. The letter explains,

> Some people want to protect the status quo, to preserve the traditional family, to make society strictly egalitarian, or to never take any risks at all. Throughout discussions, our one

guiding question is this: What's in the best interest of the people to come? It doesn't matter what parents want, what society wants, or what the current fashion is, what matters is what is best for 'our grandkids to come,' you (Pence 2000) (p. 96).

Offering illustrations of contemporary cultures that actively try and reduce genetic disease by preemptively suggesting who can and should reproduce with whom, Pence draws attention to the widely known case of Tay-Sachs in the community of New York City Ashkenazi Jews. Tay-Sachs is a rare condition that affects the neurons in the brain leading to childhood seizures, muscular loss, blindness, and early death (childhood). As a community governed by their own culture and customs, a subsection of the Ashkenazi self-monitored in ways that they felt acceptable to their worldview, personal behaviors and beliefs. The outcome of self-monitoring was a reduction in the number of Ashkenazi Jews born with Tay-Sachs and a better understanding of how the disease could spread if carriers of the genes reproduced *together*.

However, the same letter is also critical of the Amish and Mennonite cultures that have a relatively high incidence of Crigler–Najjar syndrome. With this condition children lack an important liver enzyme and jaundice ensues. To overcome the jaundice the children spend "ten to twelve hours a day in a mirrored bed with lights that break down the…[chemical causing the condition]. The children hate sleeping this way, and the therapy loses its effectiveness as the children become adults, but the alternative is death" (Pence 2000) (p. 98). Pence writes with stern candor: "The tragedy was that all these cases were preventable. By using family trees and genealogy maps, by testing adults for the genes they carry, and by doing *preimplantation diagnosis (PGD)* in embryos when using in vitro fertilization, no Crigler-Najjar baby need have been born." (Italics added) (Pence 2000) (p. 98).

Caplan's observation of the ways in which parents and families are already crafting their children through use of outside influences, and Pence's argument that we owe it to future generations to fix deleterious genetic traits, including not implanting an embryo that will have a genetic disorder, rest on a fine balance of ensuring individual liberty to reproduce versus a social contract in which societies minimize pain within existing communities (on the importance of considering how cultural contexts define good parenting, c.f. Malek 2011). Although both theorists are well intended in elucidating what is currently the case and what could occur in the future, these arguments are not without concerning implications. Caplan's observation that good parenting incorporates involvement of the parent with the child pre- and post-birth leads to a question of equity. Who deems who has access to goods and services that are beneficial to the unborn and what conditions are considered acceptable? More vexing is that Pence's argument largely ignores the cultural environment (i.e., conditions or differences are only deleterious when they carry negative meanings within their contexts). To illustrate, Pence argues that the "tragedy" of Crigler–Najjar could be controlled if parents took the steps to prevent it from spreading, including "…family trees and genealogy maps, by testing adults for the genes they carry, and by doing *preimplantation diagnosis…*" (Pence 2000) (p. 98). According to his letter, Crigler–Najjar is affecting the self-described "Plain People" who are Amish and Mennonite in Lancaster County, Pennsylvania. Many questions emerge.

Do cultures closed off from larger segments of US societies understand a family tree that is based on genetics and not kinship? Do the religious underpinnings of the culture allow followers of the faith to alter pregnancies and, in the case of PGD (a highly technologized approach to birth that necessitates in vitro fertilization and genetic screening), are these interventions permissible under the teachings of the church? Even if one were to find a clinic that offers the treatment, a way to pay for it, and be willing to act on the outcome (e.g., discarding affected embryos, abortion), would the experience be accepted by the community or would the individual be ostracized? In closely knit cultures the choice or *decision* to use or not use reproductive technologies (including prenatal diagnosis and PGD) may be one that is highly visible and suspect, carrying with it grave implications within the larger cultural beliefs of health, illness, and the body (Rapp 2000).

A New Stop on the Conveyor Belt of Reproductive Diagnosis or New Hope for Women? Preimplantation Genetic Diagnosis (PGD)

One of the more illuminating feminist concerns over the uncritical use of reproductive technologies is that at some point an individual's decisions will become meaningless in the face of social and cultural pressures to create healthy (and even superior) children (McGee 2000). Similar to Niccol's imaginings of a bifurcated world in which enhanced embryos lead to a new racism of the genetic haves and have-nots, some researchers ask if we are entering a technological *slippery slope* in which one small step takes us to the decision regarding which technologies should and which should not be used to create preferred embryos and babies. Will this then lead to normalization of the technology and greater ease of accepting other technologies, technologies which at an earlier point in time would have been seen as unreasonable and unacceptable? The slippery slope metaphor is one that hinges on a negative view: it is a slope downhill—a slippery one that is difficult, if not impossible, to scale once one has descended.

The metaphor of the slippery slope stands alongside an equally compelling metaphor within women's reproductive decision-making: the conveyor belt. Although at first glance the term suggests an ill intended mechanization of the gestational process, its power to bring this image to mind is its strength and, based upon some feminist critiques, is not too far from reality. In this metaphor, the conveyor belt moves less refined materials through stations of quality control and observation to arrive at an end good, packaged and ready for market: the item, the commodity, is complete. When holding this metaphor to contemporary pregnancy, the conveyor belt expresses a deeply rooted feminist concern: once the pregnant or would be pregnant woman is on the conveyor belt, how free is she to get off? What happens when a blood test leads to multiple ultrasounds, amniocentesis, and additional investigations of the fetal patient within? Considering the Western pregnancy as a condition which passes milestones (e.g., trimesters and measurements), what happens when women no longer want to partake of such a mechanized view of their bodies? What other options might exist? And, if she decides to no longer partake of the advantages afforded by this mechanized view of pregnancy, how will her family and community receive her? At what point is it possible that the decision to undergo this form of pregnancy is no longer a decision but a process through which she must demonstrate her willingness to be a good mother? When considering these perspectives, it is helpful to explore some of the historical routes leading to contemporary reproductive technology development, prenatal diagnosis and PGD.

One of the most prolific visual technologies to diagnose an in utero fetus is ultrasound. Developed as a medical spin off of the technology required to guide submarines, ultrasound has found great use in many forms of medical diagnosis, including obstetrics (Arney 1982). With the emergence of ultrasound, obstetrics turned from a tradition of monitoring the pregnancy at a distance, demarcated by the skin of the mother-to-be, to being able to visualize and monitor the fetus inside the woman. The physician could now bypass the woman and see the new patient directly: *the real patient*. As ultrasound became commonplace in many Western pregnancies, and its images were recognizable to lay audiences, feminist concerns were voiced over the very "public" visuals that were making their way into the American conscious (Petchesky 1987; Taylor 1993). Although from a medical standpoint viewing the fetus was a tremendous advantage, the cultural myths also grew as individuals completely removed from the fetus began to assert their values on it. By literally removing the woman from the picture the fetal patient could be intellectually removed from the environment in which it was located and people other than the pregnant woman could—and did—assert claims over its rights and meanings. Ultrasound images set the stage for what has become a long-time feminist concern: as the fetus is seen as separate from the woman who carries it, some individuals assert that it has rights (even personhood) and thus argue that the fetus may be at odds with the woman who conceived and carries it (Blizzard 2007; Mattingly 1992). Although ultrasound proved worthwhile to many, its ability to bring new information and decisions to pregnant women and to the public who peered in opened the door to questions of patient autonomy and informed consent: Did the pregnant woman know what the ultrasound could suggest? Did it occur to her that such knowledge could lead to unanticipated complex decision-making? Did she realize she might be in the middle of cultural debates on acceptable maternal and civic behavior? What could be done to alter such tensions even if she did not support the arguments?

As ultrasound clarity improved and small diameter sampling needles were developed, additional information could be sought on the developing fetus. Of particular note are the sampling technologies, amniocentesis and chorionic villus sampling (CVS).[4] Though both technologies sample cells from the in utero environment, neither can determine the severity of many conditions or the ways in which the potential child may or may not be received into its community (e.g., school, church, town, and family). Women, now armed with even more information on specific traits, face excruciating dilemmas regarding whether to keep, end, or try to aid a developing,

[4] Because CVS can be performed earlier in gestation than can amniocentesis, it is an important indicator of technology development and the desire to continuously know more about a pregnancy earlier in gestation.

infirm, fetus. To illustrate, one of the best-known conditions diagnosed by amniocentesis is Down syndrome. Although the test can identify if the fetus has the condition, it cannot predict the severity of its expression. Down syndrome is well known for its variation in severity. At one end of the spectrum, individuals with Down syndrome can learn well and live almost independent lives. At the other end, individuals with Down syndrome may have severe physical and mental impairments and require extensive assistance and lifelong care. Both the condition and the environment in which the person with Down syndrome lives contribute to the life the individual may lead. Although amniocentesis can confirm that the condition does exist, it cannot offer insight into what this may mean for the family or future child (including how it is understood within the community) (Rapp 2000). The woman is still left with troubling decisions: what could or should she do to alter the troubled pregnancy, and, for that matter, how troubled is it?

Although amniocentesis and ultrasound have become entrenched reproductive technologies in contemporary medicine, other technologies waxed and waned. Of note was the aforementioned fetoscopy (Blizzard 2007; Quintero 2002). Beginning in the 1970s and still in use today, though not as popular or readily available as ultrasound, amniocentesis, CVS, and other diagnostic technologies, fetoscopy utilized an endoscope to enter the womb and give the physician relatively clear views of the developing fetus and the region around it such as the umbilical cord and placenta. Although fetoscopy was a near futuristic technology that lent itself well to popular culture,[5] the technology was hampered by relatively large diameter endoscopes and unfortunately led to a higher than acceptable rate of fetal loss. Thus, fetoscopy fell out of favor until the smaller diameter endoscopes of the 1980s and 1990s allowed for its reemergence (Quintero 2002). Today fetoscopy has gained purchase in some few hospitals and clinics and is both a diagnostic and therapeutic tool (i.e., diagnostic and operative fetoscopy). However, unlike amniocentesis and ultrasound and more in line with PGD, fetoscopy is currently a boutique medical procedure with limited use. Nevertheless, under the correct circumstances what was once a rarely used medical device may possibly move closer to the mainstream. Time will tell (Blizzard 2007).

The technologies noted above have a considerable history and literature within medical and social scientific publications. Each brings with it hope and concern and can be seen as part of the medical conveyor belt moving women through technologies. Some have been adopted into nonmedical settings, e.g., ultrasounds performed by nonphysicians in shopping malls, while others require skilled practitioners to implement, e.g., a detailed ultrasound, amniocentesis, CVS, and others. From one view, the emergence of these technologies is a boon; with more information physicians and their patients have more options and more potential ways to care for troubled pregnancies. From another perspective, these same technologies and the

[5] For example, an image of a free-floating fetus is seen at the end of the 1968 film *2001 A Space Odyssey*. Stanley Kubrick's work brought the idea of the public fetus into theaters and the minds of moviegoers, who while being entertained were also faced with a new way to see the unborn.

timelines they represent may be seen as a trap whereby one seemingly innocuous test that is abnormal suggests and may even necessitate further testing with different and more invasive technologies that may not resolve the problem but rather create more confusion. Thus the slippery slope of technology development and the conveyor belt moving a woman from test to test is of considerable concern to many feminists.

One of the newest technologies in reproductive medicine is preimplantation genetic diagnosis (PGD). To accomplish PGD, in vitro fertilization (IVF) must occur: an egg and sperm are brought together outside a woman's body, resulting in fertilization in a controlled environment. Historically, IVF has been used when individuals cannot conceive or maintain a pregnancy on their own, or when a surrogate is used to carry a fetus that a woman is unable to gestate herself. IVF, dubbed creation of *test tube babies*, presented a considerable medical and cultural hurdle in the 1970s. However, with the healthy and very visible births of Louise Joy Brown and Elizabeth Jordan Carr (1978 England and 1981 USA, respectively), IVF became another potential reproductive technique, yet it was also special. Unlike ultrasound and amniocentesis that are now seen as normal parts of a pregnancy experience, IVF is not. IVF is not average, nor is it commonplace; like fetoscopy and PGD it is boutique and signals a different approach to conception and gestation. Even before conception, IVF creates a high-tech birth. It is not surprising then that the use of IVF has also ushered in other high-tech solutions to troubled pregnancy contexts. One of the most dramatic is PGD.

PGD, similar to *prenatal* diagnostic techniques, is designed to give women and their families more choice in their reproductive experiences. However, unlike the aforementioned reproductive technologies that are used on conceived and gestating fetuses, PGD takes advantage of the environment afforded by IVF: PGD takes place outside of the woman, after facilitated conception, and before uterine implantation. In short, it takes place during the window in which an embryonic form has been created but its possibility for further development is not yet determined. At this point diagnosis that does not occur on or through a woman's body is possible. This diagnosis takes place in the laboratory under the scrutiny of geneticists and other medical professionals who, acting on the desires of the parents-to-be, screen the embryo for deleterious genetic traits. Of concern to many feminist scholars, however, is what constitutes a "defective embryo" with a genetic trait that should be excluded from transfer back to the woman. What makes a condition unbearable to the mother-to-be or family in which the baby will reside? What makes a *genetic trait* a *medical condition*? When does a genetic trait need medical diagnosis, treatment, and if possible, a cure.

Philosopher John Davis (2008), shares the concerns offered by some feminists and argues that when we use PGD we may be entering an environment in which what counts as a potentially threatening or unwanted medical condition may become more and more liberally defined. As PGD offers more choice of what genetic traits a potential child can and should carry will there be implicit or explicit attempts to make the child both healthy and possibly better than average, in essence to create the "perfect baby" (McGee 2000)? Described by bioethicist and philosopher, John Davis,

> …some prospective parents are becoming more finicky, and this *is* controversial. Some wish to avoid creating children with genes that are either mildly undesirable or not defective at all, or even to select *for* children whose genetic traits are above average. I call this *selection drift* – the standard for accepted children is creeping upwards as we get better at selecting potential children on genetic grounds (Davis 2008) (p. 258–259).

As genes and their expressions are better understood, it is possible to view genetic illness as falling along a spectrum. At one end of the spectrum exist conditions so benign that they are not visible or recognizable to nonmedical observers. At the other end are genetic traits that are definitely associated with a reduced life span, chronic pain, and need for medical intervention. Davis explains that "as we gain greater genetic knowledge about potential children, our notion of an acceptably healthy baby inches upwards, and children who would have once been considered normal may be seen as unsatisfactory" (Davis 2008) (p. 259).

When combining a technological slippery slope with genetic selection drift we are faced with a complex foundation for understating how individual women and their caregivers make decisions regarding their bodies and those of the unborn. Feminists and bioethicists alike ask, as new methods of *prenatal* diagnosis develop and are refined, will the same type of development happen with PGD?

How one reacts to the concept of PGD and potential fetal therapy may depend on how the issue is framed. Is PGD a weeding out approach akin to negative eugenics in which ill or other "less than normal" individuals are sought out and removed from the population able to reproduce, or is it akin to positive eugenics whereby the best traits are identified and, like other forms of animal husbandry and breeding of purebreds, are actively sought and created through assisted reproductive technologies?

Two examples that highlight different arguments for and against the use of PGD are those of genetic deafness and family balancing. In light of the critiques of prenatal diagnosis and the concepts of autonomy, informed consent and risk, deafness and family balancing will be discussed below.

Medical and Nonmedically Based Selection Drift: Individual Rights and Social Limits—The Cases of Deafness and Family Balancing

Deafness

One popularly discussed but little understood case is selection for deafness (Fahmy 2011). The question of whether or not to use PGD to exclude or actively pass on genetic deafness is a battleground that demonstrates the flexibility of naming (or *creating*) a disease and understanding the cultural context in which a trait is expressed. Recent US statistics report that 11, 074, 450 out of a general population of 311, 591, 919 US citizens consider themselves deaf or hard of hearing, approximately 3.6 % of the population (2011 statistics).[6] Each of these individuals faces

[6]For excellent statistics on deaf and hard of hearing individuals in the USA see the National Technical Institute for the Deaf Collaboratory and the American Community Survey from the US Census Bureau.

their deafness in different ways and interacts within their families and kin through a variety of mechanisms. While many use American Sign Language (ASL), others use Oral means whereby they interpret the facial and lip gestures of others and, in response, answer in spoken English. Still others use a form of Total Communication in which they blend ASL and Oral communication, as needed. From a political and policy standpoint these individuals are seen as having a disability and are covered under the Americans with Disabilities Act (ADA). Although the ADA can offer some individuals access to interpreters, captioning, and other technologies to ensure their access to communication, not all individuals diagnosed as deaf identify with the term *disabled* and in fact many refuse the label and do not consider their deafness a negative condition.

Deafness, as a medical condition, has been depicted in popular culture through movies and television in which deaf characters and actors (e.g., Marilee Matlin) sometimes challenge viewers to rethink how to identify and define disability. To understand the arguments for and against passing on genetic deafness it is paramount to understand the differences between medicalized deafness and Deaf culture. The former, *medicalized deafness*, is a condition found within Western medicine and is defined by the amount of a person's hearing loss, as measured by a medically trained audiologist. This measurement implicitly frames deafness as a loss. It is not how much you can hear but the inability to hear at a certain level defined as the hearing norm. Technological fixes such as hearing aids and cochlear implants have been created to bring hearing ability more in line with that of the average hearing person. A second way to understand deafness is by understanding Deaf culture. In Deaf culture, individuals value their deafness and see within it their own language (ASL), cultural patterns (including conversational styles), and kinship (how one sees relationships with others like themselves). Deaf culture and deafness cannot be separated; however, one can be deaf and not identify with Deaf culture. Thus one of many problematic aspects emerge: Those who belong to and value Deaf culture do not want it to be eliminated via policies and medical processes that seek to "fix" deafness.

Within Deaf culture, as with many cultures, those who belong to it, or identify with it, are generally in partnership with one another and value their traits and families (however defined and experienced) (Foster 1989). For example, in Deaf culture to be *deaf of deaf* is highly valued[7]. Deaf of deaf denotes a deaf child born to a deaf family. Immediately, a bond can form as the dreaded language barrier does not exist between parents and child. Signing at home, going to known schools, familiarity with social and medical policies, and being born into a world where some family, friends, or relatives also share in Deaf culture suggests (not always correctly) to others that the child has the opportunity to grow and be protected within the community of like individuals who see positive life enrichment with and through their shared trait and culture.

[7] For detailed explanation of the social construction of Deafness as medicalized disease and the desire of Deaf parents to create Deaf children see the case of Duchesneau and McCullough in Regulating Preimplantation Genetic Diagnosis (2005).

Because most hearing individuals do identify medical deafness as a disability, many see the birth of a deaf child as a potential burden to the child, and perhaps to the family. Thus in the Western medical model hearing parents of a deaf child generally seek technologies and intervention services to assist the child (and family) in living as a deaf person in a largely hearing world. In this light it is reasonable to assume that hearing parents who identify an embryo carrying a genetic trait for deafness through PGD may not want this embryo transferred back to the woman's uterus. The hearing family thus recreates itself with likeness in the child and in this particular case, the ability to hear *normally*.

But what is normal has long been problematized by feminist scholars. What is normal from a cultural and historical standpoint can often be seen as a pattern of power over others, imperialism, and patriarchy. As those with power, through numbers or political (medical) access, define normal, they implicitly and explicitly substantiate what is normal and thereby acceptable within the larger community. Through these means the status quo continues and those who are different often cannot gain the spoils of the advantaged. Furthermore, when the latter do succeed or gain advantage, they may be held up as hyper visual examples indicating that the system is not biased toward or against any particular group (Kimmel 2012). As long as there are some marginalized individuals who succeed within the social system it is possible to highlight them and imply that it is not the system that promotes or rejects limitations, thus demonstrating the inherent equity of the system.

The case of deafness is an example in which the norm or average hearing is seen as preferred as it is assumed it will lead to a life of more opportunities and fulfillment. Many within Deaf culture take issue with this assumption. What is a life worth living and what leads to personal fulfillment? Living in a community and culture (Deaf) that accepts them from birth and maintains its own customs and language, may be preferable to being hearing and living in a hearing world that lacks a local culture that celebrates one's family history.

The benefits of Deaf culture for some individuals are clear, but within a larger hearing world that may not understand it or sees it as a separatist community or an economic burden on federal, state, and local governments, its claim to be an advantage may fall short. Nevertheless, it should not be shocking that some deaf individuals would select embryos *for* genetic deafness to continue their family traditions and culture. The child, who is thought by its parents not to be medically harmed by being deaf, is brought into a family and culture that is positioned to support and care for the child both within the smaller family unit and in a larger cultural structure where ties of kinship and likeness are highly valued. Thus the question of which approach is right: medical deafness that views deaf children as being deficient yet technologically fixable or the Deaf culture approach that identifies deafness as a valued trait for full existence, is near impossible to answer.

Family Balancing

Different from the case of deafness is the nonmedical case of preferential sex selection. Better understood in popular culture than genetic deafness, the issue of sex selection through PGD leads to political and moral discussion and questions the acceptable use of PGD technology (such selection also occurs with prenatal technology and will be noted below). Yet similar to the case of deafness, a critical examination of the context and the cultural reasons why the technology might be used creates discussions in which feminist scholars highlight social equity and sexism.

Although in some cultures one gender is preferred over another due to historical forms of kinship, economic trade, and cultural worth (e.g., China and India), in the USA most often sex selection is driven by sociomedical legitimacy: family balancing or reducing sex-linked disease. The arguments for reducing sex-linked diseases are fairly clear and can be followed in the reasoning of Caplan, Pence, and others who argue that to pass on traits when we know that they lead to pain, suffering, hardships, and possible early death is not in and of itself wrong, but many may wish to avoid this as well as any parental blame associated with doing so. Family balancing, however, is a concern for feminist theorists, as many of its negative outcomes have already been seen in parts of world in which structural violence and patriarchy frame the context in which women conceive, give birth, and live their lives.

For example, in China and India (two of the most populated countries in the world), abortion and infanticide has led to a decrease in female children. These countries now face the unintended consequence of how to repopulate when there are not enough female partners. China and India are dealing with gender bias in the generation that is charged with both repopulating their country and taking care of aging family members, roles which have been attached to the feminine gender in their respective countries (Kimmel 2012). Yet these and other countries are also founded on patriarchal notions of control over the family unit. Male children are valued as the more worthwhile with the ability to work and carry on a family business and/or finances. Beyond the capital the male child will bring to the family, the cultural capital of having a son can be immeasurable. Although this is seen as a problem primarily in the rural countryside, it also occurs in urban areas.

While it is relatively easy to look at China or India as considerably different cultures from those in the USA, there are similarities in how sex disparities occur. Sex selection is not only the purview of China, India, and other countries, sex selection of embryos is also practiced in the USA, though it is often stated for different reasons. (see The Economic Survey, which measures standard of living, like expectancy, and education level between men and women) (Gender Diparity 2010). Sex selection of embryos is also practiced in the USA, though it is often *stated* for different reasons. These practices are linked to the use of prenatal diagnosis including PGD and IVF. Bioethicists McGowan and Sharp explain, "…reproductive technologies for non-medical sex selection has generated a great deal of debate within bioethics, feminist studies, and medicine" (McGowan and Sharp 2012) (p. 272). They continue,

> One justification for sex selection that has provoked controversy is family balancing, a term used in the biomedical sector to characterize the practice of selecting spermatozoa or embryos on the basis of sex to 'balance' the ratio of girls to boys in a family (Sauer 2004). Critiques of family balancing focus on the presumption that families with uneven sex ratios are somehow abnormal and how such rhetoric masks the many prejudicial implications of sex selection by couching decisions within the realm of family planning and reproductive choice (Ettorre et al. 2006; Sauer 2004).

Many feminist critiques that examine the rhetoric of family balancing and its outcomes question the assumption of the desirability of balanced gender ratios within a family unit, and further ask, what are the social implications of these personal decisions? This raises questions similar to the case of deafness, when individual desires are placed primary without consideration of their social implications. How do laws and policies allow for the individual to make personal decisions such as pursuing certain genetic conditions or family balancing? If genetic deafness can be identified, and, with proper intervention, be (somewhat) fixed, can and should the same be said for family balancing? Is an unbalanced family a condition needing fixing or intervention?

Although there is considerable debate over the true number of sexes in human physiology (e.g., intersexuality), in general, Western culture dichotomizes sex into male and female, and gender into masculine and feminine (Fausto-Sterling 2012). As noted above some countries such as India and China have cultural, economic, and historical reasons for preferring one sex to another in the birth of a child. Technologies such as ultrasound, amniocentesis and PGD offer parents and others a glimpse of the baby-to-be and what sex (and implicit gender) that baby will represent to the family and community. In the USA, such technologies can also be used for sex selection and may promote sexism. However, the frequency of the use of medical technologies in the USA to identify the nonlethal and nonmedical condition of sex is largely unknown and, in fact, can be camouflaged by the use of PGD and other reproductive technologies to look for other medical conditions while also *happening* to diagnose sex.

In the USA, the effect of medical technologies on sex ratios has not been scrutinized, but concerns are growing both within feminist scholarship and amongst professionals tasked with implementing reproductive procedures, namely obstetricians, perinatologists, and others, who adhere to the ethical parameters set forth by the American Society for Reproductive Medicine (ASRM). According to the Ethics Committee of the ASRM the use of IVF and PGD solely for sex selection is not an appropriate use of the technologies and place a woman in danger of medical harm for no medical reason (McGowan and Sharp 2012). However, in their study on family balancing McGowan and Sharp state, "Though professional recommendations discourage IVF-PGD for sex selection and family balancing, there is no formal regulation of the practice. And data on the incidence of IVF-PGD for sex selection in the United States are limited" (McGowan and Sharp 2012) (p. 272). Feminists interested in the use of PGD or sex selection and its cultural implications have discovered that even though the Ethics Committee of the ASRM indicates that statistics are difficult to find, some studies show that

> IVF-PGD for nonmedical sex selection increased from 2007 to 2008 by over 5 percent (Ginsberg et al 2011). These reports suggest that, despite professional recommendation to the contrary…sex selection via IVF-PGD is available and incidence may be increasing in the United States, though overall incidence is still infrequent (McGowan and Sharp 2012) (p. 273).

In light of these statistics, feminist perspectives are growing and concerns appear warranted.

When considering PGD and its role in sex selection, a number of issues arise in the larger global context, i.e., non-implantation of female embryos, increased incidence of female abortions, and female infanticide. While in no way should the global use of medical technologies for sex selection be minimized, it is also important to investigate the ways in which similar practices are being used in the USA. As many feminists have argued it is often easier to see the gross injustices of mistreatment of females through limiting access to education, social freedoms, and rights to decide how they want their bodies touched or reconfigured in cultures different from the USA than to make a reflexive turn to ask the same of our own culture and subcultures.

Conclusion

Feminist discussions of prenatal and preimplantation diagnosis rest on a number of concepts that are difficult to agree upon because of the need to balance individual desires within the larger contexts in which the individual lives. Western health care, practiced within the ethical ideals of justice, beneficence, nonmaleficence, and autonomy, when mixed within the reality of lived experience which includes personal desires, histories and needs, can easily become entangled in slippery slopes of medical technology use and selection drift decision making.

Feminist studies of prenatal and preimplantation diagnosis with a focus on patient autonomy and informed consent problematize the ideals of personal decision-making within a larger social context that defines acceptability through cultural beliefs, laws, and policies. In these cases autonomy, informed consent and risk, and even the definition of what constitutes a medical condition merge into a crucible of confusion, hope, limited access, and intended personal, and unintended social, consequences. Reproductive technology and diagnostic tests beg examination of how "we" are reproducing ourselves, under what circumstances, and with what goals.

Critiques of prenatal and preimplantation genetic diagnosis have led many to caution the limits of value free decision-making, coercion, and the ability of the individual to define what type of child they wish to reproduce and what child they are able or willing to rear and under what circumstances. When debating what prenatal and preimplantation genetic diagnosis can and should identify and how women make decisions about how to respond to these technologies, two intriguing types of cases emerge: whether or not to pass on a medicalized genetic condition and whether to pass on a non-medicalized genetic condition that is nevertheless seen as important to the future family. By utilizing the controversial cases of genetic deafness and of family balancing, it is clear that the moral ground on which prenatal and preimplantation diagnosis and decision-making occurs is constantly shifting. Feminist theorists have addressed similar concerns over a variety of reproductive technologies for decades and PGD has joined the list of nuanced political and personal debates. In a world of evolving objectivities, realities, and desires, the rightful use of future prenatal diagnosis and PGD in medical and nonmedical situations will likely continue to be debated. Feminist scholars may be the best positioned to identify and ask the most salient questions, taking into account the provocative, political, personal, and morally infused contexts in which these practices occur.

Although no clear answer will likely guide the way, this should not dissuade practitioners, users, and those who critique the practices from continued cautious use of these technologies.

References

Alper J, Ard C, Asch A, Beckwith J. The double-edged helix: social implications of genetics in a Diverse Society. Baltimore, MD: Johns Hopkins University Press; 2004.

Annas GJ, Grodin MA. The Nazi doctors and the Nuremberg Code: human rights in human experimentation. Oxford: Oxford University Press; 1995.

Arney WR. Power and the profession of obstetrics. Chicago, IL: University of Chicago Press; 1982.

Blizzard D. A trying experience: fetoscopy and maternal decision making. Clin Obstet Gynecol. 2005;48(3):562–73.

Blizzard D. Looking within: a sociocultural examination of fetoscopy. Cambridge: MIT Press; 2007.

Caplan, AL. If I were a rich man could i buy a pancreas? And other essays on the ethics of health care (medical ethics). Bloomington, IN: Indiana University Press; 1992.

Casper M. The making of the unborn patient: a social anatomy of fetal surgery. New Brunswick, NJ: Rutgers University Press; 1998.

Crasnow S, Waugh J. Philosophical feminism and popular culture.

Davis J. Selecting potential children and unconditional parental love. Bioethics. 2008;22(5):258–68.

Ettorre E, Rothman BK, Steinberg DL. Feminism confronts the genome: introduction. New Genet Soc. 2006;25(2):133–42.

Fahmy MS. On the supposed moral harm of selecting for deafness. Bioethics. 2011;25(3):128–36.

Fausto-Sterling A. Sex/gender: biology in a social world. London: Routledge; 2012.

Feyerabend P. Against method. New York, NY: Verso; 2010.

Foster S. Social alienation and peer identification: a study of the social construction of deafness. Hum Organ. 1989;8(3):226–35.

Gender Diparity still wide; India ranks 114th globally. 2010 February 26.

Harding S. Whose science? Whose knowledge?: thinking from women's lives. Ithaca, NY: Cornell University Press; 1991.

Harding S. "Strong objectivity": a response to the new objectivity question. Sythese. 1995;104(3):331–49.

Harding S. The feminist standpoint theory reader: intellectual and political controversies. London: Routledge; 2003.

IMDb Gattaca Quotes. [Online]. http://www.imdb.com/title/tt0119177/quotes.

Jones JH. Bad blood: the Tuskegee syphilis experiment. revisedth ed. New York, NY: Free Press; 1992.

Kimmel M. The gendered society. Oxford: Oxford University Press; 2012.

Malek J. Use of refuse reproductive genetic technologies: which would a 'good parent' do? Bioethics. 2011;27(2):59–64.

Mattingly SS. The maternal-fetal dyad: exploring the two patient obstetric model. The Hastings Center Report. 1992 Jan–Feb; p. 13–18.

McGee G. The perfect baby : parenthood in the new world of cloning and genetics. Lanham, MD: Rowman & Littlefield Publishers, Inc.; 2000.

McGowan MR, Sharp RR. Justice in the context of family balancing. Sci Technol Hum Val. 2012;38(2):271–93.

Munson R. Intervention and reflection: basic issues in bioethics. Boston, MA: Cengage Learning US; 2011.

National Technical Institute for the Deaf. Collaboratory: D/HH Population – 2011. [Online]. http://www.ntid.rit.edu/research/collaboratory/demographics/deaf_hh_population.

Pence GE. Re-creating medicine: ethical issues at the frontiers of medicine. Lanham, MD: Rowman & Littlefield Publishers, Inc.; 2000.

Petchesky R. Foetal images: the power of visual culture in the politics of reproduction. In: Stansworth M, editor. Reproductive technologies: gender, motherhood, and medicine. Minneapolis, MN: University of Minnesota Press; 1987. p. 57–80.

Preimplantation Genetic Diagnosis: The Pathologization Problem. Harvard Law Review. 2005;118(8):2770–2791

Quintero RA. Diagnostic and operative fetoscopy. New York, NY: The Parthenon Group; 2002.

Rapp R. Testing women, testing the fetus: the social impact of amniocentesis in America (the anthropology of everyday life). London: Routledge; 2000.

Restivo S. Science, society, and values : toward a sociology of objectivity. Bethlehem: Lehigh University Press; 1994.

Sauer M. Gender selection: pressure from patients and industry should not alter our adherence to ethical guidelines. Am College Obstet J. 2004;191(5):373–5.

Taylor J. The public fetus and the family car: from abortion politics to a Volvo advertisement. Sci Cult. 1993;3(4):601–18.

The National Commission. The Belmont report: ethical principles and guidelines for the protection of human subjects of research. Bethesda, MD: The National Commission; 1978.7For detailed explanation of the social construction of Deafness as medicalized disease and the desire of Deaf parents to create Deaf children see the case of Duchesneau and McCullough in Regulating Preimplantation Genetic Diagnosis (2005).

Part IV
Psychosocial Perspective

Chapter 13
Critical Aspects of Decision-Making and Grieving After Diagnosis of Fetal Anomaly

Judith L.M. McCoyd

> *I can't decide! If I have this baby, all it'd do is suffer- and so would I. I can't be the mother of a baby that never really grows up and who suffers all his life. But I can't have an abortion- I'm not the kind of woman who has an abortion. Ann*
>
> *I know I can't bring 7 children to fruition in this little body of mine- but how can I decide to not have some of them? And how will I tell the two who survive that they are only here because I let their brothers and sisters be killed? Betty*

Women sit with me in my clinical social work practice and say things like this to me regularly. They agonize over how to respond when a fetal anomaly is found or when a pregnancy with multiple fetuses means that the pregnancy is unlikely to yield a healthy child unless selective fetal reduction occurs. In this chapter, the process and factors that frame these types of decisions are delineated and the latest research describing the medico-psychosocial context within which women[1] make such decisions is included.

The Finding of Elevated Risk for Fetal Anomaly (via Prenatal Screenings)

The decision to engage in prenatal screening to detect fetal anomalies is generally viewed as self-evident, particularly in Westernized nations (Santalahti et al. 1998). Although some women refuse such testing (Markens et al. 1999; Rapp 1998), most professional obstetrics organizations encourage screening of most pregnant women

[1] Throughout, I will refer to the (pregnant) woman as the decision-maker, but I will also assume that she is likely to include her partner or other support people in her decision-making and grieving processes.

J.L.M. McCoyd, Ph.D., L.C.S.W. (✉)
School of Social Work, Rutgers University, 217 N. 6th Street, Camden, NJ 08102, USA
e-mail: jmccoyd@ssw.rutgers.edu

J.P. Galst, M.S. Verp (eds.), *Prenatal and Preimplantation Diagnosis*,
DOI 10.1007/978-3-319-18911-6_13

(ACOG 2007). Even though advancing maternal age is known to increase the risk of trisomy conditions, obstetricians encourage widespread screening of all pregnant women due to the possibility of detecting other fetal anomalies (cardiac and neural tube defects for example). Because they account for the great majority of births, the number of pregnant women under age 35 whose fetus has an anomaly is greater than the number of "older" women with an affected pregnancy (Choi et al. 2012). This means that many women who receive the news that their fetus is at higher risk for an anomaly have not previously considered this possibility (McCoyd 2007, 2013).

Once a woman is told that her fetus has a higher risk for an anomaly or condition, a group of decisional processes is set in motion that leads the woman into greater and greater use of medical diagnostic technology (McCoyd 2009b) and that requires more decision-making. Often, the distinction between screening and diagnosis must first be clarified. When a greater risk for anomaly is identified (via screening), the medical provider generally encourages testing that can diagnose the suspected condition. If the screening indicates a higher likelihood of Down syndrome, the woman may be encouraged to have either a chorionic villi sampling (CVS) or an amniocentesis. CVS gathers placental cells and amniocentesis grows fetal cells to examine fetal karyotype for purposes of diagnosis. Notably, new technologies are enabling examination of fetal DNA in maternal blood, making it likely that screening and possibly diagnostic testing for certain conditions will soon transition away from the invasiveness of CVS and amniocentesis to a simple blood draw from the mother (Bianchi et al. 2014; Norton et al. 2012). Should the prenatal screening indicate a neural tube defect, a high resolution ultrasound may be prescribed. Sometimes, the decision about whether to intervene in a pregnancy may stem from the presence of multiple fetuses which may require a decision about whether to selectively reduce the number of fetuses to enhance the likelihood of a healthy child/healthy children (Evans and Britt 2005).

Therefore, the first decision a woman must make is whether to pursue diagnostic testing to determine if the fetus actually has the condition in question. Many women describe this as the beginning of a roller coaster ride that may end with a reassuring test outcome indicating that the condition is not present. Alternatively, testing may show that the suspected diagnosis is present in the fetus (or that another condition is present). Occasionally, a condition may be diagnosed in the fetus that is amenable to fetal surgery (e.g., spina bifida; congenital cystic adenomatoid malformation of the lung (CCAM); congenital diaphragmatic hernia (CDH); twin–twin transfusion Decisions about whether to pursue fetal surgery include uncertainty about the success of the surgery, and the difficulties of traveling to a fetal surgery center, and spending a long time on bedrest near the fetal surgery center after completion of the surgery (Farrell and Howell 2012; Zamora et al. 2013). It is outside the scope of this chapter to examine fetal surgery decisions in detail, but many of the aspects of decision-making noted below will be applicable to these decisions as well.

If diagnostic testing indicates a disorder not amenable to fetal surgery, the woman must then decide whether to (1) plan to raise the child with the condition/s, (2) carry the pregnancy for as long as possible and pursue palliative care or perinatal hospice if the condition is life threatening, (3) relinquish the child for adoption, or (4) terminate the pregnancy. Any of these scenarios require decision-making that incorporates synthesis of medical information about the condition/s, values clarification on the part of the woman and her partner, and research about all of the options and resources available.

Each decision carries within it another set of decisions: if carrying the pregnancy as close to term as possible, how aggressively should the neonate be resuscitated after birth and will surgeries and extensive medical care be utilized or only comfort measures (English and Hessler 2013)? If planning on raising the child, the same decisions about the aggressiveness of neonatal care will need to be made while also exploring resources for sophisticated medical care and supportive early intervention services. If the neonate is expected to die, a pediatric palliative care/hospice agency must be contacted; if the decision is to relinquish for adoption, neonatal care will need to be decided upon and the adoption plan determined, including whether to use a public or private agency in a closed or open adoption. Finally, if pregnancy termination is the decision, this will then also require decision-making about how to end the pregnancy (i.e., induced early delivery or surgery to remove the fetus (Kerns et al. 2012)). In short, the finding of an elevated risk for fetal anomaly pitches the pregnant woman into a myriad of decisions that must be made quickly, under a level of uncertainty as to the severity of many fetal diagnoses (i.e., the level of cognitive delay of a fetus with Down syndrome cannot be determined prenatally, although mosaicism and presence of comorbidities may be indicative of lesser or greater delays respectively), and in a social context where many of the options are stigmatized (Kumar et al. 2009; McCoyd 2010).

Factors Affecting Women's Decisions About Continuing or Terminating an Affected Pregnancy

One of the more critical aspects of women's decisions about whether to continue a pregnancy affected by a fetal anomaly/disorder is whether the condition is life-threatening. Sandelowski and Jones (1996) observed that women often viewed lethality of a fetal condition as "nature's choice," absolving them of responsibility for making a decision to terminate the pregnancy. This criterion is weighed differently by different women and is also subject to changing circumstances. Although anencephaly clearly is incompatible with life as little to no brain tissue is present, there are (a few) individuals with trisomy 18 or trisomy 13, previously deemed incompatible with life, who have survived for up to a decade (Rasmussen et al. 2003). Some women find it easier to make the decision to terminate the pregnancy when they know the condition is lethal, whereas others carry to term and plan on palliative or hospice care after the birth.

Another major factor in framing a woman's decision is her willingness to consider abortion as an option. Women who identify themselves as "pro-life" and against abortion in any circumstances may have the courage of their convictions and maintain a pregnancy under any and all circumstances. That said, there is widespread recognition that what women believe hypothetically bears little resemblance to what women actually do when confronted with a pregnancy affected by fetal anomaly (Choi et al. 2012). Indeed, even high ranking officers in "Right to Life" organizations have been known to have pregnancy terminations after diagnosis of a fetal anomaly (McCoyd 2003). However, for women who adhere to an anti-abortion stance, Sandelowski and Jones found that there was a sense of "disowned" choice and they viewed pregnancy termination as "not their choice to make" (1996: p. 357), seemingly comforted in not having to actively engage in decision-making as the option of abortion was not viewed as possible for them.

More recent reviews have indicated that women who feel strongly about their values (in either direction) find that commitment to be "a source of ease" in the decision, while those who perceive a lack of information or some inconsistency in their values feel this creates "sources of difficulty" (St-Jacques et al. 2008). They note the fact "that the same factors may be perceived as a source of difficulty for some and as a source of ease for others highlights the need to develop tailored interventions addressing the personal decisional needs of the people involved in decision-making" (St-Jacques et al. 2008: p. 1202). In my practice with couples who are making decisions, those who have considered the possibility of an abnormal fetal diagnosis and who have made tentative decisions about what they would do in various circumstances before an abnormality is diagnosed, often cope with their decision more effectively when they have to make it, seemingly feeling that the decision was already made and they just need to implement it. This makes sense as they have thought through the decision before having to cope with the short time frames and emotional duress *after* an abnormality has been diagnosed in the fetus.

Botti et al. (2009) considered the "tragic choice" of stopping futile treatment of neonates in the NICU through the lens of autonomy of decision-making. This type of decision-making mirrors that of women and their partners after the diagnosis of a fetal anomaly as they too are essentially making a "tragic choice" to "remove life support"[2]—the woman's body being that life support. These researchers examined data from an ethnographic study (Orfali 2004) comparing decisions to withdraw life supporting care in NICUs in the USA and France. The researchers found parents in the USA preferred to maintain their role as the "chooser" (in contrast to France where the physician chose whether to continue treatment) even when it was also clear that the role of "chooser" led them to experience more negative emotions such as guilt and prolonged grief (Botti et al. 2009). They then ran simulations of parental decision-making (with Cornell University undergraduates) in choice and non-choice conditions with the no-choice (physician decided) treatment including information provision or no provision of information. They found that "choosers" preferred to choose despite a higher sense of "perceived causality" (meaning that they felt responsible for the death of the neonate) and the negative emotional toll that took; they were also less likely to want to change to the non-choice condition. Notably, the preferred condition (as defined by having lower levels of negative emotion) actually came when the case was presented to the simulated parents as a

[2]This phrase comes from a client I worked with who used this understanding to support her decision to terminate a pregnancy affected by triploidy (triplication of all chromosomes).

strong recommendation by the physician and/or as medically futile treatment, yet still given to them as a choice. This becomes an ethically tricky outcome as the value among physicians (and patients) in the USA is to preserve autonomy of decision-making. Many women have reported dissatisfaction with genetic counselors and physicians who strongly encourage termination after the finding of an anomaly (McCoyd 2009b; Parens and Asch 2003), or indeed, any strong opinion conveyed to the woman from the provider while the woman is still deciding (Helm et al. 1998; Skotko 2005).

Choi et al. (2012) reviewed 11 studies about decision-making after diagnosis of Down syndrome (DS) published between Jan 1999 and Sept 2010 and identified many of the framing factors noted above. They identified the demographic factors that framed decisions as religion (with church attenders less willing to consider termination); maternal age (with mixed findings among studies); and the presence of other children in combination with estimated gestational age (EGA) (those under 16 weeks EGA with living children were 26 times more likely to terminate for a DS diagnosis than those 17 weeks EGA and above with no children). They identified psychosocial factors influencing decisions as: (1) the perceived burden/reward of parenting a child with DS (although many studies noted increased sense of burden, others noted the rewards of caring for a child with DS); (2) quality of life for a child with DS (again, research findings were mixed); (3) attitudes towards individuals with disability (IWD); termination of pregnancy for fetal anomaly [TOPFA] was elected much more frequently when attitudes about disability were more negative; (4) personal comfort with IWD (where good relationships with IWD existed, women were less likely to elect TOPFA); and (5) level of support from others (partners and religious providers tended to have the most influence). It is notable that this review did not address the choice of continuing the pregnancy and relinquishing the baby for adoption. Very few research studies mention the possibility of relinquishing for adoption; historically, babies with disabilities were viewed as difficult to place (Glidden 2000). Nevertheless, there is a literature about how these placements work out in the adoptive families. In Great Britain, there is even a special group of social workers involved with this type of placement (Gould 2010). Clinically, I have found that religiously affiliated adoption agencies often have families who are quite willing and able to adopt children with disabilities of many types, and some are willing to foster children who are expected to die shortly after birth.

Women whose fetus has a condition that is likely to affect the child's quality of life (but not an inherently lethal condition) often struggle with their decisions more than do those with a fetus with a lethal disorder as they must weigh their views of what a "quality life" is (Garcia et al. 2009; Rapp 2000; Vailly 2014), their views about individuals with disability (Bryant et al. 2005; Lawson 2001), the ethical imperatives of pregnancy (Miller et al. 2012), and what they believe they and their family can manage in terms of care for a child with a disability (McCoyd 2008). In addition, these decisions are also population based, both in terms of the diagnosis of the fetus (Schechtman et al. 2002) and the demographic characteristics of the mother. The diagnostic category of the fetus is a population level variable. Schechtman et al. (2002) found that the severity of the condition (how likely to cause death or ongoing illness) and central nervous system (CNS) involvement both positively correlate with a decision to terminate the pregnancy. The demographics of the mother also influence the decision: religious women are less likely to terminate than secular women, and women with lower levels of education and minority status are less likely to make use of prenatal screening, testing or termination (Dormandy et al. 2005; Jackson et al. 2014). Yet a recent systematic review suggested that rates of termination for various fetal diagnoses (and in particular DS) may be lower than previously suggested due to geographical differences, younger women now being included in more universal prenatal screening, and more women feeling comfortable using prenatal screening even if they have no intent to terminate an affected pregnancy (Natoli et al. 2012).

Yet these population level variables cannot tell the story of the decision-making process for any particular woman. For instance, decisions are known to be affected by heuristics and inherent biases, one of which is availability bias (Kahneman et al. 1982): in the case of prenatal diagnosis, this means that a woman who has experience with people who have the same diagnosis as the fetus is both more likely to believe that it is possible that her fetus will have the condition, but also that she will have a similar type of experience with the condition as the other (known) individual (Schild and Black 1984). In clinical practice, I explore these availability biases and the valence they have for the woman as they can strongly influence the woman's decision. Farrelly et al. (2012) strongly encourage counselors to include the following areas when discussing decision-making about affected pregnancies: (1) the social aspects of the quality of life for individuals with disability; (2) the client's experiences and perceptions of IWD; (3) the resources available to support IWD (including introduction to people living with that disability); and (4) exploration of all options.

Women often "Google" the diagnosis and develop availability biases based on feeling they know individuals encountered on-line who faced these decisions, who have children with these conditions, or who have the condition themselves. Together with gathering medical information by "doctor-shopping" on- or off-line, prenatal counselors often encounter people who have been very busy gathering as much information as possible, yet who are somewhat paralyzed in terms of making a decision because they believe that one more piece of information will make the decision clearer or easier. This may mirror the finding that "maximizers" (those who seek to maximize their information gathering rather than be satisfied ["satisficers")] continue to seek information in ways that do not lead to better decisional competence, outcomes, nor lessened regret (Parker et al. 2007; Schwartz et al. 2002). Gigerenzer (2007) found that this type of information gathering is a common, yet ineffective strategy for making medical decisions and that use of heuristics/biases that yielded "gut" decisions may actually work better in assuring that one's values are incorporated into the decision-making. Durand et al. (2011) also suggest that "Take the best" and tallying approaches to a patient decision aid incorporate the notion that information to decision-making effectiveness operates as an inverted U shape with increasing information actually impairing decision-making. Pieterse and de Vries (2011) question this, noting that these attenuated decisions may work better for decision makers like physicians who make repeated decisions and who can check the accuracy of those decisions in the outcome of a case over time. They note that people making decisions about amniocentesis (and by extrapolation, prenatal diagnosis) will not be making these decisions multiple times and have no way of contrasting their decision with an alternate outcome, so they seldom have any way of determining if it was "correct," even with themselves as the adjudicators of the correctness. Yet Pieterse and de Vries (2011) agree that research needs to incorporate the use of intuitive forms of decision-making. In my practice, I have known many women who agonize for a period of time, but report waking up one morning, "knowing" what they need to do. It appears the intuitive form of decision-making can function actively in some women. Although some may argue that this is a form of retrospective rationalization (see Haidt 2001), my sense is that women who have this experience feel both surprised and relieved when these decisions come intuitively.

A final factor involved in many women's decisions is stigma (McCoyd 2008). As Ladd-Taylor and Umansky (1998) demonstrated, women are held responsible for the outcomes of their child bearing lives: when children have disabilities or poor behavior (often for reasons of genetic developmental delays) and are seen in public spaces, women are stigmatized. Yet termination/abortion is also laden with high levels of stigma, particularly in the USA (Kumar et al. 2009; Major and Gramzow 1999; McCoyd 2010). Even though I have found no literature supporting this observation, I have seen women who relinquished children for adoption after an abnormal fetal diagnosis whose frequent self-degradation for not feeling able to care for the child was freighted with fears of stigma. Ebaugh (1988) alludes to the societal disapproval that often comes with "becoming an ex" of any type and notes that role exit for mothers is particularly disdained. Kumar et al. (2009) build on this idea and note that the feminine ideals of perpetual fecundity, the inevitability of motherhood and the idea of instinctual nurturing are all violated when a woman terminates a pregnancy, leading to high levels of stigma. It can be seen that no choice allows women to avoid stigma; each woman must weigh which type of stigma feels most damaging to her.

Ultimately, each woman weighs and balances the fetal condition, her beliefs about abortion, her beliefs about what constitutes a quality life in connection with her beliefs about disability, her availability biases about the diagnosis, her ability to understand the information provided to her by her medical providers as they explain probabilities and severities of medical conditions, and her sense of support from her partner, her family and her community. Each decision is made under highly emotional circumstances which are known to interfere with decision-making, provoke anxiety and depression (Paulus and Yu 2012) and challenge coping. In light of this highly contextualized, very individualized decision-making process, there is no one correct way to assist women in their decision-making process.

Decision-Making Assistance

Decision aids have been somewhat successful in helping women consider the various facets of their decision-making; they provide a visual representation of the risks and decision points (with benefits and consequences specified where possible) and an explicit discussion of the individual's values, beliefs, and attitudes as they relate to each decision point and option (Bekker et al. 2003). Bekker et al. (2003, 2004) randomly assigned pregnant women to routine care (counseling but no structured decision aid) or to the intervention group with a structured decision aid used in the counseling session. They found that using structured decisional aids and guided evaluation discussions led to more negative emotions in the short term despite fewer long-term negative emotions; yet patients expressed more dissatisfaction with decision analysis consultations (and had higher attrition rates from the study). It may be that the structured approach felt less supportive (and raised more difficult material to process) than is typical in routine care. Durand et al. (2011) and Pieterse and de Vries (2011) show that the gathering of information and the use of various structured decision-making strategies have varied levels of satisfaction (as reported by the mothers) and effectiveness (as measured by time-to-make a decision and confidence in the decision) in perinatal contexts. Although structured decision aids are available, many who work with women/couples during decision-making prefer to conduct the sessions more like typical counseling sessions with values clarification and attention to each of the decisional factors noted above.

Another dynamic operating when assisting decision-making is how much the individual actually wants to participate in decision-making. In a review of medical decision-making, Brom et al. (2014) found only 60 % congruence between what patients wanted in terms of their own participation in decision-making and what actually occurred. Most of the non-congruence group preferred to be more involved with the decision, yet a substantial sized group (about a fifth) preferred to be less involved or more passive. Since its inception, the model for genetic counseling is very much one of providing information about levels of risk and the conditions the fetus may have and relying on the woman/couple to make the decision—with focus on the patient's autonomy (Kessler 1997; Marteau 1995). This mismatch between what parents want and what the typical genetic counseling/perinatologist encounter may offer calls us to attend to the needs of women/couples during the decision-making process and to recognize the needs women have for personalized counseling that helps them weigh their own values and judgments. Some women are monitors who prefer more information and others are blunters who prefer to avoid discomforting information (Miller 1987). Either requires time for reflection, consideration of all options, and psychosocial assessment and support, a set of conditions that are often hard to provide in the typical busy perinatal clinic.

Many have asserted that a value neutral, non-directive stance is an ideal not achieved in practice (Farrelly et al. 2012; Parens and Asch 2000), failing most often in discussions of how one might parent a child with a disability (Farrelly et al. 2012). A critical feature of working with women throughout their decision-making process is to help them assess each possibility, clarify their value set, and determine how each option might fit within their family. Women are clear that they do not want to be coddled or misled. In the words of one of the participants in my dissertation research (McCoyd 2003):

> *Be honest about everything. Don't let your personal views come into the picture- either way. I knew from the first word that came out of our doctor's mouth what his opinion was- abort. Even though I chose that, I think it placed unfair weight on one side. If I had wondered about the possibility of carrying to term, he is not the person I would have asked because I felt he would think we were crazy. Being truly unbiased and ACTIVELY supportive of both choices is the best gift you can give your patients.*

Likewise, women appreciated having the choice they finally made affirmed by their medical providers as noted in the same research report:

> *That's when I said, "you know, I'm probably terminating" and he said "Well, I think you're making the right decision." And that meant a lot to me because for somebody to say "Oh whatever you do is fine" is one thing, but for somebody to say "I really think you're making the right decision" meant a lot.*

In short, women making difficult decisions do not need to be protected from consideration of all the choices; they need to be protected from judgment and allowed to consider all options through the lenses of their own values, social supports, and beliefs about what constitutes quality of life. They need to be given accurate information about the fact that they are likely to feel grief regardless of their choice—that is to say, they will mourn, there is no choice that will yield them the healthy child they had hoped for.

Carrying Through with Decisions

Once a decision is made, women often report a brief period of relief as they are no longer agonizing over the decision. For those who have elected to continue the pregnancy, there are many reports that friends, family, and medical providers continually question the decision in ways that are extremely invalidating (Helm et al. 1998; Skotko 2005). Some who have decided to continue the pregnancy and relinquish the baby for adoption may find their decisions questioned to the point that they change their mind and raise the child themselves. Helm et al. (1998) report a case where the fact that other families were so interested in adopting a baby with Down syndrome led the biological parents to reconsider their decision and keep the baby after all. Others who have elected to keep a child after a prenatal diagnosis may have to justify their decision to family members and medical providers (Beck 1999/2000; Vitez 2001; Zuckoff 2002). A reported coping strategy is to surround themselves with people who support their decision (or in Beck's case, with the "puppeteers" she imagines around her). Often women have relied on their religious beliefs in making the decision to continue a pregnancy; religious communities are often a source of support, both instrumental and emotional.

Most parents continuing pregnancies report that the single most important intervention they received was a referral to speak with other parents who were raising a child affected by the same condition (Helm et al. 1998). Many found that early referral to a support group for that condition was particularly helpful as they began to learn about resources they could mobilize to assist them once the child was born. Many had been told the old canard that parents who have children with a disability end up divorced, yet this is not accurate (McCoyd et al. 2010). When the decision is to continue a pregnancy that will be affected by a life threatening condition, referral to a pediatric hospice or palliative care agency is important in assuring that the family can have support at the time of birth and for as long as the neonate lives (English and Hessler 2013). Such services help create the memories that will assist the parents in preserving a bond with their baby (Klass et al. 1996), as well as instrumental support and comfort care for the baby until its death. English and Hessler (2013) provide extensive guidance for developing an Advanced Care Birth Plan to guide the birth and neonatal experience when there is a diagnosis of a fetal abnormality. The literature currently available indicates that most parents electing pediatric hospice are confident that they have made the best decision (English and Hessler 2013; Lathrop and Vandevusse 2011).

As noted earlier, there is a paucity of literature about women who make the decision to relinquish a baby with a diagnosed disability/condition. The stigma attached to this decision likely keeps women from speaking about this experience in much the same way that women are silenced for exiting the role of "mom" or violating norms about motherhood more generally.

For women making decisions about a pregnancy with multiple fetuses, the options are much more limited because after a certain point (generally triplets), most medical providers will be concerned about the wisdom of continuing the pregnancy and anticipate a very premature delivery. Most physicians now recommend reducing (aborting one or more of the fetuses/embryos in a multifetal pregnancy) a triplet or higher order pregnancy in order to maximize the possibility of having a "take home" baby (Evans and Britt 2005). Even having twins risks higher chances for fetal demise, stillbirth, and prematurity with the ongoing complications of prematurity. The same authors utilized three different but intersecting "frames" to analyze the decision to reduce multiple gestation and the angst associated with that decision (Britt and Evans 2007). Using frames labeled (1) "conceptional" (life begins at conception and is valued in and of itself), (2) "medical" (risks for viability justify taking some fetal life to reduce the risk to the pregnancy as a whole and promote the welfare of a particular fetus) and (3) "lifestyle" (which incorporates the woman's attempts to balance family and career), they found that the conceptional frame led to the most difficulty in decision-making. The difficulty of decision-making was mediated when the medical frame was prioritized. Lifestyle frames seldom intersected with conceptional frames. Mirroring the Botti et al. (2009) findings, women and couples who felt that the decision was not really theirs to make (it was due to medical necessity) fared better in carrying out and coping with their decision.

For those making a decision to terminate a pregnancy for fetal anomaly (TOPFA), there is no doubt that having to make an active decision to end the pregnancy with perceived causality (Botti et al. 2009) adds to the grief (McCoyd 2009a, 2010). Zeanah et al.'s (1993) classic study asked, "Do women grieve following termination of pregnancy for fetal anomalies?" and answered a resounding "yes." Many have confirmed this, expanding the original finding by observing that grief increases with lack of supportive medical providers and friends/family, high levels of self-blame, being childless, strong religious beliefs, and lack of confidence in the decision (Geerinck-Vercammen and Kanhai 2003; Kersting et al 2004; Korenromp et al. 1992; Lafarge et al. 2013; McCoyd 2007). Others have noted that grief also occurs when a baby is diagnosed with an anomaly at birth (Macinnes 2008; Vailly 2014); that grief may lead to changes in future childbearing choices and to a sense of guilt. Several research studies suggest that women who see and hold their babies after TOPFA (where induced delivery is the method of termination) may experience less intense levels of grief (Geerinck-Vercammen and Kanhai 2003; Kersting et al 2004). Further, quantitative analyses of grief scores on both the Perinatal Grief Scale (PGS; Toedter et al. 1988) and the Perinatal Bereavement Scale (PBS; Theut et al. 1989), comparing women who had experienced a miscarriage vs. those who had experienced TOPFA showed no difference in the level of grief of the two groups (Keefe-Cooperman 2004/5). PGS scores for the women who had experienced TOPFA did not differ significantly from the norms for miscarriage in my own dissertation data, as well (McCoyd 2003).

Nevertheless, certain factors are found to correlate with higher levels of grief: time elapsed since the loss (negative correlation [−]), counseling intervention [−], employment outside the home [−], feeling responsible (positive correlation [+]), maternal age, if a source of guilt [+], and gestational length of the pregnancy [+] (Keefe-Cooperman 2004/5). Typically, women are not in a position to compare their own loss experiences, so women may enhance their sense of responsibility for their own grief by assuming that the intensity of their grief indicates that they "made the wrong decision" (McCoyd 2007). Yet they are actually experiencing similar levels of grief to women with miscarriage in which there was no decision to be made.

Another decision that often needs to be made is whether to have surgery (dilation and evacuation) to remove the fetus, or to have an induced delivery (Lyus et al. 2014). Availability of each option differs geographically in the USA (McCoyd 2003). Yet most research indicates that, although surgical termination has lower levels of associated physical complication/morbidity, women benefit from considering which method better fits their needs (e.g., having the surgery done more quickly vs being able to hold the baby (Kerns et al. 2012)). This research reiterates the frequent finding that women need emotional support and continuity from their health care providers throughout the diagnosis, selection of termination method, and aftermath of termination.

Discussion about whether the fetal body will be intact and what needs the family has for a ritual such as a memorial service or burial must be part of preparing for TOPFA. Although these are difficult discussions, avoiding them leaves the woman and her support network in a position of once again needing to make a quick decision about the disposition of the fetal body. Clinical experience has taught me that women are aided in carrying through with the decision to TOPFA when they are given time to assess their own need for a ritual of some type. They will likely still anticipate the actual termination procedure with great trepidation, yet they will also know what they will do after that procedure (e.g., see the baby [or not] if termination is by induction; chose a funeral home for cremation or burial; arrange to consult with clergy). Discussions of death are challenging but necessary with people preparing for typical end of life (Abba et al. 2013), and are just as necessary when end of life is occurring at the typical beginning of life.

Grieving After Fetal Diagnosis

For women making the choice to continue an affected pregnancy, anticipatory grieving during the rest of pregnancy allows the family to begin to move through the grief that their child will not be born healthy as they had originally anticipated (Goff et al. 2013). This may offer the family the opportunity to gather resources (both instrumental and emotional) that will enable adjustment to a new family member who needs additional support. Anticipatory mourning will likely occur during the same time the parents may be meeting families who have children with the same diagnosis and may allow gradual adaptation. There is much debate in the disability studies world about the validity of Olshansky's assertion (1970) that families with a child with a disability live with chronic sorrow. Others focus on the lessons of empathy and caring that are learned when a family member has a disability (Green 2007). The truth likely lies between those positions, yet grief over not having the child one expected happens even under the best of circumstances. Even when families are authentically happy about the impending birth of a child who has a diagnosed condition/disability, they must mourn the change from the expected healthy newborn to one who will require more support.

For families who decide to continue a pregnancy knowing that the fetus has a life threatening condition, the preparation will ideally entail connection with a perinatal hospice. Although research in this area is in its infancy, the support women and their families feel as their parenting and emotional needs are validated (Lathrop and Vandevusse 2011) is invaluable. Perinatal hospice allows the woman and her family to build memories and to receive ongoing bereavement services with a team who often have been part of the antenatal period and the birth. Such continuity of care and knowledge provides comfort as grief is processed. When referral to hospice is made during the pregnancy, the family is able to create realistic expectations, get to know the care team that will attend them after the birth, and receive guidance in creating an Advanced Care Birth Plan (English and Hessler 2013).

When the decision is made to continue the pregnancy with the intent to relinquish the child for adoption, early referral to an adoption agency that specializes in special needs children helps to ensure that a birth and transition plan is in order. Additionally, agencies provide counseling to all sides of the adoption triangle to assist in the adaptation, grief and ongoing coping. Parenting a special needs child can result in parental burn out, as can parenting a typical child if expectations of oneself are unrealistic (McCarthy 2007). Follow-up support for the adoptive parents as well as the biological parents allows the latter to know that they have provided a supportive home for the child. The National Down Syndrome Adoption Network (www.ndsan.org) has a respectful booklet, "A Loving Choice," for parents considering relinquishment for adoption of a child with Down syndrome that acknowledges the legitimacy (and pain) of this decision. Counseling for women continuing affected pregnancies must include the recognition that they will mourn the child they wished to have had, yet they will likely also mourn a self-image that must undergo revision as they come to understand their own limits. Addressing the ways she will share information (or not) with family, friends, and work colleagues, will help the woman consider various facets of the experience and allow her to process any internalized stigma she may be experiencing.

In considering the needs of women and their partners after decision-making and with grief due to a decision to TOPFA, the similarities and differences between the loss of a pregnancy to miscarriage (SAB) versus to TOPFA are important in considering grief recovery. The similarities between SAB and TOPFA are: both groups need validation of their loss; both need opportunities for memory-building (ultrasound pictures, locks of hair); both experience a heightened sense of vulnerability (as is typical in most experiences of loss [Walter and McCoyd 2009]); both often experience a sense of social judgment and lack of support (internalized stigma); both feel the loss of the dream of the idealized pregnancy and baby; and both experience anxiety in subsequent pregnancies. Yet the differences reveal part of the challenge for moving through the grief experience. For women who experience a TOPFA, decision-making is involved (often inspiring self-blame due to perceived causality), the sense of responsibility is heightened, there is often a waiting period between when a decision is made and when it is implemented during which fetal movements can be emotionally agonizing; there is a political climate that stigmatizes and even prohibits TOPFA in some geographic areas; and genetic issues may have implications for parents and their future children. Identifying and discussing these similarities and differences are ways counselors can help women and their partners process their experience and identify strategies for becoming more confident of their decisions. Helping them to recognize that the pain is caused by the fetus' diagnosis (and only secondarily by the decisions that have to be made and implemented) is one strategy for helping parents cope with their grief. They need help realizing that they have "made the wise choice even where there was no right choice," as a client once said to me.

As women come to see that the choices they must make as a result of anomaly or a higher order multiple gestation are the result of a set of medical conditions—not due to something they themselves have done—they are often more able to perceive the experience as one in which the decision is self-evident (like Britt and Evans "medical necessity" frame). At that point, they can decrease their feelings of self-blame and castigation. When women learn that intense grief is part of any pregnancy loss, they can use this information to help validate their right to grieve and move through their grief. Although grief is a part of any decision after the finding of a fetal anomaly or condition incompatible with good health, it is important to work with the woman and her partner to recognize the ways they can continue a bond with the baby they bore in their hearts (when this is comforting to the couple). Working with them in the ways described in Chaps. 15 and 16 to process their grief and share their experiences with friends and family is a critical follow-up to the decision-making process that will enable them to recognize this event as a chapter in their life which will undoubtedly change them in some ways, but which does not need to inspire grief forever.

References

A loving choice: making an adoption plan for a child with Down Syndrome. http://www.ndsan.org/adoption-process/birth-parents/. Accessed 2 June 2014.

Abba K, Byrne P, Horton S, Lloyd-Williams M. Interventions to encourage discussion of end-of-life preferences between members of the general population and the people closest to them – a systematic literature review. BMC Palliat Care. 2013;2013:12(40). doi:10.1186/1472-684X-12-40.

ACOG Practice Bulletin. Screening for fetal chromosomal abnormalities. Obstet Gynecol. 2007;109(1):217–27.

Beck M. Expecting Adam. New York, NY: Berkley Books; 1999/2000.

Bekker HL, Hewison J, Thornton JG. Understanding why decision aids work: linking process with outcome. Pat Ed Counselor. 2003;50:323–9. doi:10.1016/S0738-3991(03)00056-9.

Bekker HL, Hewison J, Thornton JG. Applying decision analysis to facilitate informed decision making about prenatal diagnosis for Down syndrome: a randomized controlled trial. Prenat Diagn. 2004;24:265–75. doi:10.1002/pd.851.

Bianchi DW, Parker RL, Wentworth J, Madankumar R, Saffer C, Das AF, Craig JA, Chudova DI, Devers PL, Jones KW, Oliver K, Rava RP, Sehnert AJ. DNA sequencing versus standard prenatal aneuploidy screening. N Engl J Med. 2014;370(9):799–808. doi:10.1056/NEJMoa1311037.

Botti S, Orfalik K, Iyengar S. Tragic choices: autonomy and emotional responses to medical decisions. J Consum Res. 2009;36(3):337–52.

Britt D, Evans M. Sometimes doing the right thing sucks: frame combinations and multi-fetal pregnancy reduction decision difficulty. Soc Sci Med. 2007;65(11):2342–56.

Brom L, Hopmans W, Pasman HW, Timmermans DM, Widdershoven GM, Onwuteaka-Philipsen BD. Congruence between patients' preferred and perceived participation in medical decision-making: a review of the literature. BMC Med Inform Decis Mak. 2014;14(1):1–27. doi:10.1186/1472-6947-14-25.

Bryant L, Hewison JD, Green JM. Attitudes towards prenatal diagnosis and termination in women who have a sibling with Down's syndrome. J Reprod Infant Psychol. 2005;23:181–98.

Choi H, Van Riper M, Thoyre S. Decision making following a prenatal diagnosis of Down syndrome: an integrative review. J Midwifery Womens Health. 2012;57(2):156–64. doi:10.1111/j.1542-2011.2011.00109.x.

Dormandy E, Michie S, Hooper R, Marteau TM. Low uptake of prenatal screening for Down syndrome in minority ethnic groups and socially deprived groups: a reflection of women's attitudes or a failure to facilitate informed choices. Int J Epidemiol. 2005;34:146–352. 10.109.1093.

Durand M, Wegwarth O, Boivin J, Elwyn G. Design and usability of heuristic-based deliberation tools for women facing amniocentesis. Health Exp. 2011;15(1):32–48. doi:10.1111/j.1369-7625.2010.00651.x.

Ebaugh HRF. Becoming an ex: the process of role exit. Chicago IL: U of Chicago Press; 1988.

English NK, Hessler KL. Prenatal birth planning for families of the imperiled newborn. J Obstet Gynecol Neonatal Nurs. 2013;42(3):390–9. doi:10.1111/1552-6909.12031.
Evans MI, Britt DW. Fetal reduction. Sem Perinatol. 2005;29(5):321–9.
Farrell J, Howell L. An overview of surgical techniques, research trials, and future directions of fetal therapy. J Obstet Gynecol Neonatal Nurs. 2012;41(3):419–25. doi:10.1111/j.1552-6909.2012.01356.x.
Farrelly E, Cho M, Erby L, Roter D, Stenzel A, Ormond K. Genetic counseling for prenatal testing: where is the discussion about disability? J Gen Couns. 2012;21(6):814–24. doi:10.1007/s10897-012-9484-z.
Garcia E, Timmermans DRM, van Leeuwen E. Reconsidering prenatal screening: an empirical-ethical approach to understand moral dilemmas as a question of personal preferences. J Med Ethics. 2009;35:410–4. doi:10.1136/jme.2008.026880.
Geerinck-Vercammen CR, Kanhai HHH. Coping with termination of pregnancy for fetal abnormality in a supportive environment. Prenat Diagn. 2003;23:543–8.
Gigerenzer G. Gut feelings: the intelligence of the unconscious. New York: Viking; 2007.
Glidden LM. Adopting children with developmental disabilities: a long term perspective. Fam Relat. 2000;49(4):397–405.
Goff BSN, Springer N, Foote LC, Frantz C, Peak M, Tracy C, Veh T, Bentley GE, Cross KA. Receiving the initial Down syndrome diagnosis: a comparison of prenatal and postnatal parent group experiences. Intellect Dev Disabil. 2013;51:446–57. doi:10.1352/1934-9556-51.6.446.
Gould J. Disability: breaking down the barriers to child placement – report of BAAF Health Group Conference. Adopt Foster. 2010;34(4):79–82. doi:10.1177/030857591003400412.
Green SE. "We're tired, not sad": benefits and burdens of mothering a child with a disability. Soc Sci Med. 2007;64:150–63.
Haidt J. The emotional dog and its rational tail: a social intuitionist approach to moral judgment. Psychol Rev. 2001;108(4):814–34. doi:10.1037//0033-295X.108.4.814.
Helm DT, Miranda S, Chedd NA. Prenatal diagnosis of Down syndrome: mothers' reflections on supports needed from diagnosis to birth. Ment Retard. 1998;36:55–61.
Jackson JM, Crider KS, Cragan JD, Rasmussen SA, Olney RS. Frequency of prenatal cytogenetic diagnosis and pregnancy outcomes by maternal race-ethnicity, and the effect on the prevalence of trisomy 21, Metropolitan Atlanta, 1996–2005. Am J Med Genet A. 2014;164A(1):70–6. doi:10.1002/ajmg.a.36247.
Kahneman D, Slovic P, Tversky A. Judgment under uncertainty: Heuristics and biases. New York: Cambridge University Press; 1982.
Keefe-Cooperman K. A comparison of grief as related to miscarriage and termination for fetal anomaly. OMEGA. 2004/5;50(4):281–300.
Kerns J, Vanjani R, Freedman L, Meckstroth K, Drey EA, Steinauer J. Women's decision making regarding choice of second trimester termination method for pregnancy complications. Intl J Gynecol Obstet. 2012;116:244–8. doi:10.1016/j.ijgo.2011.10.016.
Kersting A, Dorsch M, Kreulich C, Klockenbusch W. Coping with termination of pregnancy for fetal abnormality. Prenat Diagn. 2004;24:70–2. doi:10.1002/pd.770.
Kessler S. Psychological aspects of genetic counseling. VII. Thoughts on directiveness. J Gen Couns. 1997;1(1):9–17.
Klass D, Silverman PR, Nickman SL. Continuing bonds: new understandings of grief. Philadelphia, PA: Taylor & Francis; 1996.
Korenromp MJ, Iedema-Kuiper HR, Van Spijker HG, Christiaens GGML, Bergsma J. Termination of pregnancy on genetic grounds; coping with grieving. J Psychosom Obstet Gynecol. 1992;13:93–105.
Kumar A, Hessini L, Mitchell EMH. Conceptualising abortion stigma. Cult Health Sex. 2009;11(6):625–39. doi:10.1080/13691050902842741.
Ladd-Taylor M, Umansky L, editors. "Bad" mothers: the politics of blame in twentieth century America. New York, NY: New York University Press; 1998.

Lafarge C, Mitchell K, Fox P. Perinatal grief following a termination of pregnancy for foetal abnormality: the impact of coping strategies. Prenat Diagn. 2013;33:1173–82. doi:10.1002/pd.4218.

Lathrop A, Vandevusse L. Affirming motherhood: validation and invalidation in women's perinatal hospice narratives. Birth (Berkeley, CA). 2011;38(3):256–65. doi:10.1111/j.1523-536X.2011.00478.x.

Lawson KL. Contemplating selective reproduction: a subjective appraisal of parenting a child with a disability. J Reprod Infant Psychol. 2001;19:73–82. doi:10.1080/02646830020032400.

Lyus R, Creed K, Fisher J, McKeon L. Termination of pregnancy for fetal abnormality. Brit J Midwifery. 2014;22(5):332–7.

MacInnes MD. One's enough for now: children, disability, and the subsequent childbearing of mothers. J Marriage Fam. 2008;70(3):758–71.

Major B, Gramzow RH. Abortion as stigma: cognitive and emotional implications of concealment. J Pers Soc Psychol. 1999;77:735–45.

Markens S, Browner CH, Press N. "Because of the risks": how US pregnant women account for refusing prenatal screening. Soc Sci Med. 1999;49:359–69.

Marteau T. Towards informed decisions about prenatal testing: a review. Prenat Diagn. 1995; 15(13):1215–26.

McCarthy H. Parent burn out. 2007. http://www.rainbowkids.com/ExpertArticleDetails.aspx?id=276&title=Parent Burn-out. Accessed June 13 2014.

McCoyd JLM. Pregnancy Interrupted: non-normative loss of a desired pregnancy after termination for fetal anomaly. Unpublished dissertation, Bryn Mawr (PA): Bryn Mawr College; 2003. p. 281. Available from: Proquest, Ann Arbor, MI; 3088602.

McCoyd JLM. Pregnancy interrupted: loss of a desired pregnancy after diagnosis of fetal anomaly. J Psychosom Obstet Gynecol. 2007;28(1):37–48.

McCoyd JLM. "I'm not a saint": burden assessment as an unrecognized factor in prenatal decision making. Qual Health Res. 2008;18(11):1489–500.

McCoyd JLM. Discrepant feeling rules and unscripted emotion work: women terminating desired pregnancies due to fetal anomaly. Am J Orthopsychol. 2009a;79(4):441–51.

McCoyd JLM. What do women want?: experiences and reflections of women after prenatal diagnosis and termination for anomaly. Health Care Women Int. 2009b;30(6):507–35.

McCoyd JLM. Women in no man's land: the U.S. abortion debate and women terminating desired pregnancies due to fetal anomaly. Br J Soc Work. 2010;40:133–53. doi:10.1093/bjsw/bcn080.

McCoyd JLM. Preparation for prenatal decision-making: a baseline of knowledge and reflection in women participating in prenatal screening. J Psychosom Obstet Gynecol. 2013;34(1):3–8.

McCoyd JLM, Akincigil A, Peak EH. Pediatric disability and caregiver separation. J Fam Soc Work. 2010;13(3):251–68.

Miller SM. Monitoring and blunting: validation of a questionnaire to assess styles of information seeking under threat. J Pers Soc Psychol. 1987;52(2):345–53.

Miller C, Hewison J, Morley S. A comparison of decisions about prenatal diagnosis and preimplantation genetic diagnosis. J Reprod Infant Psychol. 2012;30(4):377–87. doi:10.1080/02646838.2012.725128.

Natoli JL, Ackerman DL, McDermott S, Edwards JG. Prenatal diagnosis of Down syndrome: a systematic review of termination rates (1995–2011). Prenat Diagn. 2012;32:142–53. doi:10.1002/pd.2910.

Norton ME, Brar H, Weiss J, Karimi A, Laurent LC, Caughey AB, et al. Non-invasive chromosomal evaluation (NICE) study: results of a multicenter, prospective cohort study for detection of trisomy 21 and trisomy 18. Am J Obstet Gynecol. 2012;207:1371–8.

Olshansky S. Chronic sorrow: a response to having a defective child. In: Nolen R, editor. Counselling parents of the mentally retarded. Springfield, IL: Charles C Thomas; 1970.

Orfali K. Parental role in medical decision-making: fact or fiction? A comparative study of ethical dilemmas in French and American neonatl intensive care units. Soc Sci Med. 2004;58:2009–22. doi:10.1016/S0277-9536(03)00406-4.

Parens E, Asch A. Prenatal testing and disability rights. Washington, D.C.: Georgetown University Press; 2000.

Parens E, Asch A. Disability rights critique of prenatal genetic testing: reflections and recommendations. Ment Retard Dev Disabil Res Rev. 2003;9(1):40–7.
Parker AM, Bruine de Bruine W, Fischoff B. Maximizers versus satisficers: decision-making styles, competence, and outcomes. Judge Dec Mak. 2007;2:342–50.
Paulus MP, Yu AJ. Emotion and decision-making: affect-driven belief systems in anxiety and depression. Trends Cogn Sci. 2012;16(9):476–82. doi:10.1016/jtics.2012.07.009.
Pieterse A, de Vries M. On the suitability of fast and frugal heuristics for designing values clarification methods in patient decision aids: a critical analysis. Health Exp. 2011;16:73–9. doi:10.1111/j.1369-7625.2011.00720.x.
Rapp R. Refusing prenatal diagnosis: the meanings of bioscience in a multicultural world. Sci Technol Hum Val. 1998;23(1):45–70.
Rapp R. Testing women: testing the fetus. New York: Routledge Press; 2000.
Rasmussen SA, Wong LY, Yang Q, May KM, Friedman JM. Population-based analyses of mortality in trisomy 13 and trisomy 18. Pediatrics. 2003;111(4 Pt 1):777–84.
Sandelowski M, Jones LJ. Healing fictions': stories of choosing in the aftermath of the detection of fetal anomalies. Soc Sci Med. 1996;42:351–61.
Santalahti P, Hemminki E, Latikka A, Ryynaen M. Women's decision-making in prenatal screening. Soc Sci Med. 1998;46(8):1067–76.
Schechtman KB, Gray DL, Baty JD, Rothman SM. Decision-making for termination of pregnancies with fetal anomalies: analysis of 53,000 pregnancies. Obstet Gynecol. 2002;99:216–22.
Schild S, Black RB. Social work and genetics. New York: Haworth; 1984.
Schwartz B, Ward A, Monterosso J, Lyubomirsky S, White K, Lehman DR. Maximizing versus satisficing: happiness is a matter of choice. J Pers Soc Psychol. 2002;83:1178–97.
Skotko B. Prenatally diagnosed Down syndrome: mothers who continued their pregnancies evaluate their health care providers. Am J Obstet Gynecol. 2005;192(3):670–7. doi:10.1016/j.ajog.2004.11.001.
St-Jacques S, Grenier S, Charland M, Forest J-C, Rousseau F, Légaré F. Decisional needs assessment regarding Down syndrome prenatal testing: a systematic review of the perceptions of women, their partners and health professionals. Prenat Diagn. 2008;28(13):1183–203. http://dx.doi.org/10.1002/pd.2059.
Theut SK, Pedersen FA, Zaslow MJ, Cain RL, Rabinovich BA, Morihisa JM. Perinatal loss and bereavement. Am J Psychol. 1989;146(5):635–9.
Toedter L, Lasker J, Alhadeff J. The perinatal grief scale: development and initial validation. Am J Orthopsychol. 1988;58:435–49.
Vailly J. Genetic testing, birth, and the quest for health. Sci Technol Hum Val. 2014;39(3):374–96. doi:10.1177/0162243913509413.
Vitez M. Knowing her baby will die, she chooses to give birth. The Philadelphia Inquirer. 2001: A1–A14.
Walter CA, McCoyd JLM. Grief and loss across the lifespan: a biopsychosocial approach. New York: Springer Publishing; 2009.
Zamora IJ, Ethun CJ, Evans LM, Olutoye OO, Ivey RT, Haeri S, et al. Maternal morbidity and reproductive outcomes related to fetal surgery. J Pediatr Surg. 2013;48(5):951–5. doi:10.1016/j.jpedsurg.2013.02.010.
Zeanah CH, Dailey J, Rosenblatt MJ, Saller N. Do women grieve following termination of pregnancy for fetal anomalies? A controlled investigation. Obstet Gynecol. 1993;82:270–5.
Zuckoff M. Choosing Naia: a family's journey. Boston: Beacon; 2002.

Chapter 14
Helping Patients Cope with Their Decisions

Joann Paley Galst

Give sorrow words; the grief that does not speak knits up the o-er wrought heart and bids it break. William Shakespeare, Macbeth

> Melissa and Tom entered my office. She looked stunned. He kept glancing over at her anxiously, apparently checking to see if she was all right. When asked what brought them in, they looked at each other and he started talking, seemingly to protect her from the painful narrative. He explained how they recently lost their baby at 23 weeks. He reported Melissa was not eating or sleeping well and was overwhelmed with guilt. She quickly took over to explain in greater detail. As she revealed more of what happened to their baby, she tentatively acknowledged that they made a decision to terminate this pregnancy, their first, because of a diagnosis of a serious chromosomal anomaly with heart defects. Melissa carefully watched for my reaction to this disclosure.

In the past, when a woman became pregnant she typically gave birth to a baby unaware of any problems that the infant might have until after delivery. Prenatal testing has rapidly expanded and consequently, women (and their partners, if part of a couple) have been increasingly provided with information during a pregnancy indicating the viability and well-being of their fetus. Currently the power to diagnose fetal conditions exceeds the power to treat them. Thus, when presented with the identification of fetal anomaly, parents[1] face a Herculean task in deciding between continuing a pregnancy with a fetus that may not survive the pregnancy, have a shortened life expectancy or a compromised quality of life, or interrupting the pregnancy with limited time and limited information about the severity of

[1] The terms patient, client, and parent are used interchangeably in this chapter to refer to pregnant individuals (or their partner) facing a decision to continue or terminate a pregnancy with a fetal anomaly.

J.P. Galst, Ph.D. (✉)
30 E. 60th Street, Suite 802, New York, NY 10022, USA
e-mail: jgalst@aol.com

J.P. Galst, M.S. Verp (eds.), *Prenatal and Preimplantation Diagnosis*,
DOI 10.1007/978-3-319-18911-6_14

the problem(s). Parents, riddled with uncertainty, may feel torn between their connection to their unborn child and a desire to prevent the child's suffering, with most parents uninformed of resources available to raise a child with special needs.

Parents who become pregnant with high order multiple fetuses, usually after experiencing infertility and the use of assisted reproductive technology, may also be faced with making a decision to reduce the number of fetuses being gestated to improve the chances of a healthy pregnancy and outcome for the remaining fetuses, a particularly ironic dilemma after having faced infertility and the possibility of never conceiving any children. Additionally, through preimplantation genetic diagnosis and screening of embryos after an in vitro fertilization (IVF) cycle, embryonic quality can be determined, with doctors discarding abnormal embryos and transferring only chromosomally healthy embryos to the woman's uterus.

The strong cultural bias in the western world toward technological control of our environment may create a conflict when prenatal screening and diagnosis is offered to parents, as it may make quality control of offspring feel less like an option and more an obligation of responsible parenting (Boss 1999). Although limitless choices may be an ideal for some, for others it can feel like a burden. Furthermore, one cannot undo the knowledge of prenatal diagnostic testing results. Therefore, women and their partners must be made aware of the nature of the results they may receive so they can give fully informed consent to proceed with testing. No matter how well-informed patients may seem, however, parents are rarely prepared to be told they are carrying an imperfect fetus.

Pregnancy loss, a nonnormative loss, is a jarring deviation from most individual's assumptive world. A pregnancy termination due to fetal anomaly replaces the expectation of a normal healthy baby with a pregnancy defined by risk and/or the anticipation of death. It entails multiple losses, i.e., a wanted baby, future dreams, hopes, and possibilities, the parenting role, and the natural innocence embodied in the "just world belief" (i.e., if I follow the rules good things will happen). Additionally, parents' self-esteem suffers (biological for creating a pregnancy that ends in failure, moral for being responsible for ending the pregnancy, and social for feeling inadequate to take on the role of parenting a disabled child and alienated from others [White-Van Mourik et al. 1992]). Receiving a diagnosis of serious fetal anomaly and a subsequent decision to terminate are traumatic. Initially, parents may react with acute posttraumatic stress and later suffer from posttraumatic stress disorder (PTSD), depression, and/or persistent complex bereavement disorder (American Psychiatric Association 2013). Subsequent pregnancies may be marked by uncertainty as patients come to view them through the lens of risk, conditioned to expect loss.

Parents who choose to terminate their pregnancy must come to terms with the untimely death of their fetus (before birth), the role they played in determining it (if the pregnancy was viable), and what this means about themselves as the self-expected protectors of their child. Separation from their normal support systems often occurs, as parents rarely have exposure to others in similar circumstances. Pregnancy termination continues to be a politically charged and oftentimes stigmatized issue in our society, and parents often anticipate condemnation by others. Thus, many present the loss to others, if shared at all, as due to a spontaneous miscarriage (France et al. 2013). This secret grief makes it more difficult to reduce their feelings of shame regarding the termination. Parents, performing few rituals and without tangible memories, are frequently left on their own to grieve, often wondering whether they have the right to grieve and express their emotions because of their role in ending the pregnancy.

Prevalence of Termination Rates After Diagnosis of Fetal Anomaly

Termination rates for fetal anomaly vary by severity and type of anomaly. Schechtman et al. (2002) found that 72.5 % of pregnancies were terminated when the anomaly was likely to have a serious impact on the fetus's quality of life. Fetuses with central nervous system involvement were more likely to be terminated. Mansfield et al. (1999) compared five fetal anomalies (Down syndrome, spina bifida, anencephaly, Turner and Klinefelter syndromes), and found the highest termination rates for Down syndrome and the lowest for Klinefelter syndrome. Johnson et al. (2012) found that pregnancy termination rates were 83 % after a diagnosis of anencephaly and 63 % after spina bifida. Natoli et al. (2012) reviewed articles published between 1995 and 2011 and found an average of 67 % termination rates for Down syndrome in population-based studies and an 85 % rate in hospital-based studies, suggesting parents do not always report a termination when queried by researchers.

Termination rates for sex chromosome anomalies also vary depending on the diagnosis, from 42.9 % for mosaic sex chromosome abnormalities to 58–74 % for Klinefelter syndrome and 72–100 % for Turner syndrome (Hamamy and Dahoun 2004; Johnson et al. 2012; Mezei et al. 2004). Together, these studies demonstrate that the majority of patients receiving a diagnosis of serious fetal anomaly do make the decision to terminate rather than to continue the pregnancy.

Psychological Sequelae of Decisions After the Diagnosis of Prenatal Fetal Anomaly, Multifetal Pregnancy, or Preimplantation Genetic Diagnosis

A spontaneous pregnancy loss of a desired pregnancy can be experienced as a traumatic event, with 25 % of women at 1 month post-loss and 7 % at 4 months meeting criteria for PTSD. There is also an increased risk of comorbid depression with no decline between 1 and 4 months post-loss (Engelhard et al. 2001). Between 10 and 20 % of all bereaved individuals develop a complicated grief disorder, with the loss of a child, in general, being a very high risk factor (Kersting et al. 2011).

Most studies of parental reactions to terminating a pregnancy after a diagnosis of fetal anomaly (TOPFA) have, in fact, concluded it is experienced as an emotionally traumatic life event, as devastating, if not more so, than a spontaneous pregnancy loss. A TOPFA results in posttraumatic stress symptoms and intense grief reactions for a substantial number of women, especially when the decision to terminate takes place in the second or third trimester (Iles and Gath 1993; Kersting et al. 2007; Kersting and Wagner 2012; Korenromp et al. 2009). An unanticipated diagnosis, the responsibility for decision-making, waiting for labor, and delivering a dead fetus can all contribute to the trauma. Korenromp and her colleagues reported approximately 44–46 % of women meet criteria for PTSD and 28 % for depression at 4 months post-TOPFA. Sixteen months post-TOPFA, although rates declined to 20 % for PTSD and 13 % for depression, high degrees of psychological morbidity continued (Korenromp et al. 2007, 2009). Davies et al. (2005) found even higher levels of emotional distress. At 6 weeks post-termination, 67 % of their sample of women screened positive for posttraumatic stress, 47 % for grief, and 30 % for depression. Women's distress at 6 months were 50, 31 and 39 %, respectively, and, although rates declined at 12 months, to 41 % for PTS and 27 % for grief, these figures are quite substantial. At 12–14 months after a TOPFA, 14–20 % of women meet full diagnostic criteria for a complicated grief disorder (Kersting et al. 2007; Korenromp et al. 2009). It is important to note, however, women who received a diagnosis of fetal anomaly were reported to experience intense grief, whether they chose termination, palliative care, or perinatal hospice care for their pregnancies (Wool 2011).

Although men's emotional reactions are often ignored in favor of their wives' distress, men also show high degrees of psychological morbidity post-termination. While generally lower than women, 22 % of men post-TOPFA demonstrated symptoms of posttraumatic stress and 16 % showed depressive symptomatology (Korenromp et al. 2007), highlighting the importance of including both parents in psychological counseling.

Approximately 75 % of women stated they "just wanted to die" after experiencing a TOPFA (while not the equivalent of suicidality, suicidal intent should be investigated in this population). Most female patients felt totally unprepared for the protracted emotional pain that they experienced following the termination (McCoyd 2007). Yet, despite enduring levels of posttraumatic and emotional distress for upwards of 1 year or more post-termination, only 2–2.7 % of women and 1 % of men regretted their decision (Korenromp et al. 2005a, 2007).

A multifetal pregnancy (MFP), often thought of as an abundance of riches to a couple who has experienced infertility, can quickly become another burden of choice to parents if a high-order (three or more fetuses) MFP is diagnosed on ultrasound. Parents often are faced with the decision to reduce the number of fetuses that the woman is carrying in an attempt to ensure the best chance of a positive outcome for their pregnancy. Despite attempts to reduce the frequency of multiple births around the world by educating both physicians and patients of the risks (ESHRE Task Force on Ethics and Law 2003; Practice Committee of the American Society for Reproductive Medicine 2012), most parents report being relatively unaware of the risks of multiples as they undergo IVF. Although it is possible some may not have received adequate information before the decision regarding intrauterine insemination or number of embryos to transfer during an IVF cycle, it is also important to understand that a diagnosis of infertility in and of itself appears to make it difficult for people to fully contemplate the possibility of getting pregnant with too many babies when they have lived with the fear of never having any children.

There are relatively few studies regarding the psychological ramifications of multifetal reduction (MFR) on parents. Studies have generally concluded most parents find the procedure quite stressful and emotionally distressing, with both women and men frequently experiencing initial feelings of sadness, guilt, grief, and fear for the well-being of the remaining fetuses. However, no serious long-term adverse effect on parents' mental health has been reported after a MFR when the pregnancy outcome was successful (Garel et al. 1997; Maifeld et al. 2003; McKinney et al. 1995; Schreiner-Engel et al. 1995). Additionally, the vast majority of patients undergoing a MFR reported believing they made the right decision or would make the same decision again. The levels of reported anxiety and grief both on the day of the procedure and at follow-up have been reported to be higher for parents who terminate for fetal anomaly than for those who reduce one or more fetuses in a MFP (Maschiach et al. 2013). Nevertheless, there is a subgroup for whom negative feelings may increase at the time of delivery or not resolve until approximately 2 years post-MFR, particularly if the woman had prior psychological problems, was more religious, younger, or saw the fetuses multiple times on ultrasound (Maifeld et al. 2003; Schreiner-Engel et al. 1995). Note, however, that women continuing a triplet pregnancy reported high levels of anxiety and depression and more difficulty relating to their children than mothers of pregnancies reduced to twins at 2 years after birth (Garel et al. 1997).

If an anomaly is discovered in one or more of the fetuses, the decision of which to reduce becomes less agonizing for parents. If not, the decision can be experienced as a more intense moral dilemma, and the fact that the physician usually chooses which fetus(es) to reduce takes some of this burden from parents' shoulders.

Parents reducing a MFP face the same dilemma as those terminating a pregnancy for fetal anomaly, that is, whether or not to tell their surviving children of the reduction. While there is no guidance in the literature, parents experiencing MFR are concerned that these children may develop feelings of survivor guilt or come to view their parents negatively (see Chap. 15).

Preimplantation genetic diagnosis (PGD) offers known carriers of a genetic disease the opportunity to avoid passing this disorder on to their children. Preimplantation genetic screening (PGS) allows parents undergoing IVF, usually for infertility, to detect chromosomal anomalies in embryos before an embryo is transferred to the woman's uterus. Both PGD and PGS require a woman to undergo one or more IVF cycles to obtain adequate numbers of embryos for testing. However, even after PGD/PGS, prenatal diagnostic testing is recommended to check for accuracy. Moreover, despite this testing, there remains the same 3 % baseline risk for other congenital abnormalities that do not stem from a single-gene defect or chromosomal aberration (e.g., spina bifida, anencephaly) as in the general population. Affected embryos will be discarded and this decision usually lies with the medical professionals and not the patient. For many women these procedures can eliminate the necessity to end a pregnancy and reduce the psychological trauma of a termination.

Most individuals, particularly those who have already given birth to a child with a genetic anomaly or undergone a TOPFA, favor PGD over prenatal diagnosis (Kalfoglou et al. 2005; Katz et al. 2002; Lavery et al. 2002), although many patients report the treatment cycle to be stressful and voice concern about potential damage to embryos, low success rates, and high costs (Lavery et al. 2002). Whether to test for adult-onset diseases or to transfer embryos that are carriers of a disease but will be unaffected themselves remains controversial (Bodkin 1998; Kalfoglou et al. 2005), and one wonders at which point screening for inherited diseases may turn into selecting for superior traits.

At present, there is no data to inform us of the parental psychological implication of discarding affected embryos and transferring others. Questions remain about the effect parents' ability to control for medical conditions, psychological qualities, or physical characteristics may have on the parent–child relationship. Once again, technology has outpaced our consideration of the relevant ethical issues.

Risk Factors After Termination of Pregnancy for Fetal Anomaly

Being confronted with a decision as to whether to terminate or continue a pregnancy with a known fetal anomaly is considered traumatic for most people. Individual risk factors for long term distress after a TOPFA include: high levels of decisional conflict; high distress levels immediately after the termination; low self-efficacy; lack of support from one's partner or incongruence between partners' grief and coping; low perceived social support; advanced gestational age; a diagnosis compatible with life; a prior history of trauma and/or mental health issues; having no other children; and coping through avoidance of one's emotions and memories (Kersting et al. 2007; Korenromp et al. 2005a, 2007, 2009; LaFarge et al. 2013). Although regrets about the decision are rare, parents at high risk are likely to benefit from intensified support.

It is wise for clinicians to assess a patient's coping skills with prior losses, as this may indicate the need for additional support. If patients are experiencing any concurrent stressors or crises (e.g., having undergone infertility treatment to become pregnant), ancillary assistance may be required.

Gender Differences and Impact on the Couple Relationship

Parents typically appear equally devastated upon receiving the diagnosis of fetal anomaly. However, discordance between partners in grieving and the pace of recovery often emerges after only a few weeks post-TOPFA. Many men have been socialized to be strong, protective, and exhibit no weakness in times of distress (Doka and Martin 2010), and they can internalize this gender role socialization as their mandate. Receiving the news they are pregnant, many women alter their behaviors (e.g., eliminate caffeine and alcohol intake), center their lives on the well-being of the child, and take complete responsibility for the child's welfare long before birth. Pregnancy is a more abstract experience for men. This lack of synchrony between partners may contribute to the 12 % of couples separating after a TOPFA (Seller et al. 1993).

The requirement that women provide informed consent for a pregnancy termination may result in feelings of greater responsibility for the decision. A man often defers to his partner, respecting a woman's right to make decisions involving her own body. However, this abdication can create an excessive burden on women with resulting exacerbated guilt. It has been reported that women experience higher levels of pathological posttraumatic stress after a TOPFA, recover more slowly than their male partners, and may have more frequent emotional setbacks over the first few years after a termination, e.g., resurgence of grief on anniversary dates (Korenromp et al. 2005b; Sandelowski and Barroso 2005). In general, when confronted with loss, women's grief tends to be more loss-oriented, while men's is more restoration-oriented (Stroebe and Schut 1999). However, a man's stoicism can be misunderstood as being uncaring and unaffected. Men do, in fact, have negative feelings after a TOPFA. But fathers more quickly internalize their feelings and focus on practical tasks (e.g., arranging a funeral, caring for other children when their wife is unable, and returning to work [Kaasen et al. 2013; Locock and Alexander 2006; White-van Mourik et al. 1992]). Additionally, clinical experience suggests that men fear that if they should express their emotions, their wife's sadness would be exacerbated. Losses experienced by men typically are not acknowledged by others. Rather, people usually inquire how their wives are faring after a loss, which further reinforces the idea that men should be concerned with their wives and not themselves. Thus, if a man accepts his gender socialized role to be stoic, he risks alienating his wife because she may wish to emotionally experience their loss together.

It is important to educate grieving mothers and fathers about these common gender differences in processing and coping with loss to reduce misunderstanding of incongruent grief. Clinically, it is helpful to include both members of a couple in counseling and to encourage a man to listen and validate his wife's feelings and also to express his own feelings and need for support, as this gives women the opportunity to discover the strength still residing within her, as the wife, in turn, provides support to her spouse.

Emotional Support for Parents Confronting Decisions After Diagnosis of Fetal Anomaly

Medical personnel are the front line of support to parents confronting a fetal abnormality. Patients have reported even years later their appreciation for a kind word or gentle touch from their doctor or nurse. The following human elements of care have been reported as highly valued by patients both before and after a TOPFA (Asplin et al. 2014; Korenromp et al. 2005a; Lalor et al. 2007; McCoyd 2009):

- Good communication: private, nonjudgmental, without jargon and at a level patients can understand; prompt referral to specialists for diagnostic confirmation; and sensitivity to language (i.e., pregnancy termination or interruption, as opposed to "abortion" which is stigmatizing).
- Attentive listening: giving adequate time to patients, including answering their questions, and allowing their expression, often intense, of feelings; scheduling appointments when the physician has sufficient time and when fewer pregnant patients are in the waiting room; mirroring the terminology used by the patients for their baby, including using the baby's name if one had been given.
- Genuine compassion: empathy, sensitivity, supportive gestures such as therapeutic touch; acknowledgement of men's experiences not merely as supporters of their wives.
- Creating and collecting mementos for the parents: giving them to parents or keeping them for later, as many parents later change their minds and return to try to collect these keepsakes.
- Continuity of care: designate one person with whom patients can stay in touch to prevent patients' feeling abandoned by medical professionals.
- Providing written materials: adequate explanation of the procedure patients will undergo and the common physical and emotional reactions during recovery.
- Scheduling follow-up meetings: allow time for further questions. As it is common for patients to think you will expect them to be healthy both physically and emotionally at the first follow-up visit, it is important to disabuse them of this expectation, and inform them of the common long-term course of healing from their loss.

If the anomaly is compatible with life and parents choose to continue their pregnancy, health-care professionals should leave parents' hope for their children intact, i.e., they will be able to participate in many normal childhood activities. If appropriate, information regarding options for adoptive or foster care placement of the baby can be offered (Sheets et al. 2011), although these choices are made less frequently than termination of the pregnancy (National Council for Adoption 1999).

If the pregnancy is nonviable, the patients will need reassurance that medical personnel will be available to support them throughout the pregnancy and birth, as well as afterwards. Appropriate referral to resources for perinatal palliative or hospice care can also be made.

Although a subsequent pregnancy can contribute to the emotional healing process for patients, the pregnancy itself may provoke mixed emotions and intensified anxiety. Due to the potential deleterious effects of negative maternal mental health on self-care during a pregnancy and on an infant's emotional and cognitive development (Kinsella and Monk 2009; O'Connor et al. 2002), referral for additional support may be beneficial. Patients who have undergone a prior TOPFA report a need for reassurance that all is going well in their pregnancies. Furthermore, they want others to understand, not pathologize, their intensified anxiety. Many report emotionally cushioning, or holding back from attaching to the fetus, in an attempt to protect themselves emotionally from the impact of another trauma (Cote'-Arsenault and Donato 2011).

When to Consider Referral to a Mental Health Professional (MHP)

Grief is a normal, albeit challenging, part of life and most patients will recover from their grief and won't need professional help. However, when applied to grieving individuals who developed elevated and persistent distress, psychotherapeutic intervention did result in more significant and enduring improvement compared to the outcome in those who did not receive psychotherapy (Neimeyer and Currier 2010). Thus, it is important for medical personnel to identify those parents who are at increased risk of pathological reactions and who would benefit from referral to psychological services.

The following symptoms can indicate a need to refer to a MHP: (1) Evidence of a major depressive episode: lack of self-care, indication of active suicidality, chronic insomnia, anorexia, poor grooming, and inability to care for other children in the household. (2) Symptoms remain at severe levels 4 months after loss. Posttraumatic stress symptoms 4 months after a TOPFA were associated with maladjustment later (Korenromp et al. 2009). (3) Persistent symptoms with intensity increasing 6 months after a TOPFA, and evidence of PTSD symptoms on a daily basis (e.g., continuing flashbacks, intrusive thoughts, guilt, ruminations). An encouraging and supportive referral to a MHP with whom the health-care provider has a collaborative relationship can reduce patients' negative stereotypes and ambivalence about the therapeutic process.

Psychotherapeutic Treatment for Parents After Termination of Pregnancy for Fetal Anomaly

The loss of a child during pregnancy, particularly after termination due to fetal abnormalities, may be particularly difficult to grieve as there is no dramatic absence of a person to signal the loss and confirm its reality. It is difficult to recollect the unborn child because there are few concrete memories shared with others. Both PTSD and complicated grief reactions by parents have been documented in parents after undergoing a TOPFA (Kersting et al. 2007; Korenromp et al. 2009). In contrast to a typical grief reaction, the traumatically bereaved individual tends to be preoccupied with the circumstances of the death, although he/she often tries to avoid reminders of their loss, and hypervigilantly oriented to threat as the world seems unsafe to them. The experience of prior pregnancy loss may also affect subsequent pregnancies, as close to 30 % of women have been found to develop a posttraumatic stress disorder during the pregnancy following a stillbirth (Turton et al. 2001).

Given the similarity of some symptoms of PTSD and complicated grief, for example intrusions, avoidance, and maladaptive appraisals (American Psychiatric Association 2013), and because trauma, grief, and depression interface in multiple ways in many parents after a TOPFA, it may not always be possible to distinguish between them in the typical clinical practice. For those clinicians interested in assessment, useful and well-validated measures include, the Complicated Grief Inventory (Prigerson et al. 1995), Perinatal Grief Scale (Toedter et al. 1988), Edinburgh Postnatal Depression Scale (Cox et al. 1987), Impact of Event Scale (Horowitz et al. 1979), Clinician-Administered PTSD Scale for DSM-5 (Weathers et al. 2014), and Posttraumatic Stress Disorder Checklist (Weathers et al. 1991). The Grief and Mourning Status Interview and Inventory (GAMSII) is also useful in guiding the clinical interview of these parents (Rando 1993).

Although most individuals eventually grieve losses successfully, the intensity of emotions after a TOPFA can be overwhelming. Often mothers are frightened by their emotions and fathers report being afraid of their wives' reactions. Thus, there may be greater need for support and outside intervention for this traumatic loss.

There is currently no robust empirically validated treatment protocol for parents who have lost a child after a TOPFA nor for women pregnant subsequent to this loss. Rather than using a stage model of bereavement, the present author has been guided by Rando's (1993) proposed six nonlinear, overlapping "R" processes of mourning (1993), including recognizing the loss (avoidance phase), reacting to the separation, recollecting and reexperiencing the deceased and the relationship, relinquishing the old attachments to the deceased and the old assumptive world (confrontation phase), readjusting to move adaptively into the new world without forgetting the old, and reinvesting in their life (accommodation phase), although some of the processes are particularly difficult for this population to navigate as there are so few tangible experiences and memories of their pregnancy and their baby available to these parents.

The author's psychotherapeutic treatment of these parents has been guided by an integration of research regarding treatments for both grief and trauma. Empirical studies have demonstrated trauma-focused cognitive behavioral interventions, including psychoeducation, imaginal exposure to counter avoidance and reduce the arousal and distress associated with memories of the trauma, anxiety management to cope with stress, cognitive behavior therapy (CBT) techniques to address automatic distorted thinking patterns that often perpetuate PTSD symptoms, and between-sessions home practice are effective in addressing symptoms of acute stress, PTSD (Bisson and Andrew 2007; Bryant et al. 2013; Foa et al. 2009; Mendes et al. 2008; Powers et al. 2010; Resick et al. 2002; Seidler and Wagner 2006), and complicated grief (Shear et al. 2005). In my experience, adding specifics relevant to traumatic loss in this particular population, including addressing guilt, self-blame, feeling betrayed by one's body and G-d, and grappling with the meaning of this loss is also essential.

Recently, a brief Internet-based intervention for pregnancy loss, incorporating exposure techniques, cognitive reappraisal, and social sharing was found to significantly reduce symptoms of posttraumatic stress, prolonged grief, depression, and anxiety relative to a wait-list control group (Kersting et al. 2013). This approach via the Internet may prove particularly useful for those who do not have access to a MHP familiar with this therapeutic orientation. Thus, including elements of CBT seems reasonable to recommend at this time (Bradley et al. 2005; Koopmans et al. 2013; Wittouck et al. 2011). Furthermore, eye movement desensitization and reprocessing (Shapiro 2001) may also be beneficial for processing traumatic memories.

First phase of psychotherapeutic support. Despite undergoing prenatal screening, most parents expect confirmation of a healthy pregnancy, not indication of any abnormality. The majority of parents with whom I have worked have sought psychological support within a matter of weeks post-TOPFA. Some patients worried about how they would react with the passage of time, but others present with acute stress reactions. Early presentation to a MHP may also reflect the sensitivity and concern of medical personnel.

I highly recommend seeing both members of a couple after a TOPFA, especially for the initial session, as a way of supporting and validating their common loss and giving the clinician an opportunity to determine how both members are coping. During this session, psycho-education regarding the normal course of bereavement and the variable grief reactions and coping techniques often presented by women and men is provided to the couple. This is particularly important so as not to pathologize the grief process.

The role of the MHP in the early stages of traumatic grief for a TOPFA is to engage in a skilled, supportive manner, acting as a crucible for the individual's intensely painful feelings, helping to stabilize the patients and minimize the anxiety and stress brought on by the trauma, and providing information and guidance to assist him or her to understand their grief and mourning needs.

I have found the following goals useful when patients come to therapy within the first month or 2 after a TOPFA:

- Establish rapport and trust. A strong therapeutic alliance can begin to be built by showing an empathic, nonjudgmental attitude, addressing the baby by the term the parents use or the name they have given their baby, as well as containing the intensity of the feeling expressed in the first session. Demonstrating respect for individual diversity in grief, for the deceased child, and for the difficult position the parents have encountered is crucial in developing trust and reducing the real or perceived stigma parents may feel for having terminated their pregnancy. Being sensitive to culturally diverse approaches to grief and independently researching or inquiring about the patients' customs, traditions, and rituals, when necessary, is paramount.
- Ensure patients are stabilized. Assess their sleep patterns and ability to consume adequate nutrition for sustenance, suicidality, and ability to take care of other children, if present (and help arrange support if needed). Assessment may result in more urgent intervention prior to beginning therapy. Many patients, however,

express a passive wish to die after this trauma (McCoyd 2007), which can be differentiated from an actual suicidal threat. Continue to monitor vegetative and functional behaviors during treatment. Suggestions for self-care (e.g., sleep hygiene, nutritional intake, and light exercise) should be provided. Additionally, ask about prior or concurrent traumas and stressors to determine if immediate intensive care is needed.

- Provide the opportunity for parents to share their story in your presence. Validate the significance of this loss. Let parents know you are willing to witness with them their experience of decision-making, the days leading up to and including the termination, the details of their procedure, and whether they were able to or chose to see/hold/spend time with their baby, which supports their right to their feelings about this experience. Additionally, soothing and containment may be offered as affect-evoking techniques need to be cautiously used at this point to avoid premature termination from psychotherapy.

  Later, you may ask parents to share tangible mementos they have, often in the form of a memory box given to them at the hospital. However, many patients may be reluctant to share a photo, fearing you may have a negative reaction to their baby's appearance. Thus, if parents do take the risk and share a picture with you, it is important to note and positively comment on certain features (e.g., their baby's perfectly formed fingers or a sweetly shaped mouth). Sharing these mementoes further validates their experience of losing a baby for whom they had dreams of a very different outcome.
- Determine how the couple is coping. Are both having symptoms of trauma and/or grief? Are there opportunities for each to express his or her feelings as well as provide support to the other? Is one member of the couple frightened and overwhelmed by the emotions of the other and suggesting the other is abnormally reacting or is mired in grief and should be moving on? Have either turned to self-destructive behaviors to avoid their emotional pain?
- Psycho-education. This is an opportunity for the MHP to provide normative information about the traumatic grief process (symptoms, adaptation, and recovery), and common gender differences in coping with loss. Patients are often surprised once the initial emotional shock passes to find they feel much worse. Men often worry that instead of getting better, their wives feelings are intensifying. Family and friends often want a woman to put this experience behind her as quickly as possible. Thus, it is important to educate the grieving couple about common feelings after this type of loss and validate they will not just "get over" their traumatic loss. While this experience will likely change the couple, frequently in positive ways, it takes time for these changes to evolve and intense feelings typically last for one or more years, especially for women.

  Help patients comprehend the many losses of this experience (e.g., a much wanted baby; innocence and a sense of personal invulnerability; a belief in a just and fair world, and the loss of faith that things will work out well). Inform patients of symptoms of major depression, PTSD, and complicated grief that may indicate that additional psychological help may be needed. I introduce the dual process model of adaptive coping (Stroebe and Schut 1999), explaining the oscillations between a loss focus (i.e., reflections about their loss which often generate sad and painful emotions) and a restoration focus (i.e., creating and executing concrete plans for moving toward valued life goals and restoring pleasant activities). This validates patients' experience as they will reestablish some balance in their lives as time passes, and can remove some of the guilt women, in particular, feel when they are able to experience even momentary glimpses of happiness again. I encourage patients after the first month or so following their loss to allow themselves some daily time to think about their baby and set time boundaries of approximately 20–30 min. Furthermore, I address coping techniques (e.g., cognitive restructuring techniques, differentiating possibility and probability, grounding techniques). I also prepare patients for the fact that while spousal, family, and community support may be quite strong in the first few weeks after loss, this support may continue for too brief a period of time (Geerinck-Vercammen and Kahai 2003).

- Offer practical help:

The couple relationship: Facilitate communication, stress the individual's needs for solitary time; help them find ways to work through their potentially disparate desires for communication, physical intimacy, and a sexual relationship. Help them accept differences in grieving and coping behaviors.

Return to work: Patients benefit from some specific input regarding when and how to return to work (e.g., suggest people at work be notified by one colleague about the reason for their absence; walking into work with a friend from work helps patients tolerate the stares from others; advise returning to one's place of employment mid-week so the mourner does not have to work a full week their first week back), and help the parent accept she or he temporarily will be unlikely to function at their prior level of capability because of difficulties in focus and concentration.

Follow-up medical visits: Planning a return to their doctor is also stressful for patients. MHPs can suggest clients request to be seen when fewer pregnant women are in the office. Patients find sensitively being taken to a private room upon entering helpful. Assist them in creating a list of questions to ask their physician and to accept they may experience emotion in the presence of the doctor.

Negotiating the social context: One's partner may be unable to provide all of the support needed after a loss. Helping patients identify a range of social support is beneficial. Managing patients' expectations of others also helps. Friends, family, and coworkers may provide relief and comfort when one experiences intensified emotional states. However, some will not be supportive and others may say nothing at all to the patient. Lack of adequate social support is commonly reported by patients and usually attributed by grieving parents to insensitivity. Regrettably, family and friends may minimize the loss, ask inappropriate questions, or make simplistic or dismissive suggestions. For example, telling parents they can have another child tends to discount the attachment the parent may feel and suggest that one can simply replace one baby or one pregnancy with another. Those who may not have been informed of the true nature of the loss may view miscarriage as a common occurrence. Others may have no experience with traumatic loss and incorrectly assume parents will recover quickly. Alternatively, the powerful emotions which parents demonstrate may overwhelm friends and family who may feel awkward and not know what to say to the grieving parents. On the other hand, this loss may evoke intense feelings of personal vulnerability in other young individuals and/or couples who are also in their childbearing years. It is important to validate the mourner's feelings and MHPs should support their need to distance from some people for self-protection. Their view of others, however, can often be softened by gently having clients acknowledge that before this loss, they, too, would not have understood what others in the situation were feeling. It has been my experience that this can reduce their sense of isolation and estrangement from others. In addition, since people often take their cues from the bereaved individual, discussion of how to transmit the signals they want to express to others (i.e., to approach them or not) can be helpful.

Supporting the grieving process in an unsympathetic social context: Some people indicate to the parent that she should be "moving on." However, the mourner may resent this as she can erroneously believe sustaining her sorrow is respectful of the deceased child. Initially, the parent may only know how to maintain the bond with the lost fetus/child through sadness and tears, actually feeling disloyal when she is not crying. It is therapeutic to help parents find other ways to remember and honor their baby. Additionally, I have found after a TOPFA, parents tend to exclusively focus on what might have been the best possible outcome for their baby, not the most likely based on the diagnostic information they have received (one reason consulting with various specialists prior to making their decision is important). This is an example of a hindsight bias which makes it easy to believe the decision was unjustified and one should have made a different decision. It will be important for the MHP to contextualize the decision-making process under traumatic circumstances, helping patients rediscover what they were thinking or feeling as they were making their decision. Often parents had limited time, yet still typically did enormous amounts of research to inform their decision. Frequently, parents come to believe they feel such deep and agonizing pain because they made the wrong decision. Patients can be helped to recognize they are crying for the existence of the abnormality in their baby and having been forced to make such a difficult decision rather than for the actual decision, painful though it remains.

Needs of surviving children: If there are other children in the household, helping parents understand the grief and mourning needs of surviving children is important (see Chap. 15). Many parents do not believe their young children know anything unusual is happening within the family. This may reflect parental denial, a desire to protect their children from emotional pain, or a lack of understanding young children's developmental needs for security and safety, which results in their acute sensitivity to the emotional environment around them, especially in their parents, who are their source of security.

Most parents who tell their child of the death of the baby, do not inform them of the termination decision, however (France et al. 2013).

- Teach self-soothing techniques (e.g., breathing retraining, grounding techniques, distress tolerance skills [Linehan 1993]). These can help patients who struggle with intense emotions, but should not be used to direct all of the patient's attention away from their grief.
- Provide relevant resources including books, reputable online resources, local support groups addressing a TOPFA, facilitating contact with others who have gone through a similar experience (see Appendix). Before referring to support groups, determine if it would be beneficial for the couple, i.e., they appear able to tolerate hearing others' stories, receive support from others and usefully process it, and offer support to others even as grieving themselves. Often women's natural tendency to "tend and befriend" under stress (Taylor et al. 2000) means that they will more naturally gravitate to others during difficult times, whereas men may feel more comfortable handling things independently and need encouragement to attend a support group with their wives. I have found this beneficial to both members of the couple.
- Facilitate rituals. Many rituals have likely been completed, but helping parents consider their wishes for future milestone dates (e.g., due date, anniversary date of loss, Mother's/Father's Day) can be introduced briefly at this juncture along with informing parents of emotions that commonly arise on these occasions. Help the couple create daily time, with boundaries, to discuss their experiences, thoughts, feelings, and needs so as to keep lines of communication open between them.

Parents and the MHP may determine collaboratively that this is sufficient intervention at this time. A follow-up call is often appreciated with a reminder that the MHP will remain available for consultation and support should it be requested.

Middle phase of psychotherapeutic support (after approximately 2 months post-loss). The role of the MHP at this time becomes that of expert companion, one who guides patients through the aftermath of a highly stressful event. The MHP can help parents face and manage their emotional distress, facilitating a new understanding of the world, their beliefs, and their goals. Moreover, MHPs can assist their patients to revise their life narrative as a result of the changes imposed by this experience, and, hopefully, guide them from "merely suffering to suffering meaningfully" (Tedeschi and Calhoun 2009). A collaborative relationship between the MHP and client empowers parents to face their feelings and can allow the return of some sense of control as parents help guide the pace of the therapy.

PTSD and prolonged grief after a TOPFA show a good deal of symptom overlap, as both can involve intrusive thoughts and avoidance behavior. At this stage of traumatic grief, three aspects of the loss may need to be addressed by a MHP: (1) intrusive thoughts, emotions, and sensory experiences and the tendency to try to avoid these (addressed through exposure work), (2) extreme guilt (cognitive restructuring and reappraisal), and (3) isolation and feeling stuck in grief (rebuilding one's life, relationships with others, and preparing for the future). Treatments including imaginal reliving, in vivo exposure, and cognitive processing therapy have shown promise in effectively reducing the intensity of grief and PTSD symptoms (Resick and Schnicke 1993; Shear et al. 2005). In addition, the author has found Stroebe and Schut's (1999) dual process model of bereavement effective in helping patients to: (1) focus on their loss and concomitant feelings at times, and (2) titrate their pain by setting aside difficult memories and feelings to allow for replenishment of their emotional strength at other times.

I have found the following goals useful for patients who are approximately 2 months or more post-TOPFA:

- Provide a rationale for the treatment of PTSD and traumatic grief the MHP intends to use, including the benefit of exposure, the relationship between thoughts and feelings, the importance of meaning attached to events, and building one's internal and interpersonal resources.
- Assess patients' resources, coping skills, and attachment history, as they are relevant to the ability to manage both the experience and the therapy for traumatic bereavement. Coping strategies will be utilized to help patients focus on their loss, tolerate their strong feelings, and focus on restoration. Teach techniques of distress tolerance and emotional regulation (if not already introduced). Techniques of dialectical behavior therapy are useful to help patients learn how to tolerate and modulate their affect, and soothe themselves after they have completed the proposed therapeutic exercises (Linehan 1993).
- Loss focus. Exposure to traumatic, often intrusive, memories in a safe environment has been demonstrated to be a key element in effective psychotherapy both for PTSD (Bradley et al. 2005; Foa et al. 2009; Resick and Schnicke 1993) and complicated grief (Bisson and Andrew 2007; Boelen et al 2007; Shear et al 2005; Wittouck et al. 2011). If a patient avoids thinking of their painful memories, they may not really look at the full context of what happened, i.e., what they did and why. If avoidance is part of the patient's symptom presentation, I have incorporated suggestions involving prolonged exposure, from Resick and Schnicke (1993) cognitive processing therapy for trauma, i.e., having parents write an *Impact Statement* giving a full account of their experience of this trauma and its impact on them (from learning of a problem through the termination procedure and after), or Shear et al.'s (2005) *Imaginal Revisiting* of the trauma, which is audio recorded in session. For both, patients are asked to write (by hand) or speak their account of the traumatic events in the first person, present tense, with the inclusion of as many sensory details, thoughts, and feelings that they had at the time that they can handle. Moreover, patients are encouraged to experience their current emotions as fully as possible to allow the affective elements of the stored trauma memory to be revised and distress lessened over repeated exposures. The therapist can insert questions to help patients remember why they made the choices they made, e.g., What were you thinking as this was happening? What were you feeling? What were you thinking right before you made the decision? What information did you actually have at the time of the decision?

Self-soothing techniques may be used before and after the exposure, but not during the exposure so as not to reinforce avoidance of their emotional experience. It is important for the MHP to normalize the tendency to want to avoid this aspect of the therapy, while emphasizing its effectiveness in decreasing long-term distress. Reinforcing the parent's capability to experience intense emotions without being disabled by them allows individuals to regain feelings of control over their emotions. This exercise will be repeated, encouraging the client to add more sensory and emotional details, if deemed appropriate for patient progress.

Parents are asked to read or listen to their account in session, giving the MHP an opportunity to periodically determine the level of distress by asking the patient to rate their distress level at various times in retelling their story, and to determine some of their problem areas. These might include "stuck points" or "hot spots," i.e., detailed memories of peak emotional distress, distorted interpretations about the trauma, or unrealistic beliefs about themselves and others that are keeping them from being able to effectively process the trauma. They are asked between scheduled appointments to read or listen to this account daily during the time they have set aside to think about their loss. When thoughts of their loss arise outside of these time-bounded periods, the patient is advised to change their focus to something else and postpone focusing on these thoughts until their chosen time to concentrate on or address the loss. This can help patients regain some sense of control over their intrusive thoughts and reduce their overwhelming feelings of sadness, anxiety, or guilt. Impact statements are rewritten or revisiting experiences rerecorded throughout therapy as processing of the trauma progresses. If patients are avoiding specific situations, a hierarchy can be created which allows gradual in vivo exposure to avoided situations, beginning with the situation that is least distressing to the client. Note that fear may be more responsive to exposure techniques whereas guilt may respond better to cognitive reappraisal techniques (Rothbaum et al. 2000).

- Cognitive restructuring and reappraisal: These CBT techniques have been used to rebuild the shattered assumptions of the self and the world (Janoff-Bulman 1992) and address the self-blame and guilt typically demonstrated by individuals after a TOPFA. Positive reappraisal has been associated with less intense grief in parents who terminate for fetal abnormality (LaFarge et al. 2013). Reinforce the fact that information regarding a severe fetal anomaly during pregnancy does, in fact, rupture expectations about pregnancy, parenthood, and family, as these losses and the lingering shame of this experience are often unrecognized by patients and others within their environment. As part of the process of cognitive restructuring, patients need to actively incorporate updated information ("I know now") into the worst moments of their trauma memory, and be helped to discriminate between stimuli present during the trauma ("then") and the current retriggering stimuli of reexperiencing symptoms ("now"), recognizing that experiences can be transformed from a more distant perspective (Ehlers et al. 2004). Socratic questioning is used to challenge examples of distorted cognitions about the trauma parents may have, especially those of self-blame, hindsight bias, and other guilt cognitions (for example, offering the following questions to challenge their automatic thoughts: What is the evidence for/against this idea?; Are you thinking in all-or-nothing terms or in extreme or exaggerated terms?; Are your judgments based on feelings rather than facts?; How would you react to a good friend thinking this way if they experienced the same situation?). Parents taught to use this method will learn how to challenge their own cognitive distortions when they arise outside of the therapy session.

Address feelings of guilt. Parents often express self-doubt about whether they made the right choice, whether they should have made a different decision, whether they are properly grieving, remembering the baby properly, wallowing, or making others uncomfortable. They need help to discover that they had no good option, that they made the decision that they determined was the least bad one, and that now they would be suffering whatever choice they made. Guilt can be alleviated by recognizing that when all available options have negative outcomes, the least bad choice can be a highly moral choice (Kubany and Watson 2003).

They also need to be reassured there is no right or wrong way to grieve. Feelings of guilt or betrayal of their lost child when a parent is not showing intense sadness or the belief that if her pain diminishes she will lose her only attachment to the baby must also be addressed. I try to help patients realize with time they will remember and honor their unborn child in ways other than tears, and explain that with time, they will develop practices that are meaningful to them. I have found that wearing symbolic jewelry often reminds mothers and others of how much their child is loved.

Intense guilt for having been instrumental in the decision to end this wanted pregnancy (emotional culpability) differentiates this experience from that of a spontaneous pregnancy loss and may compromise the grieving process. Patients may see themselves as active agents versus tragic recipients of a spontaneous loss. Parents may feel guilty for having felt relief in having prevented the birth of a severely disabled child. Guilt may lead to self-punishment or self-destructive behavior, or be projected onto others (e.g., spouse) which can disrupt relationships. However, when both having the baby and not having the baby felt wrong and parents are responsible to make a decision, guilt may be inescapable. Cognitive Processing Therapy has been found to be effective in reducing trauma-related guilt cognitions (Nishith et al. 2005). Although women having a spontaneous loss often blame themselves, believing they "might have" done something wrong or "could have" done something differently to avoid the loss, parents after a TOPFA know they actively made a decision that resulted in ending the life of their unborn baby.

Women often state with intense pain, "*Mothers are supposed to protect their children, but I killed my baby.*" MHPs should not try to remove guilt feelings too quickly, but rather determine their cause (e.g., the personal value or belief that patients deem they violated; denial of the sense of helplessness the parent feels; a belief that bad outcomes should be punished) and help patients accept their feelings. However, if these thoughts continue, the MHP will try to help the patient transform guilt to regret by reframing the belief from "*I am a murderer/I shouldn't have done this,*" to "*I did make the decision to end my baby's life and I wish I would have had a different option that would have allowed my baby to lead a full life without ongoing physical pain, suffering, or a life-limiting condition.*" Asking patients what their intent was (i.e., to harm or protect), what positive aims the decision served, and what evidence contrary to the overgeneralized belief, "I am a murderer," they have, can help them develop a more balanced view of what they did, why they did it, and who they are, else they may continue to believe that they don't deserve to feel better because of what they did. Patients come to recognize that although they did end the life of their baby, the decision was made from love, based on their assessment of the quality of life this baby would have and the impact this would have on their family. MHPs help patients come to accept that without intention to do harm, blame is not appropriate.

Other reasons patients experience guilt include: normal ambivalence about the pregnancy; wishing the baby would have died on his or her own; having felt relief immediately after the decision was made or termination completed; one's body and/or genes failing to create a healthy baby; and falling short of one's self-image. It may be necessary to alter parents' unrealistic standards and role responsibilities—teaching that we do not always have the control we desire. Having made a termination decision, women and men often wonder if they can be good parents to a healthy child (i.e., loss of trust in self). Noting that US culture tends to believe good mothers do not have bad babies (Ladd-Taylor and Umansky 1998) can help parents recognize the emotional bind they confronted. Guilt can also be mitigated by doing something constructive which helps others or contributes to society, for example, donating to or founding a charitable organization in their child's name or offering support to other parents facing a similar dilemma. The therapist may maintain a list of open-minded and compassionate clergy people of various religions with whom these parents may speak to help them with their feelings of guilt, as well. Moreover the MHP can help parents create a therapeutic ritual to say good-bye to guilt (e.g., letting it go into the universe through a helium balloon or casting it into the ocean), but, if guilt cannot be expiated, one must learn to live with it and not perpetuate self-punishment (e.g., build self-compassion for having been in a no-win situation).

Using cognitive reappraisal to address other faulty beliefs. "*If I follow the rules* (e.g., take folic acid, don't drink alcohol), *I will be safe and good things will happen.*" Holding this just and benevolent world belief results in feelings of betrayal by the world and the medical community. It reflects the failure to recognize that this belief is not an absolute but rather a probability statement. A more accurate, realistic belief is: "If I follow the rules, my risk of something bad happening will be reduced, but not completely eliminated as we can never completely eliminate all risks in life (or in pregnancy)."

A just world belief often leads to attempts to control everything. Superstitious beliefs can run rampant as a result (e.g., wearing certain underwear to prenatal visits to ensure a subsequent fetus is all right). Through Socratic questioning, the MHP attempts to help parents reframe to, for example: "I cannot control everything, but I can take reasonable and proven precautions (e.g., folic acid, no medications without checking with my obstetrician, etc.) to reduce the likelihood of future traumatic events."

Self-blame is often an attempt to regain control in the future. However, parents can be encouraged to offer self-forgiveness and accept they do not and cannot have control over everything.

"*I am having a bad day or flashbacks so I am back where I started.*" Teach patients to recognize all-or-nothing thinking and to differentiate between a lapse and a relapse. Learn from a lapse, e.g., what were the triggers, how can I help myself cope with a temporary backslide? Having a cry is not a sign of a relapse. It is a sign of having feelings, which is normal.

"*No one understands or still cares.*" Through Socratic questioning, teach the patient to ask him- or her-self whether everyone has been unsupportive. Then help them to reframe to: "Though some people are unsupportive, many have been wonderful. I have examples of supportive, nonjudgmental people, even some who I would not have expected. Therefore, I cannot conclude that everyone is unsupportive." The MHP can emphasize that trust is not an all-or-nothing concept, but rather falls on a continuum. Some people will be more trustworthy than others.

"*It wouldn't hurt this much if I made the right decision.*" This is an example of emotional reasoning. It can be dangerous to use one's emotions as a barometer for the rightness or wrongness of a decision, as wise decisions can cause pain. Help patients consider that the existence of the anomaly is causing the emotional pain and pain would exist whether they terminated the pregnancy or had a baby who had to cope with medical and social challenges (McCoyd 2007).

"*I should have thought about the choices more or longer.*" Help patients remember the process they went through (typically, a thoughtful process of decision making). Assist patients to recognize they did the best they could, with the information they had, and within the time frame which they were given to decide.

"*I have no right to feel happiness. I will never feel happy again.*" Socratic questioning can guide parents to conclude the length and amount of suffering does not constitute proof of love or remembrance of the baby and that a fulfilled life may be the best tribute they can offer to their baby.

"*I could never handle this again,*" implying the patient needs a guarantee that this will never happen again. No one can promise this (as lightning, unfortunately, does sometimes strike twice), but patients can learn they do not have to behave as if it were a high probability. However, most parents believe if they fell into an atypical statistical category once, they can (and predict they will) fall into such an unlikely category again. A good Socratic question to pose to these parents is: Although it could happen again, does anyone always have improbably bad luck? Also, asking the catastrophizing patient to predict the worse/best/and most likely outcome may help put some fears in perspective. Help patients recognize that when we are anxious we are also more likely to perceive perils or interpret ambiguous situations as threatening (Mogg and Bradley 1992).

The above examples are intended to demonstrate how Socratic questioning can help patients develop a balanced and realistic belief about themselves, the world, other people, and about what happened to them so they can feel their feelings about the trauma, create their own ways to effectively address cognitively distorted thinking, and then move on.

- Restoration focus: Work to rebuild the patient's life, couple's relationship, and social relationships. Help the couple build support for themselves through assertion and education of potential supporters about traumatic bereavement and the type of support the parents find helpful. Restore activities that generate positive emotions (pleasure/mastery), satisfying relationships, and social activities. Reintroducing social activity may confront patients with decisions regarding attendance at baby-related events (e.g., baby showers, brit, and christenings). The MHP needs to encourage parents to behave in accordance with what feels right to them, i.e., to take care of themselves, to realize there will be others to share the joyful events with their friend or family member, or, if they choose to attend, to help them to mitigate the situation by, for example, coming late or leaving early, preparing food in the kitchen, developing an exit strategy in advance, and forgiving and not berating themselves if they become emotional. MHPs can assist patients to set reasonable goals and increase their exposure to pleasurable activities through behavioral activation, activity scheduling, and increasing their exercise level. I encourage clients to begin incrementally, guiding them to experience just 5 min of happiness each day and gradually adding to this. Hopefully, all of the above will contribute to rebuilding patient resilience.

I have patients rewrite their impact statement or rerecord their imaginal revisiting of the trauma at the end of this phase of treatment, noting changes that have occurred. Individual differences in symptom presentation suggest that therapeutic protocols should be flexibly applied in response to each patient's needs, values, resources, and experiences, keeping in mind the social and cultural context in which they are embedded. There is no one-size fits all therapy for anyone, and certainly not for individuals who have undergone a TOPFA.

Late phase of psychotherapy and working with patients during a subsequent pregnancy. Rather than quickly dismissing their loss and immediately trying to become pregnant after a TOPFA, parents who have reached this stage of adjustment have already effectively worked on processing their traumatic loss and are beginning to look towards their future. One remaining factor may make it difficult for some patients to give themselves adequate time to process their loss. Those who are of advanced age and/or who have used assisted reproductive technology to conceive their prior pregnancy often feel an urgency to conceive again as soon as possible. However, feeling either numb or emotionally raw from a recent TOPFA makes it very difficult to move forward and navigate the myriad of conflicted feelings of sadness, fear, and hope that a subsequent pregnancy is likely to present.

MHPs can help patients achieve the following goals for this phase of psychotherapy:

- Prepare for the future: Apprise patients of the likely upsurge of negative feelings around anniversary dates or milestones (e.g., due date, holidays). Help clients prepare for these and find positive ways to remember their loss, assisting them to identify and reflect on the memories they still cherish, especially on significant dates.

  Redefine priorities and identify future goals consonant with their values, including a possible future pregnancy. Help parents identify what matters most so they can regain a sense of purpose and direction, delineate strategies for reaching their goals, readjust to a new normal, and reinvest in their lives. Have patients imagine themselves a year or two from now, remembering the loss, but with reduced intensity, and asking themselves, what might have occurred in the intervening time that enabled them to do this? This question conveys the therapist's confidence in the parents' ability to recover and that it is acceptable for them to be experiencing less grief. Although they are unlikely to feel fully emotionally ready to undertake another pregnancy, explain they need to be prepared to tolerate the range of mixed emotions that are likely to be triggered.
- Find meaning in their loss experience: Broaden parents' perspective by acknowledging strengths they have realized within themselves and/or their partner (e.g., a deepening of their compassion for others who feel isolated and set apart from the course of "normal" life, trusting in the solidity of their strengthened relationship). Discuss what they would say to someone else experiencing the same traumatic loss. Encourage involvement in tasks which enable parents to process the meaning of the loss (e.g., through writing letters, and/or poems, creating art; donating to relevant organizations in their child's name; posting online in a memorial garden, planting a tree that continues to thrive; when ready, making oneself available to others who have experienced the same type of loss). Encourage parents to reengage in meaningful relationships and a world beyond grief and mourning.

  Making sense of the event itself, finding benefit in the experience, and identity reconstruction all play independent roles in finding meaning after a loss (Davis et al. 1998). Parents who lost a child are the grieving population most preoccupied with questions about the meaning of the loss (Cleiren 1993). But it takes time to find meaning after struggling to adapt to the loss and changes in one's assumptive world, and to recognize not just what was lost but what was gained. Through this process, one can develop a new appreciation for one's life and the people in it (Keesee et al. 2008; Neimeyer et al. 2010). However, it is important that neither patients nor MHPs feel a sense of failure if finding meaning is not achieved as a significant subset of individuals after a loss do not search for meaning yet ultimately adjust well to loss (Wortman 2004).

  Determine what the patient can still enjoy and recognize the healing power and resilience of the human spirit. Many, but not all, patients experience posttraumatic growth, reemerging after a loss not simply to a return to baseline, but rather with a sense of new possibilities in life, improved interpersonal relationships, and an increased empathy for others (Tedeschi and Calhoun 2004).

- Implementing future goals. Develop future goals and concrete plans for implementation. The experience of loss informs women's next gestation as they now know that pregnancy is a hope, not a guarantee. Many patients can benefit from emotional support and anxiety management as they attempt to conceive or experience a subsequent pregnancy. Parents need information regarding their realistic risk. They need adequate time to speak about conflicted feelings with supportive and nonjudgmental health-care professionals prior to and during a subsequent pregnancy. Individuals and/or couples believe if they can do things differently (e.g., PGD, use of a high-risk obstetrician, planning for additional fetal monitoring), they may have a better outcome. Some patients may decline prenatal testing, fearing loss and/or not wanting to be put in the position to make a decision regarding a pregnancy termination. Medical personnel should not pass judgment on this choice.

Parents need to be prepared for the stress and range of emotions likely to be reactivated in a subsequent pregnancy (Forray et al. 2009; Hamama et al. 2010; Turton et al. 2009). Sometimes writing a letter to the lost baby to express their ongoing memories and their plans for coping now and in the future can help parents move forward. Mothers tend to develop emotional armor to cope with a subsequent pregnancy (Rillstone and Hutchinson 2001). They typically attempt to shield the pregnancy from public participation, delaying its announcement, and emotionally cushioning themselves by trying not to think of a future with this baby, having restrained expectations, postponing preparations for the baby, and avoiding emotional attachment as much as possible (Cote'-Arsenault and Donato 2007). Furthermore, by expecting the worst, they believe they will hurt less if everything does not work out, an erroneous belief from my clinical experience. Often women fear that they will never be able to love another baby as much. This fear can be addressed through cognitive reappraisal such that parents can come to realize that love is not finite and that loving another baby does not equate to forgetting or abandoning the baby they lost.

Long-term effects such as posttraumatic stress, depression, anxiety, etc. may be experienced in subsequent pregnancies and have been reported to remain at moderate intensities eight months post birth (Armstrong et al. 2009). Although anxiety in subsequent pregnancies is understandable, cognitive-behavioral reappraisals of unrealistic predictions of danger are beneficial. Both anxiety and stress have been implicated in poorer obstetrical and maternal–child outcomes and therefore techniques for coping with both are necessary (DiPietro et al. 2006; Federenko and Wadwa 2004; Kinsella and Monk 2009).

Help parents predict situations likely to trigger a resurgence of emotions. This may allow them to feel more in control in these situations. For example, help them anticipate the question, "Is this your first child?" Encourage them to prepare a response as their ambiguous sense of loss often emerges in this context.

It is often at the time of a subsequent birth of a healthy baby that the memory of a lost baby can take its proper place within the family. Parents often need help dealing with the rekindled memories of their prior loss and benefit from support in finding ways to differentiate their healthy newborn from memories of their deceased baby.

- Prepare for parenting after a TOPFA. Help patients develop realistic expectations of themselves to avoid their becoming unduly stressed by a compensatory need to be a perfect parent, overprotective, or controlling of future children. MHPs can normalize ambivalence both during pregnancy and when parenting children.
- Review progress and address the possibility of relapse. Consolidating and reinforcing treatment gains, strengths, and/or skills can help patients in the future as they face other life crises or losses.
- Plan for ending therapy and explore feelings. Offer parents the opportunity for follow-up or tune-ups and recognize that new life events may trigger memories and feelings about this life experience.

Support for Parents Deciding to Continue a Viable Pregnancy Diagnosed with a Fetal Anomaly

Parents who receive a diagnosis of a curable and/or surgically correctable fetal anomaly initially need information regarding the abnormality, how it can be treated, and the prognosis and likely ability of the child to function in various domains. Moreover, they will require referral to specialists to discuss a post-delivery plan. Information about available social services and local and/or national support networks should be provided to parents.

Communicating a diagnosis of fetal anomaly is not a discrete event, but a continuous one requiring further contact, clarification, and the provision of additional information to parents (Sheets et al. 2011). Parents choosing to continue their pregnancy need availability of a multidisciplinary team that provides information, access to resources, and ongoing care. Support will be essential so parents can transition through the emotional first days post-diagnosis and cope with an anxious and uncertain pregnancy (Aite et al. 2002). A recent combined quantitative and qualitative investigation in Thailand of women's experience of a continuing pregnancy after the diagnosis of a nonlethal fetal anomaly found three stages of distress: an initial intense stage of negative psychological reactions after the diagnosis in which women experienced the sense of loss of an ideal child as well as impairments in their self-worth; a subsequent healing stage in which distress gradually declined and women used various coping strategies including minimizing or discrediting the bad news, recasting hope, and stressor avoidance by not revealing the anomaly to others and limiting the information they sought out and received regarding the abnormality of their fetus; and finally, a reemergence of intense negative psychological reactions as women neared their due dates and began to worry about the uncertainty of their baby's future and their management plans for the baby (Titapant and Chuenwattana 2015). If confirmed by additional studies, MHPs may need to be aware of these changes in the nature and intensity of distress during a pregnancy in which a woman is carrying a fetus with a diagnosed nonlethal anomaly to offer effective psychological support throughout the pregnancy. Assistance is needed to help parents plan for obstetrical needs and to create a birth plan, as well. Hopefully, with help, clients will have a successful and positive parenting experience. Information about adoption and foster care can also be provided in a nonjudgmental manner to help parents understand that it is acceptable to be unable to raise a child with special needs themselves.

Asch (1999) has suggested the reasons for the high rate of termination of pregnancy for fetal anomaly include an overemphasis on the disability after diagnosis without seeing the impairment as only one characteristic of the child, parents having limited information regarding available services, and the common belief that a certain level of health is required for an acceptable life despite the fact that chronically disabled people perceive themselves as healthy and can thrive even in a less than welcoming society. Mental health professionals working with families given a diagnosis of a fetal anomaly must also examine their beliefs and emotional reactions toward various disabilities, explore how the world has informed their view of disabilities, and determine how their beliefs might influence their work.

Parents will benefit from favorable information about living with a disability, its positive impact on parents (Skotko et al. 2011a), siblings (Mulroy et al. 2008; Skotko et al. 2011b), and the disabled individuals themselves (Skotko et al. 2011c). Asch also recommends parents be offered a visit with a family raising a child with the same diagnosed disability and birth experience.

Typically, once having given birth, parents do not see the birth of a child having a medical problem or disability as tragic (Hedrick 2005; Kearney and Griffin 2001). The experience of parenting seems to change, especially for mothers, from one of fear and apprehension prenatally to one of strength and energy. Usually, the parents rise to the challenges with which they are confronted (Giuliani et al. 2014). However, most mothers require a minimum of 6–12 months to integrate and fully process their infant's health issues and disability after which most become assertive, authoritative, and ardent advocates for their child's needs (Wright 2002). This process probably contributes to the fact that by the time their infant is 6 months of age, parents report feeling more satisfied with themselves as parents and perceive parenting as easier than they had originally anticipated (Giuliani et al. 2014).

Noting parental coping skills after the birth of an infant with a diagnosed disability can help determine if there is a need for psychotherapeutic intervention. Most parents will need multidisciplinary support, i.e., medical as well as psychological, to confront and cope with the often ongoing challenges they face.

Support for Parents Choosing to Continue a Nonviable Pregnancy

Some parents when informed their pregnancy is nonviable wish neither to interrupt the pregnancy nor pursue aggressive interventions to prolong their baby's life. Rather, they choose to continue the pregnancy until a natural prenatal or postnatal demise of the baby occurs, and can be actively involved with their health-care team in decision-making and creating a perinatal advance care birth plan for what happens at birth and after birth (English and Hessler 2013). It is useful to present the concept of perinatal hospice or palliative care, including local resources. This terminology, however, may feel insensitive to a woman who is currently pregnant. Thus, reframing it as holistic care may be more easily interpreted as indicating "what we can offer" versus "there's nothing more we can do."

Perinatal palliative care can enable families to address their expectations, needs, hopes, and fears, and make meaningful plans for their baby's birth and life closure. Additionally, it addresses physical, psychological, social, spiritual, and practical issues, and includes siblings and grandparents, giving parents the opportunity to create memories of their baby (Caitlin 2005). After receiving a lethal fetal diagnosis, parents who plan to continue their pregnancy may not view this as catastrophic and report experiencing their baby as a person whom they wish to honor (Cote'-Arsenault and Denny-Koelsch 2011). Medical personnel can assist parents in so doing by having the perspective at birth of seeing a beautiful infant first and the child's disability second.

Although limited research is currently available on perinatal palliative care, parents studied thus far have reacted positively to this option, as, for some, it provides an opportunity to optimize the emotional outcome for their family (Breeze et al. 2007; Calhoun et al. 2003; D'Almeida et al. 2006). It is also beneficial to offer parents bereavement support after their baby's death.

Effects of Treatment on Medical and Psychotherapeutic Caregivers

Caring for patients who make a decision to undergo a TOPFA requires professional knowledge, empathy, and the ability to tolerate intense feelings and reflect upon one's own values as well as the ethical and moral conflicts these choices can trigger. This work can be enormously rewarding, creating positive transformation in the therapist by deepening one's understanding of human strength and resilience as well as one's own humanity. However, it is also emotionally difficult work. Treating these patients can be painful for health-care professionals who have to give bad news and/or be intimately involved with the parents through the trauma and loss experience and can have repercussions for their personal lives. Not surprisingly, those who treat these patients report experiencing their own difficult emotions, and they often feel largely unsupported by others (Andersson et al. 2014; Bernhardt et al. 2010; Menezes 2010). Awareness of countertransferential reactions, projecting the therapist's own unresolved personal losses, traumas, or conflicts onto the client, is important so these reactions may be used in a therapeutic manner on behalf of the patients, if appropriate, or addressed through the MHP's personal therapy. Vicarious traumatization can occur when one internalizes the pain and trauma of others and compassion fatigue can ensue, i.e., feeling emotionally drained and depleted. Health-care professionals may become debilitated if they have unrealistic expectations of themselves that remain unrecognized and unaddressed.

Indications of compassion fatigue include: changes in interpersonal affect management (e.g., irritability with loved ones and/or patients), depression, feeling that others (e.g., patients, staff, or family) are intentionally trying to wear you down, a decreased sense of accomplishment, a reduced ability to experience joy, a sense of isolation, sleep disturbances, workaholism, and an empathy drain wherein one loses empathy and compassion for others. Finding oneself abusing alcohol, drugs, food, or sex to escape the emotional strain needs to be immediately addressed. Awareness of one's own reactions and needs for additional support is key to being able to provide effective and ethical treatment.

Personal self-care and a healthy work-life balance are crucial for all medical, genetics, and psychological providers of care to these patients. Prioritize self-care and consider the following suggestions for rebalancing your emotional equilibrium: eat healthily, regularly exercise, and meet your needs for sleep; engage in relaxing, pleasurable, and rejuvenating activities; nourish your relationships by spending quality time with family and friends; incorporate activities into your daily routine to promote relaxation and relieve stress (e.g., mindfulness, meditation, or yoga); engage in reflective writing or other creative expression; take time off to reenergize yourself; and reach out to others, including trusted and respected colleagues, for support and help in identifying one's blind spots. Provisions for ongoing education, bereavement training, mentoring, and support from experienced colleagues are essential for professionals working with these patients.

Conclusions

Parents coping with their decision after learning of a fetal anomaly, whether that decision is to not bring a disabled child or one with a life-limiting condition into the world or to continue the pregnancy, often have a difficult time acknowledging and coming to terms with their loss. This nonnormative loss encompasses multiple losses including a shattered world view. In addition, if the decision is made to terminate the pregnancy, it can be experienced as a disenfranchised loss (Doka 2002) in that often it is not disclosed for fear of judgment or publicly mourned as there are few, if any, available rituals. Often the loss is not socially recognized or supported. The devastation of this loss can be intensified when it is not validated by others. Frequently parents feel unsure of whether their infant's death is considered a loss by others, leaving them confused about how to navigate a world that no longer feels familiar. The need to address their loss, find their own way to integrate this experience into their identity, and restructure their world view can be immeasurably aided by the sensitivity of their medical and psychological caregivers. It is hoped the information presented in this chapter will be useful in providing knowledge and tools to medical and mental health care clinicians working with these parents so they can help them mourn their traumatic losses and reengage in a meaningful life.

Challenges for the Future

The technologies of prenatal and preimplantation screening and diagnosis present multiple challenges. Future needs in this field include:

- Increasing awareness of the trauma of a TOPFA as this will inform the diagnosis and treatment of parents struggling with this experience. Additionally, to guide mental health professionals in their implementation of evidence-based practice, dismantling studies are needed to determine which components of psychotherapy are necessary for clinical improvements and whether different modalities of psychological treatment can and should be combined or sequentially offered. Male partners and diverse cultural, racial, and socioeconomic groups should be included in this research.
- Additional supports and resources provided both for parents who choose to interrupt their pregnancy after a diagnosis of fetal anomaly as well as for those who choose to continue their pregnancy.
- Policy changes for parents confronted by diagnoses of fetal anomaly in pregnancy. The complexity of the decision to terminate a pregnancy for fetal anomaly needs to be recognized and the legality of abortion in the second trimester of pregnancy must be maintained. In addition, greater economic resources and emotional supports for families raising children with disabilities must be provided. We must ensure that parents who choose not to undergo prenatal testing and those who continue a pregnancy knowing their baby carries an anomaly are not stigmatized or refused insurance to cover potentially lifelong medical costs.
- Further exploration of the ethical issues involved in prenatal and preimplantation genetic screening and diagnosis, e.g., how much control should we have in determining the biological structure of our children? Would increasing control change the way parents view their children? How will the children view their parents and themselves? If socioeconomic inequities continue in access to this technology, being genetically disabled could become a mark of social class and perpetuate a societal injustice.

Appendix: Sample of Resources

General Information on Fetal Diagnoses: www.poorprenataldiagnosis.com

FOR A TOPFA:

Brooks, C, editor. Our heartbreaking choices: forty-six women share their stories of interrupting a much-wanted pregnancy. NY: iUniverse; 2008.

Kushner, H. When bad things happen to good people. NY: Random House; 1981.

Minnick, MA, Delp, KC, Ciotti, MC. A time to decide, a time to heal: for parents making difficult decisions about babies they love. 4th ed. St. Johns, MN: Pineapple Press; 2000.

Online:
A Heartbreaking Choice
www.aheartbreakingchoice.com
www.aheartbreakingchoice.net
Baby Center open group:
http://community.babycenter.com/groups/a6325/termination_for_medical_reasons
Ending a Wanted Pregnancy:
http://endingawantedpregnancy.com
Stories for women who terminated wanted pregnancies in the second or third trimester:
www.1in10blog.wordpress.com

FOR SELECTIVE REDUCTION:

Fertile Thoughts: http://www.fertilethoughts.com/forums/selective-reduction-and-termination-due-to-health-issues/

FOR CARRYING TO TERM:

Be Not Afraid: www.benotafraid.net
Anencephaly: www.anencephalie-info.org
Down Syndrome Support: www.ndsccenter.org, www.ndss.org
www.kidsource.com/kidsource/content4/babies.down.pn.html
Heart Defects: www.littlehearts.net, www.congenitalheartdefects.com
Information on Local Perinatal Hospice and Palliative Care:
http://perinatalhospice.org/Resources_for_parents.html
Spina Bifida: www.sbaa.org, www.waisman.wisc.edu/~rowley/sb-kids/
Support groups and information on specific genetic and rare conditions:
www.kumc.edu/gec/support, www.rarediseases.org www.geneticalliance.org
Tay-Sachs and other fatal degenerative genetic disorders: www.ntsad.org
The Solace Foundation: www.thesolacefoundation.org/carrying-to-term.html
Trisomy 18 Support: www.trisomy18support.org
Trisomy 18, 13 and Related Disorders: www.trisomy.org

References

Aite L, Trucchi A, Nahom A, Spina V, Bilanchoni E, et al. Multidisciplinary management of fetal surgical anomalies: the impact on maternal anxiety. Eur J Pediatr Surg. 2002;12:90–4.

American Psychiatric Association. DSM-5. Diagnostic and statistical manual of mental health disorders. 5th ed. Arlington, VA: American Psychiatric Association; 2013.

Andersson IM, Gemzell-Danielsson K, Christensson K. Caring for women undergoing second trimester medical termination of pregnancy. Contraception. 2014;89(5):460–5. pii:S0010-7824(14) 00022-5. doi:10.1016/jcontraception.2014.01.012.

Armstrong DS, Hutti MH, Myers J. The influence of prior perinatal loss on parents' psychological distress after the birth of a subsequent healthy infant. JOCNN. 2009;38(6):654–66. doi:10.1111/j.1552-6909.2009.01069.

Asch A. Prenatal diagnosis and selective abortion: a challenge to practice and policy. Am J Public Health. 1999;89:1649–57.

Asplin N, Wessel H, Marions L, Ohman SG. Pregnancy termination due to fetal anomaly: women's reactions, satisfaction and experiences of care. Midwifery. 2014;30:620–7.

Bernhardt BA, Silver R, Rushton CH, Micco E, Geller G. What keeps you up at night? Genetics professionals' distressing experiences in patient care. Genet Med. 2010;12:289–97. doi:10.1097/GIM.Ob013e3181db82d9.

Bisson J, Andrew M. Psychological treatment of post-traumatic stress disorder (PTSD). Cochrane Database Syst Rev. 2007;18(3), CD003388.

Bodkin J. Ethical issues and practical problems in preimplantation genetic diagnosis. J Law Med Ethics. 1998;26(1):17–28. doi:10.1111/j.1748-720X.1998.tb01902.x.

Boelen PA, DeKeijser J, van den Hout MA, van den Bout J. Treatment of complicated grief: a comparison between cognitive-behavioral therapy and supportive counseling. J Consult Clin Psychol. 2007;75(2):277–84.

Boss JA. First trimester prenatal diagnosis: earlier is not necessarily better. J Med Ethics. 1999;20:146–51.

Bradley R, Greene J, Russ E, Dutra L, Westen D. A multidimensional meta-analysis of psychotherapy for PTSD. Am J Psychiatry. 2005;162(2):214–27.

Breeze ACG, Lees CC, Kumar A, Missfelder-Lobos HH, Murdoch EM. Palliative care for prenatally diagnosed lethal fetal abnormality. Arch Dis Child Fetal Neonatal Ed. 2007;92(1):56–8. doi:10.113i6/adc.2005.092122.

Bryant RA, Mastrodomenico J, Hopwood S, Kenny L, Cahill C, Kandris E, et al. Augmenting cognitive behavior therapy for post-traumatic stress disorder with emotion tolerance training: a randomized controlled trial. Psychol Med. 2013;43(10):2153–60. doi:10.1017/S0033291713000068.

Caitlin A. Thinking outside the box: prenatal care and the call for a prenatal advance directive. J Perinat Neonatal Nurs. 2005;19(2):169–76.

Calhoun BC, Napolitano P, Terry M, Bussey C, Hoeldtke NJ. Perinatal hospice. Comprehensive care for the family of the fetus with a lethal condition. J Reprod Med. 2003;48(5):343–8.

Cleiren MPHD. Bereavement and adaptation: a comparison study of the aftermath of death. Philadelphia, PA: Hemisphere; 1993.

Cote'-Arsenault D, Denny-Koelsch E. My baby is a person: parents' experiences with life-threatening fetal diagnosis. J Palliat Med. 2011;14(12):1302–8. doi:10.1089/jpm.2011.0165.

Cote'-Arsenault D, Donato KL. Restrained expectations in late pregnancy following loss. J Obstet Gynecol Neonatal Nurs. 2007;36(6):550–7.

Cote'-Arsenault D, Donato K. Emotional cushioning in pregnancy after perinatal loss. J Reprod Infant Psychol. 2011;29(1):81–92. doi:10.1080/02646838.2010.513115.

Cox JL, Holden JM, Sagovsky R. Detecting postnatal depression. Development of the 10-item Edinburgh Postnatal Depression Scale. Br J Psychiatry. 1987;150:782–6. doi:10.11921bjp.150.6.782.

D'Almeida M, Hume RF, Lathrop A, Njoku A, Calhoun BC. Perinatal hospice: family-centered care of the fetus with a lethal condition. J Am Phys Surg. 2006;11(2):52–5.

Davies V, Gledhill J, McFadyen A, Whitlow B, Economides D. Psychological outcome in women undergoing termination of pregnancy for ultrasound-detected fetal anomaly in the first and second trimesters: a pilot study. Ultrasound Obstet Gynecol. 2005;25(4):389–92.

Davis CG, Nolen-Hoeksema S, Larson J. Making sense of loss and benefiting from the experience: two construals of meaning. J Pers Soc Psychol. 1998;75(2):156–74.

DiPietro JA, Novak MF, Costigan KA, Atella LD, Reusing SP. Maternal psychological distress during pregnancy in relation to child development at age two. Child Dev. 2006;77(3):573–87.

Doka K, editor. Disenfranchised grief: recognizing hidden sorrow. Lexington, MA: Lexington Books; 2002.

Doka KJ, Martin J. Grieving beyond gender: understanding the ways men and women mourn. New York, NY: Routledge; 2010.

Ehlers A, Hackmann A, Michael T. Intrusive re-experiending in post-traumatic stress disorder: phenomenology, theory and therapy. Memory. 2004;12(4):405–15.

Engelhard IM, van den Hout MA, Arntz A. Posttraumatic stress disorder after pregnancy loss. Gen Hosp Psychiatry. 2001;23:62–6.

English NK, Hessler KL. Prenatal birth planning for families of the imperiled newborn. JOGNN. 2013;42(3):390–9. doi:10.111/1552-6909.12031.

ESHRE Task Force on Ethics and Law. Ethical issues related to multiple pregnancies in medically assisted procreation. Hum Reprod. 2003;18(9):1976–9. doi:10.1093/humrep/deg357.

Federenko IS, Wadwa PD. Women's mental health during pregnancy influences fetal and infant developmental and health outcomes. CNS Spectr. 2004;9(3):198–206.

Foa EB, Keane TM, Friedman MJ, Cohen JA, editors. Effective treatments for PTSD: practice guidelines from the International Society for Traumatic Stress Studies. 2nd ed. New York, NY: Guilford Press; 2009.

Forray A, Mayes LC, Magriples U, Epperson CN. Prevalence of post-traumatic stress disorder in pregnant women with prior pregnancy complications. J Matern Fetal Neonatal Med. 2009;22(6):522–7. doi:10.1080/14767050902801686.

France EF, Hunt K, Ziebland S, Wyke S. What parents say about disclosing the end of their pregnancy due to fetal abnormality. Midwifery. 2013;29:24–32.

Garel M, Stark C, Blondel B, Lefebvre G, Vauthier-Brouzes D, Zorn JR. Psychological reactions after multifetal pregnancy reduction: a 2-year follow-up study. Hum Reprod. 1997;12(3): 617–22.

Geerinck-Vercammen CR, Kahai HH. Coping with termination of pregnancy for fetal abnormality in a supportive environment. Prenat Diagn. 2003;23(7):543–8.

Giuliani R, Tripani A, Pellizzoni S, Clarici A, Lonciari I, D'Ottavio G, et al. Pregnancy and postpartum following a prenatal diagnosis of fetal thoracoabdominal malformation: the parental perspective. J Pediatr Surg. 2014;49(2):353–8. doi:10.1016/j.jpedsurg.2013.07.025.

Hamama L, Rauch SA, Sperlich M, Defever E, Seng JS. Previous experience of spontaneous or elective abortion and risk for posttraumatic stress and depression during subsequent pregnancy. Depress Anxiety. 2010;27(8):699–707. doi:10.1002/da.20714.

Hamamy HA, Dahoun S. Parental decisions following the prenatal diagnosis of sex chromosome abnormalities. Eur J Obstet Gyecol Reprod Biol. 2004;116(1):58–62.

Hedrick J. The lived experience of a pregnancy while carrying a child with a known nonlethal congenital abnormality. J Obstet Gynecol Neonatal Nurs. 2005;34(6):732–40.

Horowitz MJ, Wilner NR, Alvarez W. Impact of Event Scale: a measure of subjective stress. Psychosom Med. 1979;41:209–18.

Iles S, Gath D. Psychiatric outcome of termination of pregnancy for foetal abnormality. Psychol Med. 1993;23(2):407–13.

Janoff-Bulman R. Shattered assumptions: towards a new psychology of trauma. New York, NY: Free Press; 1992.

Johnson CY, Honein MA, Dana FW, Howards PP, Oakley Jr GP, Rasmussen SA. Pregnancy termination following fetal diagnosis of anencephaly or spina bifida: a systematic review of the literature. Birth Defects Res A Clin Mol Teratol. 2012;94:857–63.

Kaasen A, Helbig A, Malt UF, Naes T, Skari H, Haugen GN. Paternal psychological response after ultrasonographic detection of structural fetal anomalies with a comparison to maternal response: a cohort study. BMC Pregnancy Childbirth. 2013;13:147. doi:10.1186/1471-2393-13-147.

Kalfoglou AL, Scott J, Hudson K. PGD patients' and providers' attitudes to the use and regulation of preimplantation genetic diagnosis. Reprod Biomed Online. 2005;11(4):486–96.

Katz MG, Fitzgerald L, Bankier A, Savulescu J, Cram DS. Issues and concerns of couples presenting for preimplantation genetic diagnosis (PGD). Prenat Diagn. 2002;22(12):1117–22. doi:10.1002/pd.498.

Kearney PM, Griffin T. Between joy and sorrow: being a parent of a child with developmental disability. J Adv Nurs. 2001;34(5):582–92.

Keesee NJ, Currier JM, Neimeyer RA. Predictors of grief following the death of one's child: the contribution of finding meaning. J Clin Psychol. 2008;64(10):1145–63. doi:10.1002/jclp.20502.

Kersting A, Wagner B. Complicated grief after perinatal loss. Dialogues Clin Neurosci. 2012;14(2):187–94.
Kersting A, Kroker K, Steinhard J, Ludorff K, Wesselmann U, Ohrmann P, et al. Complicated grief after traumatic loss: a 14-month follow up study. Eur Arch Psychiatry Clin Neurosci. 2007; 257(8):437–43.
Kersting A, Brahler E, Glaesmer H, Wagner B. Prevalence of complicated grief in a representative population-based sample. J Affect Disord. 2011;131(1-3):339–43.
Kersting A, Dolemeyer R, Steinig J, Walter F, Kroker K, Baust K, et al. Brief internet-based intervention reduces posttraumatic stress and prolonged grief in parents after the loss of a child during pregnancy: a randomized controlled trial. Psychother Psychosom. 2013;82(6):372–81. doi:10.1159/000348713.
Kinsella MT, Monk C. Impact of maternal stress, depression and anxiety on fetal neurobehavioral development. Clin Obstet Gynecol. 2009;52(3):425–40. doi:10.10971GRF.060.
Koopmans L, Wilson T, Cacciatore J, Flenady V. Support for mothers, fathers and families after perinatal death. Cochrane Database Syst Rev. 2013;6:CD000452. doi:10.1002/14651858. CD000452.pub3.
Korenromp MJ, Page-Christiaens GC, van den Bout J, Mulder EJ, Hunfeld JA, Bilardo CM, et al. Long-term psychological consequences of pregnancy termination for fetal abnormality: a cross-sectional study. Prenat Diagn. 2005a;25(3):253–60.
Korenromp MJ, Page-Christiaens GC, van den Bout J, Mulder EJ, Hunfeld JA, Bilardo CM, et al. Psychological consequences of termination of pregnancy for fetal anomaly: similarities and differences between partners. Prenat Diagn. 2005b;25(13):1226–33.
Korenromp MJ, Page-Christiaens GC, van den Bout J, Mulder EJ, Hunfeld JA, Potters CM, et al. A prospective study on parental coping 4 months after termination of pregnancy for fetal anomalies. Prenat Diagn. 2007;27(8):709–16.
Korenromp MJ, Page-Christiaens GC, van den Bout J, Mulder EJ, Visser GH. Adjustment to termination of pregnancy for fetal anomaly: a longitudinal study of women at 4, 8, and 16 months. Am J Obstet Gynecol. 2009;201(2):160.e1–7. doi:10.1016/j.ajog.2009.04.007.
Kubany ES, Watson SB. Guilt: elaboration of a multidimensional model. Psychol Rec. 2003;53:51–90.
Ladd-Taylor M, Umansky L. Bad mothers: the politics of blame in twentieth century America. New York, NY: New York University Press; 1998.
LaFarge C, Mitchell K, Fox P. Perinatal grief following a termination of pregnancy for fetal abnormality: the impact of coping strategies. Prenat Diagn. 2013;33(12):1173–82. doi:10.1002/pd.4218.
Lalor JG, Devane D, Begley CM. Unexpected diagnosis of fetal abnormality: women's encounters with caregivers. Birth. 2007;34:80–8. doi:10.1111/j.1523-536X.2006.00148.
Lavery SA, Aurell R, Turner C, Castello C, Veiga A, Barri PN, et al. Preimplantation genetic diagnosis: patients' experiences and attitudes. Hum Reprod. 2002;17(9):2464–7.
Linehan MM. Skills training manual for treating borderline personality disorder. New York, NY: Guilford; 1993.
Locock L, Alexander J. 'Just a bystander'? Men's place in the process of fetal screening and diagnosis. Soc Sci Med. 2006;62(6):1349–59.
Maifeld M, Hah S, Titler MG, Mullen M. Decision making regarding multifetal reduction. J Obstet Gynecol Neonatal Nurs. 2003;32(3):357–69. doi:10.1177/0884217503253493.
Mansfield C, Hopfer S, Marteau TM. Termination rates after prenatal diagnosis of Down syndrome, spina bifida, anencephaly, and Turner and Klinefelter syndromes: a systematic literature review. Prenat Diagn. 1999;19(9):808–12.
Maschiach R, Anter D, Melamed N, Ben-Ezra M, Meizner I, Hamama-Raz Y. Psychological response to multifetal reduction and pregnancy termination due to fetal abnormality. J Matern Fetal Neonatal Med. 2013;26(1):32–5. doi:10.3109/14767058.2012.722714.
McCoyd JL. Pregnancy interrupted: loss of a desired pregnancy after diagnosis of fetal anomaly. J Psychosom Obstet Gynaecol. 2007;28(1):37–48.
McCoyd JL. What do women want? Experiences and reflections of women after prenatal diagnosis and termination for anomaly. Health Care Women Int. 2009;30(6):507–35. doi:10.1080/07399330902801278.

McKinney M, Downey J, Timor-Trisch I. The psychological effects of multifetal pregnancy reduction. Fertil Steril. 1995;64(1):51–61.
Mendes DD, Mello MF, Ventura P, Passarela C d M, Mari J d J. A systematic review on the effectiveness of cognitive behavioral therapy for posttraumatic stress disorder. Int J Psychiatry Med. 2008;38(3):241–59.
Menezes MA. Life on the front line: exploring personal and professional impacts on healthcare professionals working with fetal anomaly. PhD thesis, medicine, dentistry and health science. Department of Paediatrics, The University of Melbourne; 2010.
Mezei G, Pepp C, Toth PE, Beke A, Papp Z. Factors influencing parental decision making in prenatal diagnosis of sex chromosome aneuploidy. Obstet Gynecol. 2004;104:94–101.
Mogg K, Bradley BP. Selective attention and anxiety: a cognitive-motivational perspective. In: Dalgeish T, Power M, editors. Handbook of cognition and emotion. Chichester: John Wiley and Sons; 1992. p. 145–70.
Mulroy S, Robertson L, Alberti K, Leonard H, Bower C. The impact of having a sibling with an intellectual disability: parental perspectives in two disorders. J Intellect Disabil Res. 2008;52(Pt3):216–29. doi:10.1111/j.1365-2788.2007.01005.
National Council for Adoption. State, national and international data on adoption. In: Marshner C, Pierce WL, editors. Adoption factbook III. Waite Park, MN: Park Press Quality Printing; 1999. p. 27.
Natoli JL, Ackerman DL, McDermott S, Edwards JG. Prenatal diagnosis of Down syndrome: a systematic review of termination rates (1995–2011). Prenat Diagn. 2012;32(2):142–53.
Neimeyer RA, Currier JM. Grief therapy: evidence of efficacy and emerging directions. Curr Dir Psychol Sci. 2010;18:352–6.
Neimeyer RA, Burke LA, Mackay MM, van Dyke Stringer JG. Grief therapy and the reconstruction of meaning: from principles to practice. J Contemp Psychother. 2010;40:73–83. doi:10.1007/sl0879-009-9135.
Nishith P, Nixon RD, Resick PA. Resolution of trauma-related guilt following treatment of PTSD in female rape victims: a result of cognitive processing therapy targeting comorbid depression? J Affect Disorders. 2005;86(2-3):259–65.
O'Connor TG, Heron J, Glover V, Alspac Study Team. Antenatal anxiety predicts child behavioral/emotional problems independently of postnatal depression. J Am Acad Child Adolesc Psychiatry. 2002;41(12):1470–7.
Powers MB, Halpern JM, Ferenschak MP, Gillihan SJ, Foa EB. A meta-analytic review of prolonged exposure for posttraumatic stress disorder. Clin Psychol. 2010;30(6):635–42. doi:10.1016/j.cpr.2010.04.007.
Practice Committee of the American Society for Reproductive Medicine. Multiple gestation associated with infertility therapy: an American Society for Reproductive Medicine Practice Committee opinion. Fertil Steril. 2012;97(4):825–34.
Prigerson HG, Maciejewski PK, Reynolds 3rd CF, Bierhals AJ, Newsom JT, Fasiczka A, et al. Inventory of complicated grief: a scale to measure maladaptive symptoms of loss. Psychiatr Res. 1995;59(1-2):65–79.
Rando TA. Treatment of complicated mourning. Champaign, IL: Research Press; 1993.
Resick PA, Schnicke MK. Cognitive processing therapy for rape victims. Newbury Park, CA: Sage; 1993.
Resick PA, Nishith P, Weaver TL, Astin MC, Feuer CA. A comparison of cognitive-processing therapy and prolonged exposure and a waiting condition for the treatment of chronic posttraumatic stress disorder in female rape victims. J Consult Clin Psychol. 2002;70:867–79.
Rillstone P, Hutchinson SA. Managing the reemergence of anguish: pregnancy after a loss due to anomalies. J Obstet Gynecol Neonatal Nurs. 2001;30:291–8. doi:10.1111/j.1552-6909.20001.tb01547.
Rothbaum BO, Meadows EA, Resick P, Foy DW. Cognitive-behavioral therapy. In: Foa EB, Keane TM, Friedman MJ, editors. Effective treatment for PTSD: practice guidelines from the International Society for Traumatic Stress Studies. New York, NY: Guilford; 2000. p. 60–83.

Sandelowski M, Barroso J. The travesty of choosing after positive prenatal diagnosis. J Obstet Gynecol Neonatal Nurs. 2005;34(3):307–18.

Schechtman KB, Gray DL, Baty JD, Rothman SM. Decision-making for termination of pregnancies for fetal anomalies: analysis of 53,000 pregnancies. Obstet Gynecol. 2002;99(2):216–22.

Schreiner-Engel P, Walther VN, Mindes J, Lynch L, Berkowitz RL. First-trimester multifetal pregnancy reduction: acute and persistent psychologic reactions. Am J Obstet Gynecol. 1995;172(2):541–7. doi: 10.1016/0002-9378(95)90570-7.

Seidler GH, Wagner FE. Comparing the efficacy of EMDR and trauma-focused cognitive-behavioral therapy in the treatment of PTSD: a meta-analytic study. Psychol Med. 2006; 36(11):1515–22.

Seller M, Barnes C, Ross S, Barby T, Cowmeadow P. Grief and mid-trimester fetal loss. Prenat Diagn. 1993;13(5):341–8.

Shapiro F. Eye movement desensitization reprocessing: basic principles, protocols, and procedures. New York, NY: Guilford Press; 2001.

Shear K, Frank E, Houck PR, Reynolds 3rd CF. Treatment of complicated grief: a randomized controlled trial. JAMA. 2005;293(21):2601–8.

Sheets KB, Crissman BG, Feist CD, Sell SL, Johnson LR, Donahue KC, et al. Practice guidelines for communicating a prenatal or postnatal diagnosis of Down syndrome: recommendations of the national society of genetic counselors. J Genet Couns. 2011;20(5):432–41. doi:10.1007/s10897-011-9375-8.

Skotko BG, Levine SP, Goldstein R. Having a son or daughter with Down syndrome: perspectives from mothers and fathers. Am J Med Genet A. 2011a;155A(10):2335–47. doi:10.1002/ajmg.a.34293.

Skotko BG, Levine SP, Goldstein R. Having a brother or sister with Down syndrome: perspective from siblings. Am J Med Genet A. 2011b;155A(10):2348–59. doi:10.1002/ajmg.a.34228.

Skotko BG, Levine SP, Goldstein R. Self-perceptions from people with Down syndrome. Am J Genet A. 2011c;155A(10):2360–9. doi:10.1002/ajmg.a.34235.

Stroebe M, Schut H. The dual process model of coping with bereavement: rationale and description. Death Stud. 1999;23:197–224.

Taylor SE, Klein LC, Lewis BP, Gruenewald TL, Gurung RA, Updegraff JA. Biobehavioral responses to stress in females: tend-and-befriend not fight-or-flight. Psychol Rev. 2000; 107(3):411–29.

Tedeschi RG, Calhoun LG. Posttraumatic growth: conceptual foundations and empirical evidence. Psychol Inq. 2004;15(1):1–18. doi:10.1207/s15327965pli1501_01.

Tedeschi RG, Calhoun LG. The clinician as expert companion. In: Park CL, Lechner SC, Antoni MH, Stanton AL, editors. Medical illness and positive life change: can crisis lead to personal transformation? Washington. Washington, DC: American Psychological Association; 2009. p. 215–35.

Titapant V, Chuenwattana P. Psychological effects of fetal diagnoses of non-lethal congenital anomalies on the experience of pregnant women during the remainder of their pregnancy. J Obstet Gynaecol Res. 2015;41(1):77–83. doi: 10.1111/jcog.12504.

Toedter LJ, Lasker JN, Alhadeff JM. The Perinatal Grief Scale: development and initial validation. Am J Orthopsychiat. 1988;58(3):435–49.

Turton P, Hughes P, Evans CDH, Fainman D. Incidence, correlates and predictors of posttraumatic stress disorder in the pregnancy after stillbirth. Br J Psychiatry. 2001;178:556–60. doi:10.1192/bjp.178.6.556.

Turton P, Evans C, Hughes P. Long-term psychosocial sequelae of stillbirth: phase II of a nested case control cohort study. Arch Womens Ment Health. 2009;12(1):35–41. doi:10.1007/s00737-008-0040-7.

Weathers FW, Huska JA, Keane TM. PCL-S for DSM-IV. Boston, MA: National Center for PTSD-Behavioral Science Division; 1991.

Weathers FW, Blake DD, Schnurr PP, Marx BP, Keane TM. Clinician-administered PTSD scale for DSM-5 (CAPS-5). www.ptsd.va.gov/professional/assessment/adult-int/caps.asp. 2014.

White-van Mourik MCA, Connor JM, Fersguson-Smith MA. The psychosocial sequelae of a second trimester termination of pregnancy for fetal anomaly. Prenat Diagn. 1992;12(3): 189–204.

Wittouck C, Van Autreve S, De Jaegere E, Portzky G, van Heeringen K. The prevention and treatment of complicated grief: a meta-analysis. Clin Psychol Rev. 2011;31(1):69–78. doi:10.1016/j.cpr.2010.09.005.

Wool C. Systematic review of the literature: parental outcomes after diagnosis of fetal anomaly. Adv Neonatal Care. 2011;11(3):182–92.

Wortman CB. Posttraumatic growth: progress and problems. Psychol Inq. 2004;15:81–90.

Wright J. Transcendence: phenomenological perspective of the mother's experience of having a child with a disability. Doctoral dissertation, Widener University. DAI; 2002:63-12B.

Chapter 15
A Burden of Choice: The Ripple Effect: Parents' Grief and the Role of Family and Friends

Julie Bindeman

Background and Context

Advances in technology permeate our everyday lives and are far-reaching in the information that can ensue. It is not surprising that technology is being utilized more in the process of pregnancy, whether to attain the state of pregnancy, to analyze the raw materials necessary for pregnancy (sperm, eggs, and embryos), or to monitor and assess the health of an existing pregnancy. This technology yields information, and, as a result, more couples are finding themselves in the position of needing to make a decision regarding the pregnancy and its outcome based on health concerns for either the mother or the fetus. This chapter focuses on the termination of wanted pregnancies for medical reasons, either because of fetal anomaly or risk to the mother's health. While there is scant formal literature on medical terminations, there is even less concerning the effects of preimplantation genetic diagnosis.

Receiving an abnormal prenatal diagnosis or the knowledge that embryos are not chromosomally normal is one of the most devastating moments in a parent's life. Would-be parents must then choose a course of action based upon their beliefs, religious background, best guess at medical prognosis, economic circumstances, type of family and social support available, and other considerations that factor in such a choice for a particular couple (McCoyd 2008). The likelihood that others in their support system have encountered the same kind of decision is rare, thus exacerbating the couple's feelings of being alone in this situation. To complicate matters, the word "abortion" is very politicized in American culture, and any reference to "choice" when sharing information about this loss with others may be met with scorn and rejection rather than compassion. Sharon Covington succinctly describes

J. Bindeman, Psy.D. (✉)
Independent Practice, 5818 B Hubbard Drive, Rockville, MD 20852, USA
e-mail: drbindeman@gmail.com

J.P. Galst, M.S. Verp (eds.), *Prenatal and Preimplantation Diagnosis*,
DOI 10.1007/978-3-319-18911-6_15

how abortion due to a medical intervention differs from an unexpected loss: "if spontaneous loss is a socially isolating experience, elected loss is in a complete vacuum" (Burns and Covington 1999).

Technology has changed the ways that human beings connect with one another. The advent of the Internet and social media enables instantaneous connections: people can keep "up to the minute" tabs on others they know. "Friends" takes on a new meaning as those connected to one another via a social media platform have a variety of relationships in day-to-day life. People have different degrees of friendship ranging from relationships that have been built through various life phases to relationships based upon daily interaction. When something outside of the norm occurs, such as a perinatal loss, particularly one where a wanted pregnancy was terminated for medical reasons, communicating and receiving comfort from one's social network become critical but in some cases may be uncertain.

No amount of information from books or articles can adequately predict the trajectory of an individual's grief. Research results can suggest possible paths, but inevitably each person's grief journey is unique. Arnold and Gemma describe the uniqueness of pregnancy loss as "the loss of an adult is the loss of the past; the loss of a baby is the loss of the future" (Robinson 1999). A troubling aspect of pregnancy interruption is that, unlike an early miscarriage, which occurs in the first trimester usually prior to a pregnancy being widely announced, the decision to terminate a pregnancy for medical reasons is often made in the second trimester, when a couple has "gone public" with the fact that they are expecting a baby. Another barrier is that while there is ample literature regarding supporting patients' emotional needs after miscarriage, stillbirth, and neonatal death, very little exists focusing on terminating for medical reasons (Harris 2004).

Many theorists have looked at grief and bereavement in the hopes of understanding these universal human phenomena; however very few have addressed these issues in the context of pregnancy. From a psychological viewpoint, the task of pregnancy is to form a new attachment to the developing baby and incorporate a new identity structure (as that of a parent), both of which enhance self-esteem as the act of reproduction enables a person to experience the sense of "omnipotence" (Leon 2008). Fundamentally, all of these changes are based upon attaching to a new and unknown person and having a degree of faith in the identity that is being created simultaneously.

In taking a closer look at attachment and its role in grief, the clinician, John Bowlby, facilitates an understanding of the general grief process from an attachment perspective (Bowlby 1969). In its most simplistic form (Bowlby 1979) death and loss can be separated. Though Bowlby described the four distinct phases of grief sequentially, he acknowledged that different people might not experience them as such (Bowlby 1973).

The first phase, *Shock and Numbness*, is described by thanatologist, J. Shep Jeffreys (2005), as "an initial period of shutdown, denial, and unreality lasting for a few days to several weeks." To others, it may seem as if the bereaved are functioning at a near-normal level. For some, this phase might occur initially at the diagnosis of a chromosomal abnormality and can be maintained until further testing has been completed using the shield that "there has to be a mistake" to protect the parents-to-be from fully experiencing the devastation of losing the baby they had expected (Seller et al. 1993).

The second phase is called *Yearning and Searching*, which Jeffries describes as "a time during which the grieving person attempts to recover the person or other loss object" (Jeffreys 2005). Commonly during this phase, parents might express confusion about how to proceed with their options about the pregnancy, often vacillating between recognizing that they will be losing the baby they had been dreaming about and the need to parent this baby. Initially, this phase can be exhibited during the decision-making process and then re-experienced later once their baby has passed.

Disorganization and Despair marks the third of Bowlby's phases, and Jeffries describes it as "a sad time during which hopes for reunion fade and the mourner acknowledges that [the baby] is never coming back. Despair, fatigue, loss of motivation, and apathy are common" (Jeffreys 2005). In the case of medical termination, this phase also occurs once the pregnancy has ended and the mother must come to terms with the fact that she is no longer counting down days or weeks to the birth of a baby.

Bowlby's final phase is called *Reorganization*, which, as Jeffries explains, is when "a new definition of self is established as the grieving persons create new patterns of thinking, feeling, and acting" (Jeffreys 2005). This final phase can be a difficult one to pinpoint for many families. For some, it involves the hope and preoccupation with a successful subsequent pregnancy in order to realize the dream of being a parent. For others, it is creating meaning in their loss, whether it results in political activism, creating a lasting way to honor their child, or by assisting other bereaved parents.

Contextualizing behaviors to look for within normal bereavement is helpful for those outside of the immediate circle of loss. Applying grief, which is a vague and necessary process to the nuances of terminating for medical reasons, can be a way for others to understand how the parents are coping and where they might be within their journey.

Susan Silk and Barry Goldman (2013), both clinical psychologists, describe the roles of family and friends succinctly using the ring theory. Those in the middle of a crisis or trauma (i.e., the bereaved couple) are in the center ring. The ring immediately outside of the center is where the next closest person (or people) can be labeled. Circles are continuously drawn for those that are in the contiguous rings. This diagram (see Fig. 15.1) represents a way to conceptualize the bereaved couple's needs. Comfort measures are to be applied to each level leading into the center. For the rings going away from the center, it is appropriate to share concerns, or to "dump" out that individual's grief. Simply speaking, the rule of thumb is comfort goes into the center, and dumping comes out from the center. These rings can help family and friends understand what is expected of them both in the initial days after a diagnosis or loss as well as the weeks and months that follow (Silk and Goldman 2013).

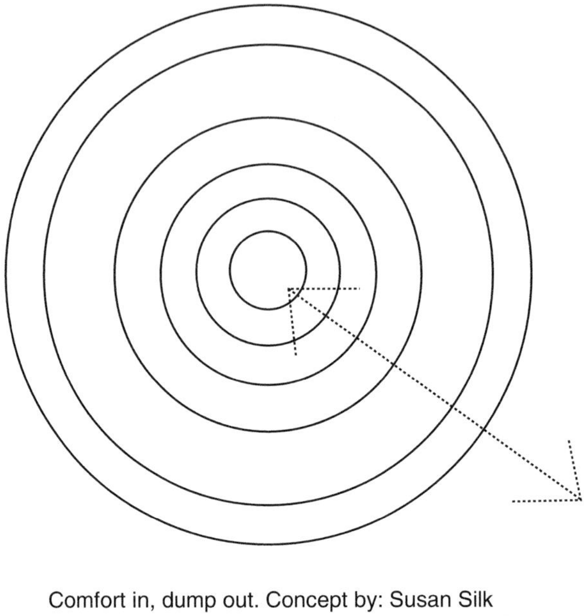

Fig. 15.1 The innermost circle represents the couple. The next circle is immediate family. The following one represents close friends. The subsequent circle represents more distant friends. The next circle is for colleagues. Finally, the last is for acquaintances. Comfort is always supposed to be directed to the circles closest to the center. Anything else gets directed outward

Grieving Couples and Their Dilemmas

Relatively little has been written about perinatal loss as compared to other aspects of pregnancy and reproduction. Even less has been studied about therapeutic abortion. Typically, the literature centers on the parents' reactions, suggesting what is normal in this type of loss, strategies for coping, and planning a subsequent pregnancy. There is limited information about how to help existing children cope with loss as well as how to assist family and friends with mitigating their reactions.

Terminating a pregnancy for medical reasons encompasses many themes similar to other types of perinatal loss as well as nuances that are unique to this specific type of loss (Sandelowski and Barroso 2005). Perinatal loss does not have widespread societal recognition or specific and universal mourning rituals, making it complicated for those outside of the loss to acknowledge or recognize the significance. In a culture that is divided on the issue of abortion, particularly those obtained later in pregnancy, couples might have additional difficulty seeking out needed support post-loss. According to a 2011 Gallup poll (Gallup 2014), 50 % of Americans surveyed think that abortion should be legal when there is evidence that the baby might be physically impaired, and 51 % if there is evidence that the baby might be mentally impaired. This is compared to 45 % of respondents who believe that abortion should be illegal where there is evidence that the baby might be physically impaired and 46 % that believe abortion should be illegal where there is evidence that the baby might be mentally impaired (Gallup 2014). Given that support for the procedure is only lukewarm, it makes sense that families that unexpectedly find themselves needing to interrupt a much-wanted pregnancy are uncertain about what is safe to communicate to others.

Such a dilemma about how and from whom to seek support creates a difficult position for grieving couples. Not only do they need to find who in their social networks can be emotionally supportive during this ordeal but also they must serve as guides for helping these allies navigate the grieving process for everyone (Lemkau 1988). Self-care and self-preservation become the immediate goals after undergoing a medical termination. For some families, this might mean not sharing too many details about the nature of their loss beyond the circle next to theirs (Bishop 1996). (Depending on a family of origin's religious beliefs, it might not be safe to disclose the details even to this ring.) The basic message can be as simple as "we lost the pregnancy." Families that have friends that are able to show understanding (i.e., keeping close contact, being thoughtful, and good listeners) report better outcomes 2 years later, according to a UK study specific to terminating for medical reasons (White-Van Mourik et al. 1992). Terminating for medical reasons is an instance when the personal *becomes* political.

In what ideally should be a private decision between a couple, along with information from medical professionals (and the optional input of a trusted religious advisor), the choice to end a much-wanted pregnancy because of genetic abnormalities becomes a matter that can be weighed in on by anyone else who might know the specifics (McCoyd 2009). On a larger scale, politicians trying to strong-arm legislation (e.g., the recent attempt to add a prohibition to access to abortion in the District of Columbia that was added to legislation about tuition assistance) (Hughes 2014) add a chorus of stigma to a decision that may have already been carried out (Boonstra and Nash 2014). Attempts at regulating access to the procedure, for example, specifics pertaining to locations in which abortion can be performed (recent TRAP laws—Targeted Regulation of Abortion Providers) (Boonstra and Nash 2014), creating abortion cutoff standards, or mandating of hospital privileges, are legislative attempts to eradicate access to abortion. All of the above perpetuate the shame that surrounds the termination of a pregnancy for medical necessity (Institute 2014). A polarized cultural climate is also exacerbated by those who have strong religious beliefs, which further inhibits couples from being able to communicate about their experience for fear of being cut off, isolated, or shunned (McCoyd 2007). Thus, a couple must disclose selectively (France et al. 2013; Friedman and Gradstein 1996; Harris 2004; McCoyd 2008).

Communicating with Children

On the other end of the spectrum, a common dilemma for couples is trying to determine how or even if to communicate to their existing children that their pregnancy will not come to fruition. Typically, medical terminations result after it is physically obvious that a pregnancy is in progress. For many couples, the news of the pregnancy has already been shared, and work has already started to prepare their living child or children for the upcoming birth of a sibling. It is human instinct to want to protect our children from sadness and loss, particularly in the form of death (France et al. 2013; Trozzi and Massimini 1999). However, children are remarkably perceptive and at the very least, without information shared, will be confused and bewildered at the expressed emotion of their parents. Since there is a decision-making process that occurs prior to the actual termination, it is possible that children will have overheard parents speak about the need to make a serious decision, noticed changes in mood, or perhaps noticed the normal inclination for parents physically to embrace them longer and closer during their everyday interactions.

How to tell a child as well as what to tell them depend on the age of the child (Trozzi and Massimini 1999). Universally it is agreed that euphemisms for death are unhelpful in communicating loss to children. Up until approximately the age of 10 (a rough estimate as development varies) children tend to be very concrete in their thinking. An abstract concept, such as death, is difficult to grasp, as the idea of death's permanence and finality does not have a reference point (Davis 1991; France et al. 2013; Seller et al. 1993; Silk and Goldman 2013). It is likely that however the loss is communicated, it will need to be done several times over the span of weeks or months in order for the child to fully understand. A person's conceptions about death begin with his or her first encounter and then evolve with each subsequent experience. After a perinatal loss, parents have the opportunity to model various expressions of grief as well as coping styles (Schwiebert and Kirk 1985).

For a child under the age of two, the conversation about loss is simplistic, as very young children possess only limited expressive language capacity. Statements like "The baby died and I am sad" will be echoed and repeated by this child who is learning how to speak. Reassurance in the form of physical closeness will be important to promote security as a parent's tears can also be frightening. As children accrue greater verbal ability, one must keep in mind their developmental phase when communicating about the loss (France et al. 2013).

Preschool children are absorbed in their own world, which includes the world of their imagination and magical thinking. Inherently, this can cause confusion and fear about death, as their imagination might create something bigger than what is being shared, including the idea that they somehow caused the loss (France et al. 2013; Leon 2008). Their questions might be limited to "how" and "why." It may not be best to share all of the details about a termination with a child, as it is a difficult enough task for the preschool-aged child to understand death itself. Often times, preschool children feel ambivalent about the idea of a sibling, so it is likely that over time, there will be ambivalence about the loss of that sibling (Leon 2008). Reassurance that they did not cause the loss (either by their thoughts or words) is of the utmost importance for this age group (France et al. 2013). In talking to a preschooler, it can be helpful to reference a known loss, such as the death of a pet or a plant: "The baby died, which is like when our cat Fluffy died, so we will not be bringing home a baby now" (Davis 1991; Trozzi and Massimini 1999). Another statement to share with a preschooler might be "The baby stopped growing."

Reiterating this story with a more concrete example can also be helpful for preschool-aged children. One idea is to plant some seeds (e.g., citrus) or a garden with your child, and demonstrate that not every seed that gets planted will grow (Davis 1991; Trozzi and Massimini 1999).

Using correct terminology helps to demystify perceptions about death. Parents need to be available for follow-up questions as they occur and to communicate to extended family the words and phrases they are using so that there is consistency in what a child hears. It can also be helpful to further conversation by responding to a child's question by asking him or her the same question, such as "How do you think the baby died?" This can help parents understand where a child is in his or her own thought process so that the answer can be tailored to correct information as necessary (Trozzi and Massimini 1999; Worden 1982).

Elementary school-aged children have a more concrete understanding of the world. They may wonder what happened to the baby after he or she died or want to know if they will die too. It is important that answers communicate that safety in the world around them is maintained, despite the fact that such an unanticipated event occurred. Elementary school-aged children can detect lies, which leads to mistrust and confusion. Thus authenticity is suggested in conversations about death. Being able to continue conversations with children, despite the pain and difficulty of the content, shows on a tangible level that they are safe, that their questions can be tolerated, and that they are loved (Trozzi and Massimini 1999).

As children near preadolescence, their ability to hold abstract concepts matures and develops, as does their understanding of death. However, this age group might approach death in a standoffish way, which might incorrectly suggest to an adult that they don't care, but the opposite is more likely. Preadolescents care a great deal and may be hurting, but do not know how to handle these intense and complex feelings. Preteens might react out of their own discomfort with insensitive jokes or comments. This is best addressed directly by indicating that the comment is not appreciated at this time, but also without suggesting that the preteen is in any way bad or a terrible person. As with any child, the parent has the best sense and understanding of what the preteen's needs and capacities might be (Trozzi and Massimini 1999).

Finally, when talking to a teenager about death, it is important to remember his or her stage of life. They are preoccupied with what others think about them, are trying to ascertain their individuality in the midst of their larger family constellation, and are envisioning themselves as adults in the near future. These tasks, on a good day, provide for stress and strife within an adolescent's life. Additionally, adolescents have the notion of immunity and immortality—death won't happen to them. Adolescents are able to struggle and wrestle with the existential question about death, namely "Why did this happen to us?", but are often unequipped with the emotional tools to fully process this problem. Teens are beginning to hone their moral compass, so going into the details around the circumstances of the loss might be difficult and can be decided on the basis of the parent's knowledge of who the teen is and what he or she is capable of handling (Schwiebert and Kirk 1985; Trozzi and Massimini 1999).

Initial conversations with children occur as the event is unfolding. Commonly, these conversations will continue over time and will even seem to arise out of nowhere as the aging child creates new meanings and understandings about his or her own life.

Parents might be conflicted about significant dates and how to handle them within the family. Some couples commemorate “angelversaries” (the anniversary of the day that the baby died) privately with their own or with specific faith-based rituals (Cardin 2007). Others include their children and perhaps extended family, and still others let the day pass unmarked. While each individual has his or her own unique process for moving through grief, if children are present, it is equally important to consider what their needs are. These occasions provide a framework for continuing a conversation about the baby that has been lost and might be more salient in the initial years post-loss than as time moves on. Oftentimes, having children acknowledge the sibling that was not born can be, for the parents as well as the children, an authentic way of expressing the totality of who is included in the family (Ilse 1990).

In time, many, although not all, couples that terminate for medical reasons are able to have a subsequent healthy pregnancy. Some families believe that it is important to impart to their existing child that this new baby is not a replacement for the baby that died, but a separate individual that will be coming into the family. Making this distinction becomes important as a way to reiterate to a child (as well as a reminder to the parents) that they too are not replaceable. For all couples, the dilemma about what to tell a “rainbow baby” (a child born after the storm of loss) about their origins is complex. On the one hand, it makes sense for mothers in particular to honor their reproductive narrative (Jaffe and Diamond 2011; Wenzel 2014) by remembering the baby that was lost. However doing so risks that the healthy child will feel like he or she is in competition with or somehow must make up for the child that was lost. The danger of this is that the lost child is memorialized and conceptualized as faultless, never having had the chance to disappoint, whereas the living child is human, and inevitably not flawless (Leon 2008). Because of these concerns, it might make sense to wait until the child is of an age of understanding to delineate the full history of their birth.

What to tell children can feel like an additional burden for couples who terminated as a result of recessive or dominant genetic factors (Kohn et al. 1993). The National Society of Genetic Counselors cautions against performing genetic testing on children to ascertain if they are carriers of known mutations prior to adulthood when they are able to fully consent (Nsgc.org 2014). Having a family history of pregnancy loss plays an important role when offspring with this type of familial loss history go on to have children of their own. The parents, now potential grandparents, will need to consider how their own reproductive history should be conveyed to their adult children as a way for them to spare the next generation from the pain of having to terminate a wanted pregnancy. Additionally, with inherited traits lies the possibility that older relatives might feel responsible for passing on these genetic variants. At this writing, there are limited ways (such as preimplantation genetic diagnosis) to prevent genetic transmission. This technology is currently limited to known genes and to inherited chromosomal abnormalities. As the field of genetics grows, more information is gained and new genes are discovered that can help guide families with complicated genetic histories.

The Grieving Couple's Role in Facilitating Support

Close social ties are imperative in healing from any kind of perinatal loss, including a medical termination. As mentioned above, the bereaved couple has multiple roles to play, one of which is to guide those in their circles in how to provide helpful comfort. This is complicated as it is new territory all around, so many couples do not know what to ask for from family and friends. Sharing the story of their pregnancy and moments that they shared with the baby are important aspects of the healing process for a couple (Kluger-Bell 2000; Bosticco and Thompson 2005). Generally speaking, supportive people have an ability to listen (White-Van Mourik et al. 1992). Most of the time, listening is fairly passive in that hearing the actual words spoken is all that is necessary. However, sometimes, to meet the needs of a couple in mourning one must listen for what hasn't been overtly stated. Listening closely can suggest what words to reflect back to the grieving parents, for example, does the couple address the baby by a specific name? Do they refer to their loss as a baby or a fetus? Adopting the language that a couple uses allows them to feel understood and heard (Bosticco and Thompson 2005).

When people mourn, the immediate job of keeping up with everyday tasks of living can be nearly impossible. A support system can be useful by assisting with household chores, doctors' appointments, keeping the mother's or parents' company, inquiring as to how they are feeling, volunteering to share the news with others, or even accompanying a parent on a walk (Davis 1991; Friedman and Gradstein 1996; Kluger-Bell 2000; Kohn et al. 1993; Wenzel 2014). An aspect that few women consider is what their postpartum visit to their doctor might feel like. Supportive friends can help in making the appointment, and in doing so can request that the grieving mother be able to wait in a separate area when she enters the office in order to be spared the pain of seeing other pregnant women or pregnancy-themed magazines. Additionally, offering company for the appointment can be a great relief for a woman who is bereft. This is by no means an exhaustive list of ways to show support in the initial days, but offers sample ideas. Many women, in particular, find that physical contact from others can be soothing. Hugging the bereaved, allowing them to cry, or even crying with them are small acts of support that can be very meaningful. Men are often not seen as active mourners, and questions posed to them typically are about how their wives are faring. Ascertaining how the male partner is feeling himself can be worthwhile and meaningful (Leon 2008).

Often, support people feel compelled to try to say the perfect thing to a grieving couple as a way of offering condolence. When a medical termination has occurred, it is important to understand that there is no ideal or magic phrase that can make the pain lessen for a couple. However, there are certain comments that can trigger a negative reaction and should be avoided. For example: "Everything happens for a reason."

"This was part of God's Plan."

"You're young and healthy—you'll have other children."

"At least you didn't lose an older child."

"I know just how you feel—my dog died last year."

"God doesn't give you more than you can handle."

"At least you have a child."

"God just needed another angel in heaven."

"At least you can get pregnant."

"Wow-that's morbid that you named your dead baby."

"You chose to end your pregnancy—why are you having a funeral/why are you sad?"

"But you're pro-choice, so what's the big deal?"

A simple, "I'm so sorry for your loss" is more than sufficient and is usually appreciated by the bereaved. Other words or acts of comfort can include the following:

"Tell me about your baby/pregnancy."

"Show me a picture."

"I'm here to listen, if you want to talk."

"I can only imagine what this is like for you."

"I wish I had words that would be helpful."

"This just sucks" (Cardin 2007; Davis 1991; Friedman and Gradstein 1996; Jaffe and Diamond 2011; Kluger-Bell 2000; Kohn et al. 1993; Seller et al. 1993; Trozzi and Massimini 1999).

Offering to educate others within one's network of support about what is likely to be well received and what is not can also be a valuable show of support to a grieving couple. Directly after a loss, most people have the benefit of friends and family willing to offer comfort and condolences. Employers might make allowances with extended bereavement leave, as the couple may feel that they are living in a surreal bubble where life is temporarily suspended. Within the span of several weeks, visitors dissipate and the support dwindles—not because of a lack of caring, but because life has a way of continuing on. This short time frame after a loss becomes challenging as the loss and its feelings have not diminished for the couple undergoing it, and yet the community of support for the most part has returned to daily life. During this time, it is particularly important for the couple to convey that support is still needed and to offer suggestions for the form that support might take. Perhaps it is remaining available to listen to them talk about and process the loss. This can be achieved simply by asking how the couple is doing and feeling. Instinctively, people feel that they should shy away from bringing up the loss as they do not want to cause pain to the couple. However, a lack of inquiring can be seen as forgetting, which may be even more painful as it might be misinterpreted as indicating that their baby and the pregnancy didn't matter. Others feel touched by family and friends using the child's name or remembering certain milestone dates such as the estimated due date or the angelversary. This shows that there was legitimacy in that child's brief presence.

Conclusion

In summation, social support is imperative to a couple's healing process after a termination due to a fetal anomaly. This support legitimizes and normalizes the feelings around the loss, provides an emotional safety net in which to process the loss in an ongoing manner, and can assist with establishing a new normal post-loss. After a pregnancy termination due to fetal anomaly, a couple has a dual role of navigating their emotions around the loss as well as facilitating support for themselves by educating others about what their needs entail. Support can be offered both in tangible ways as well as through words.

The political climate can heighten feelings of uncertainty about how to communicate the nature of the loss to others and can influence unfortunate remarks that well-meaning individuals might make. In discussing perinatal loss, others tend to feel awkward about the situation, and this is exacerbated when choice is involved. Bereaved individuals can protect themselves by selecting who is told details beyond the basics that a pregnancy loss has occurred. Additionally, managing the expectations and emotions of children is complicated both in the direct aftermath of a loss as well as in the future. Determining how much to share with children born post-loss is additionally problematic.

Recommendations

While there is a dearth of literature about coping styles, rituals, and processing a perinatal loss, there is even less specific to terminating a pregnancy for medical reasons. Feelings of loss and grief are equal to those of spontaneous loss, but the nuance of choice and the decision-making factor create additional elements that rarely are parsed out in the literature. Additional studies of this population, although a small subset of perinatal losses, are necessary.

Health care practitioners should be instructed regarding how best to communicate with couples who have terminated for medical reasons, and to address their concerns in the diagnosis and decision-making phase, the postpartum checkup, and as couples plan for and undergo subsequent pregnancies.

Other advances that would be helpful in working with this population include the following:

1. Create a societal language, such as specific words about perinatal loss in general as well as language in particular for terminating a pregnancy for medical reasons; language would give validity to all types of perinatal loss.
2. Reduce stigma by encouraging communication and education in the public forum about terminating a pregnancy for medical reasons.
3. Disseminate information about known methods of support so that family and friends have the ability to proactively assist loved ones who have experienced a termination for medical reasons.

References

Bishop S. Choosing: a double-edged sword: women's experiences with pregnancy termination after fetal abnormalities are diagnosed [Master of Science]. Toronto, ON: University of Toronto; 1996.

Boonstra H, Nash E. A surge of state abortion restrictions puts providers—and the women they serve—in the crosshairs. Guttmacher Pol Rev. 2014;17(1):9–14.

Bosticco C, Thompson T. Narratives and story telling in coping with grief and bereavement. Omega. 2005;51(1):1–16.

Bowlby J. Attachment and loss. 1st ed. New York: Basic Books; 1969.

Bowlby J. Attachment and loss. 1st ed. London: The Hogarth Press and The Institute of Psycho-Analysis; 1973.

Bowlby J. The making and breaking of affectional bonds. 1st ed. London: Tavistock; 1979.

Burns L, Covington S. Infertility counseling. 1st ed. Pearl River, NY, USA: Parthenon Pub. Group; 1999.

Cardin N. Tears of sorrow, seeds of hope. 2nd ed. Woodstock: Jewish Lights; 2007.

Davis D. Empty cradle, broken heart. 1st ed. Golden, CO: Fulcrum Pub.; 1991.

France E, Hunt K, Ziebland S, Wyke S. What parents say about disclosing the end of their pregnancy due to fetal abnormality. Midwifery. 2013;29(1):24–32.

Friedman R, Gradstein B. Surviving pregnancy loss. 1st ed. Secaucus, NJ: Carol Pub. Group; 1996.

Gallup I. Abortion/Gallup historical trends [Internet]. Gallup.com. 2014. http://www.gallup.com/poll/1576/abortion.aspx#3. Accessed 29 June 2014.

Harris A. Supportive counseling before and after elective pregnancy termination. J Midwifery Wom Health. 2004;49(2):105–12.

Hughes S. House again wants to cut tuition grants, attach abortion rider to D.C. spending bill [Internet]. DCist. 2014. http://dcist.com/2014/06/congress_again_attaches_abortion_ri.php. Accessed 29 June 2014.

Ilse S. Empty arms. 20th ed. Maple Plain: Wintergreen Press; 1990.

Institute G. [Internet]. Guttmacher Institute. http://www.guttmacher.org/pubs/gpr/17/1/gpr170109.pdf. Accessed 23 June 2014.

Jaffe J, Diamond M. Reproductive trauma. 1st ed. Washington, DC: American Psychological Association; 2011.

Jeffreys J. Helping grieving people. 1st ed. New York: Brunner-Routledge; 2005.

Kluger-Bell K. Unspeakable losses. 1st ed. New York: Quill; 2000.

Kohn I, Moffitt P, Wilkins I. A silent sorrow. 1st ed. New York: Delacorte Press; 1993.

Lemkau J. Emotional sequelae of abortion implications for clinical practice. Psychol Women Q. 1988;12(4):461–72.

Leon I. Helping families cope with perinatal loss. Glob libr women's med (ISSN: 1756–2228) 2008; doi:10.3843/GLOWM.10418. http://www.glowm.com/section_view/item/417/recordset/18975/value/417.

McCoyd J. Pregnancy interrupted: loss of a desired pregnancy after diagnosis of fetal anomaly. J Psychosom Obstet Gynecol. 2007;28(1):37–48.

McCoyd J. "I'm not a saint": Burden assessment as an unrecognized factor in prenatal decision making. Qual Health Res. 2008;18(11):1489–500.

McCoyd J. What do women want? Experiences and reflections of women after prenatal diagnosis and termination for anomaly. Health Care Women Int. 2009;30(6):507–35.

Nsgc.org. National Society of Genetic Counselors: Blogs: genetic testing of minors for adult-onset conditions [Internet]. 2014. http://nsgc.org/p/bl/et/blogid=47&blogaid=28. Accessed 29 June 2014.

Robinson M. The relationship of attachment theory and perinatal loss. Death Stud. 1999; 23(3):257–70.

Sandelowski M, Barroso J. The travesty of choosing after positive prenatal diagnosis. J Obstet Gynecol Neonatal Nurs. 2005;34(3):307–18.

Schwiebert P, Kirk P. When hello means goodbye. 1st ed. Portland, OR: Perinatal Loss; 1985.

Seller M, Barnes C, Ross S, Barby T, Cowmeadow P. Grief and mid-trimester fetal loss. Prenat Diagn. 1993;13(5):341–8.

Silk S, Goldman B. How not to say the wrong thing. LA Times [Internet]. 2013. op-ed. http://articles.latimes.com/2013/apr/07/opinion/la-oe-0407-silk-ring-theory-20130407. Accessed 29 June 2014.

Trozzi M, Massimini K. Talking with children about loss. 1st ed. New York, NY: Perigee; 1999.

Wenzel A. Coping with infertility, miscarriage, and neonatal loss. 1st ed. Washington, DC: American Psychological Association; 2014.

White-Van Mourik M, Connor J, Ferguson-Smith M. The psychosocial sequelae for a second trimester termination of pregnancy for fetal abnormality over a two year period. Birth Defects Orig Artic Ser. 1992;28(1):61–74.

Worden J. Grief counseling and grief therapy. 1st ed. New York: Springer; 1982.

Chapter 16
Postscript: A Patient's Perspective

Katherine Burns

"Pick one letter from the alphabet." I juggled a pinecone in my hands. "Come on," I said. "Please. I already have one picked out."

My husband Thomas stood a few feet away from me on a boulder. Central Park hummed with cyclists and runners, musicians and mommies, tourists and hot dog hawkers. "I don't really want to play. I don't see the point."

"The point," I said, "is to convince me that 1 in 26 is still astronomical. That one in 26 is still safe. The point is to remind me that it's ok. That the odds are still on our side. So just try. Just try to hit that one letter. Show me how impossible it is that our baby is really unwell."

"I'm sure everything will be ok, honey,"

But he frowned into the early November sunshine and sighed.

A few days earlier, bloodwork combined with the NT (nuchal translucency) scan—a routine screening—had revealed that my pregnancy had an increased risk for Down syndrome: from the normal 1 in 769 for my age group to 1 in 27. The alphabet game was the closest thing I could think of to approximate how odds like that could really play out. They were odds that held my life hostage.

The increased risk result had caught us off guard, because the ultrasound scan had gone well. It was Halloween, and to treat ourselves, we decided to splurge on an expensive Japanese dinner. As we held hands and skipped among the cavorting crowds on the way to the restaurant, I turned to my husband and beamed, "I feel like we're safe maybe," I said. "I mean, I'd rather have a perfect NT scan than perfect blood work—the blood stuff is probably highly variable and doesn't mean as much. Anyway, we'll find out about it in a day or two."

That night was the first time I'd felt a sense of ease about the pregnancy. Since the beginning, I'd felt that something was off. That sense grew with the spotting and bleeding that started at about 6 weeks. Because my progesterone levels were

K. Burns (✉)
1058 Sterling Place, Brooklyn, NY 11205, USA
e-mail: katherineburns2011@gmail.com

J.P. Galst, M.S. Verp (eds.), *Prenatal and Preimplantation Diagnosis*,
DOI 10.1007/978-3-319-18911-6_16

extremely low, my doctor put me on a synthetic dose. She assured me that it would not prevent a "bad" pregnancy from miscarrying, but that if everything else was normal, it would help me carry a healthy baby to term.

For nearly the entirety of the 12 weeks leading up to the scan, I'd fought a fatigue worse than any jetlag I'd endured during a decade of regularly flying 20-h trans-Pacific flights. The smell of food made me wretch. And the spotting never stopped.

But clutching the ultrasound picture, things felt different. I was starving. I ate hot tofu and grilled fish and fried eggplant with relish. When we arrived home, we tried to carve a jack-o'-lantern with our May due date on it. We thought we could take a picture of it and send it as a birth announcement to our families in the Midwest. But I couldn't steady my hand. The fruit was too hard. The skin was too slippery. The knife slipped time and again. By the time I'd finished all that was left was a gaping pulpy hole.

A day later, the pumpkin still sitting in the bottom of the trashcan, the nurse at my doctor's office called and told us that we should probably make an appointment with a genetic counselor. It felt like my guts were the ones that had been scraped out.

Anna, our genetic counselor, took out a binder and explained how Down syndrome (trisomy 21) manifested due to an extra copy of the 21st chromosome in all cells. She told us that if we wanted definitive results about the diagnosis, we would need to either have a chorionic villus sampling (CVS) or wait for a few weeks and have an amniocentesis. Otherwise, we could also wait for the 20-week ultrasound screen, when markers would be more apparent. Or we could adopt a wait-and-see approach and prepare for any scenario. She gave us information on Down syndrome from various Down syndrome support groups. She also gave us information about abortion and materials that included stories about women who had made that choice after a prenatal diagnosis.

In the half-week between learning about our increased risk and our meeting with the genetic counselor, my husband and I had decided to undergo the CVS—a wrenching decision in itself, as I worried about the possibility of miscarrying a healthy child. Early on in my pregnancy, I had solicited the advice of an older cousin, an MD who had her own practice, about my doctor's suggestion to take progesterone. She convinced me to take it to preserve the pregnancy. When I told her about my increased risk, she told me, "The most important question when thinking about whether or not to undertake invasive testing is what do you think you can do with the information." Despite her Catholicism, she told me frankly, "in the case of trisomy 13 or trisomy 18, abortion may be the most ethical choice." And in the case of trisomy 21? She wouldn't say.

My cousin wasn't the only one who knew about my pregnancy's increased risk. Despite my better judgment, I had told my mom and dad about my pregnancy early on, as I was struggling with the bleeding, fatigue, and nausea. We'd had our differences. My mother and father are also Catholic, but, unlike my cousin, they think that abortion is immoral regardless of the circumstance. When I was a girl, my family would stand on the street outside of our church holding "pro-life" signs. When my father spoke about abortion to my four brothers and me, his eyes welled with tears. His teeth gnashed in fury.

I considered myself a recovering Catholic, an agnostic, and I had become pro-choice in high school. Still, I was always terrified of an unplanned pregnancy and practiced birth control with the same discipline with which I once celebrated the sacraments. Once married, I heaved a sigh of relief that I'd never have to have an abortion. I'd never have to keep a poker face when my father talked about murdering abortionists and dead babies.

I had to know if Blueberry, the name we'd given our fetus, had Down syndrome. There was no way I could embark on another 27 weeks of pregnancy with such a life-altering bit of information about my future and about my potential child's future left as an unknown. But I knew that Thomas and I couldn't tell anyone in our families (his family is Catholic, too) that I would undergo a CVS, because then they would expect results, and, with results, acceptance and preparation—the only way forward. To them there was no other choice. In my heart, I knew I needed more room than that. I needed room to consider all the options. This idea rattled me.

A few years prior, when I was working abroad, a friend of mine also came back from her NT scan with increased risk. It was her first pregnancy, too.

Over tea in my apartment, she confided in me:

"Well, we'll do an amnio, and if the fetus is affected by Down syndrome, we'll terminate the pregnancy," she said.

I sucked air. I'd taken a friend for an abortion in college—I had to drive to the only city in the state that offered them—but to end a planned pregnancy because the baby had Down syndrome? Wasn't there something shallow or hubristic about that? If you went into things knowing you were trying to make a baby, shouldn't you just accept the one that comes?

My friend went in for the amnio, but it came back inconclusive. She chanced it from there, and her baby turned out to have 46 chromosomes. Today he's a perfectly healthy little guy.

Whenever I start to feel judgmental about another parent, I remember that moment. I remember the hot rush that came to my face. I remember the "how could she?" feeling. Now I pity that judgmental version of myself.

I knew I loved our Blueberry, but I was also afraid. For Blueberry. And for us. Didn't I have a responsibility for my life, for the life that was growing in me, to gain all the information at my disposal? After years of careful planning, didn't I have the right to understand what potential outcomes this pregnancy might have? I also questioned my previous assumptions: How bad was it really, to want to ensure, on some level that the human being you're bringing into the world will have the same chances as anyone else, and will have capabilities at least equal to any ordinary person and the potential to someday live independently and create his or her own life? Why did you just have to accept what you were given? Wasn't the whole point of choice to give women and families agency over their lives?

"We'll do the CVS today if you have a spot," I told Anna. Thomas squeezed my hand.

The doctor performing the procedure did it transabdominally. It didn't hurt much, but tears slid down my face for the duration of the procedure. I went home and didn't leave bed for the rest of the day. They had told me not to—I could miscarry. And that was when I started thinking a miscarriage would be the most wonderful thing. The choice wouldn't have to be mine. My body would be doing what happens with most trisomy 21-affected fetuses. I read and reread the literature that Anna had sent home with us both on parenting children with special needs and on parents who had made the decision to interrupt affected pregnancies.

Thomas remained optimistic that everything would turn out fine. I had a break with my freelance work, so I spent the next couple of days at various movie theaters, sometimes sitting through a feature twice just to kill time. I read medical studies, advocacy sites, and blogs about Down syndrome. I also read the websites aheartbreakingchoice.com and the Termination for Medical Reasons group on Babycenter.com from top to bottom. I remained conflicted about how I would proceed if the news came back that our fetus was affected by trisomy 21. I had started thinking about Blueberry that way again. I had begun to distance myself. And I baked. I baked a lot.

One evening, a friend, who was also pregnant, came over while I was making pumpkin cookies. The phone rang.

"Katherine? It's Anna. I'm sorry, your FISH results came back positive for trisomy 21."

I collapsed to my knees and screamed. To this day, the smell of those cookies makes me retch.

My first impulse surprised me: I wanted it over with. NOW. But how could I? What kind of mother would that make me? What kind of *person* would that make me? Was I vain? Had I succumbed to hubris? But what kind of life would it be for us if we carried the pregnancy to term? What kind of life would it be for the child? How bad might it be? What could be the best outcome? How would that affect the shape of our family?

How could we ever make this sort of choice?

My ObGyn called the next day.

"What are you going to do?" She asked.

"I don't know." I said.

"Are you considering terminating the pregnancy?"

"It's not out of the picture."

"Yes."

"Well, I don't know. It's surprised me. I didn't think I would ever consider it. But now that I'm here, it all feels very different."

"Well, you have to ask yourself if it's fair to bring a child into the world who's already behind the 8-ball."

My doctor had never been one for speaking gently or reserving her opinion, but I appreciated her candor.

"Yes. I wish we could just have a do-over."

"Well, you're still young. And this was a fluke. I can't tell you what to do, but if you were my daughter, I would advise you to terminate the pregnancy. You guys can try again and have a healthy baby."

"Yes."

"Do you want some numbers for doctors who will do the procedure?"

"Yes."

How was this really happening? Writing down the numbers. Calling to ask about availability. In the meantime, we stopped taking calls from family and friends. We dove into research about Down syndrome. We watched videos. We read journals. We learned some sobering statistics about heart defects, mental health difficulties, dementia, and autism dual diagnosis. We thought about what it would mean if we wanted to have a second child—would they inherit the responsibility of their older sibling upon birth? And we balked at the pro-Down syndrome literature that seemed to fetishize children with the condition as angels who teach us about life and inspire us. We also questioned the assumption that the only noble and loving decision is to bring a child into the world knowing the potential physical, mental, emotional, and social obstacles he or she would face. What if the suffering was great? Of course, to live is wonderful, but, at 13 weeks, Blueberry had no consciousness, no knowledge of his or her existence or nonexistence. We knew if we decided to continue the pregnancy we would make it work. Thomas and I had been together for a decade and had endured hardship together. We would love our child and advocate for him or her. We would be fiercely protective. But what if that became the sum of our lives? And would this be signing us up not for 20-some years of active parenting (as I would argue most people assume), but a life sentence of hands-on babysitting and management, even into our old age? And what responsibility did we have to society? And if more than 80 % of people with developmental disabilities didn't have jobs in 2011, what would that look like in a few decades when all menial work had been replaced by computers and robots? Already most stores close to where we lived were self-checkout, for example. If we devoted our lives to a child with Down syndrome, depleting all our emotional, physical, and financial resources, how much better could we make life for him or her?

I leaned heavily on my therapist. I lamented my inability to decide the next course of action. She advised us to make a decision, sleep on it, and see how it felt in the morning. If it didn't feel right, make a different decision and sleep on it. So Thomas and I drove to the Adirondacks. After depriving myself for months, I decided to drink as much coffee as I wanted on the way. I stopped taking my prenatal vitamins.

I hated the stiffness of my tiny belly. I wished Blueberry could just peacefully go. Thomas and I tramped through the woods. We howled and cursed. We talked about God—or the lack of, about chance, about morality, about parenthood, about what we wanted for our future. We talked about our family histories with depression and disability. We talked about what quality of life meant—for a potential child and for ourselves. We ranted about right-wing politicians and religionists. I screamed my parents' names and pounded a moldy log. Why couldn't they love me enough to love me through this? Why did we have to go through this alone? At times our conversation became abstract: What were the odds that any of us made it here? It could have been any other egg, any other sperm among thousands, so what made one pregnancy so precious, so irreplaceable? Humanity owed its existence to a random dinosaur's sneeze, according to one evolutionary biologist, so what was one pregnancy gone awry? Why did it matter so much?

We kicked leaves and startled squirrels. I ran hard down a hill, hoping that my body would release Blueberry and set us free. That night I took a very hot bath with the same intent. I also called my Catholic grandmother, who asked me if there wasn't anything the doctor could give me to help a miscarriage along if we discovered that the baby did indeed have Down syndrome. She didn't know that we had already confirmed it. My Catholic MD cousin had also suggested at one point that we could see a witch doctor who could induce a miscarriage. I couldn't believe the workaround. My own mother said she thought that a baby with Down syndrome would be a blessing from God, and our entire family would pitch in—but that was hard to swallow, too. That night I told Thomas that I wanted to have an abortion. He agreed.

The next morning we had breakfast with an Indian couple who had taken a weekend away. The elderly innkeepers joined us. No one knew I was pregnant. No one knew the terror that had ripped our hearts open. We ate pancakes. We laughed. That was it. Life could be normal again. This didn't have to be the way things were forever. When we got home, we made the appointment.

On the first day of the D&E I felt empowered. I had made a decision, and it was my life. This was family planning—the hardest and worst of it, but that was what it was. I believed I was making a merciful decision and protecting my life and our married life. I believed I was mitigating harm. I believed I was acting in the interest of the greatest good. I walked from the hospital after receiving the laminaria to a coffee shop. Some small angry part of me thought, "Well, mom and dad, fuck you. All your years of authoritarian parenting and moralizing and teaching me shame seem to have been for nothing." I wrote a heady message on the Termination for Medical Reasons message board, and continue to receive thanks for my post today. My username was "OwningIt," and, at that moment, I very much did.

The next day at the hospital, I tried to write Blueberry a note. But it felt too unreal. I thanked the anesthesiologist as he put me under. "I'm sorry. I'm sorry. I'm really so very sorry. I am a good person. I am."

The nurse who attended me when I came to was Filipino and had a gold cross around her neck. She was kind, even if she knew what I had done and disagreed. She didn't say anything. I was grateful for her silence. I asked her for more morphine. I told her my pain was a 10.

At home, I crawled into bed and sobbed until it felt like my ribs were broken. Thomas went to fill the prescription I had been given to control the bleeding. But there was a problem. The pharmacist couldn't read the handwriting. We tried to call the doctor who had done the procedure. He had told us that he would be at a conference for women's reproductive rights later that day, but that we could reach his mobile phone. Then we couldn't. I was frightened. We put in a call to our ObGyn, who got back to us at the end of the day after I'd been bleeding heavily for several hours. That evening, my husband called my parents and his parents and explained that I'd had a miscarriage. In the week that followed, a handful of close friends who knew what had really gone down came and visited. They brought food and flowers. I saw my therapist daily. I don't know how I would have survived any of it without her. My milk let down. We went to my parent's acreage for Thanksgiving.

No one talked about the miscarriage. One of my cousins brought along her new baby. A lovely little boy. I held him close and felt my body open up to him. I smelled him. When no one was looking, I licked his face. Later that afternoon I screamed into the woods and threw myself in the grass and kicked my legs. The why of things haunted me. My heart bubbled with rage and jealousy. Why had my cousin had four healthy children, this last one at 42, when I, a decade younger, had drawn the short straw? Why had Thomas and I had sex that 1 month that yielded this one result?

For the next several months, anger and sadness ruled me. I spent a lot of time questioning if I had made the right decision, even if, after reflection I believed that I would make the same choice again. As states rolled out abortion restrictions and right-wing politicians and pro-choice disability activists alike started publicly arguing that the use of prenatal diagnosis to determine the course of a pregnancy was a form of neo-Nazi eugenics, shame and horror filled me. I hated that I couldn't stand up for myself and my choice. I hated that these options were presented in such black-and-white terms. I spent a lot of time online reading message boards and ethics papers. The eugenics claim had a hole in it though, because I firmly believed that if scientists could come up with an inoculation women could take before becoming pregnant that would prevent Down syndrome, they wouldn't refuse it. Or if there were a shot that could turn Down syndrome children into kids with the typical number of chromosomes, they and their parents would most likely use it. So the real issue was abortion. The real issue was determinism/god's will versus an unfortunate natural fluke that doesn't have to dictate the way the rest of your life goes. Maybe I was cold and too pragmatic, but that was how I felt. It wasn't my role to make a more chromosomally different world—why did the politicians give a shit? And I didn't buy the much-bandied assertion that kids with Down syndrome make the world a better place and their family members more compassionate. I knew a handful of people with siblings with Down syndrome and they were still selfish and impatient.

Still, carrying around the anger made me sick. Grieving in secret from most people, including my family, took its toll. I found it ironic that even my parents, those right-to-lifers, saw the "miscarriage" as an unfortunate blip. It wasn't a real person until it was the woman's decision to end it, apparently. God as abortionist was fine, though. My mom told me I just needed to get over it.

The obsessive thoughts I'd struggled with my entire life intensified. And it became worse after I learned that I was pregnant again. What if, what if, what if. Even the best news after another CVS—a boy with a normal number of chromosomes—was only temporary relief. Old superstitions reared up. I knocked on wood. I blew on fallen eyelashes. I avoided cracks in the pavement. And I replayed our first pregnancy and our decision. At work, I reviewed my projects again and again, combing for mistakes and, upon finding small errors, concluded that I was a colossal failure and that any success I had enjoyed would be turned on its head when everyone realized how stupid and careless and incompetent I really was. I was a fraud. I was a loser. My therapist was patient, kind, and effective at helping me learn how to deal with destructive thinking, but she knew that I needed something more than that. She was worried that my prenatal depression would turn into a serious postnatal depression and suggested I see a psychiatrist. That doctor put me on a low dose of Zoloft. With continued talk therapy and the drug, I experienced an incredible turnaround and was able to welcome my son with happiness and a clear, anxiety-free mind.

My son is 18 months old now. He thrills me. I never thought such happiness was possible. And I'm often struck by the idea that if we hadn't gone through what we did, I never would have met him. He is not a perfect child—that is never what I wanted, despite what critics of prenatal screening might say—but he will have at least the normal intellectual capacity to someday independently navigate his world. Of course, I realize that any matter of tragedies could still befall our family—I'm all too aware—but what a wonderful start to our lives: to be healthy and strong and clever and young. This is something many take for granted, but for which I feel most grateful.

Now when I go home for a visit and hear my parents make comments about abortion, I just ignore it. I also ignore the gruesome signs on the highway by their house. And I just smile and shrug when I see propaganda suggesting that I'm a Nazi for terminating a pregnancy affected by trisomy 21. I have my lovely family, and I'm not going to change anyone else's mind. It does worry me that women's rights are being rolled back nationwide, so I donate monthly to NARAL (National Abortion and Reproductive Rights Action League) and Planned Parenthood. Maybe I'm a coward for not standing up and telling my story, but I prefer to live a happy life and quietly support others in the message groups where I first found refuge.

The choice is a burden, it's true. But thanks to it, I spent my first year with my son in parks and playrooms instead of hospitals and therapy rooms. When I think of my child's future, I imagine unlimited possibilities. Of course, it will be up to him whether or not he takes advantage of his everyday gifts to live an expansive, adventurous, and fulfilling life, but that is *his* choice, *his* responsibility, *his* freedom, and *his* life. Just as it was his mother's before him.

Index

J.P. Galst, M.S. Verp (eds.), *Prenatal and Preimplantation Diagnosis*,
DOI 10.1007/978-3-319-18911-6

J

K

L

M

N

MIX
Papier aus verantwortungsvollen Quellen
Paper from responsible sources
FSC® C105338

If you have any concerns about our products,
you can contact us on
ProductSafety@springernature.com

In case Publisher is established outside the EU,
the EU authorized representative is:
Springer Nature Customer Service Center GmbH
Europaplatz 3, 69115 Heidelberg, Germany

Printed by Libri Plureos GmbH
in Hamburg, Germany